Inpatient Dermatology

Misha Rosenbach • Karolyn A. Wanat
Robert G. Micheletti
Editors

Laura A. Taylor
Associate Editor

Inpatient Dermatology

Springer

Editors
Misha Rosenbach, MD
Department of Dermatology
Perelman School of Medicine
University of Pennsylvania
Philadelphia, PA
USA

Karolyn A. Wanat, MD
Department of Dermatology
Medical College of Wisconsin
Milwaukee, WI
USA

Robert G. Micheletti, MD
Department of Dermatology
Perelman School of Medicine
University of Pennsylvania
Philadelphia, PA
USA

Associate Editor
Laura A. Taylor, MD
Department of Pathology and Laboratory Medicine
University of Pennsylvania
Philadelphia, PA
USA

ISBN 978-3-319-18448-7 ISBN 978-3-319-18449-4 (eBook)
https://doi.org/10.1007/978-3-319-18449-4

Library of Congress Control Number: 2018941849

This Springer imprint is published by the registered company Springer Nature Switzerland AG
The registered company address is: Gewerbestrasse 11, 6330 Cham, Switzerland

We would like to thank our many mentors and colleagues, not just in dermatology, but across medicine. The emerging field of inpatient hospital-based dermatology is rapidly growing, often attracting the best and brightest dermatology residents and young physicians. Care of inpatients requires intelligence, curiosity, and interdisciplinary care and communication. We are all always learning from our patients, our students, and our colleagues who consult us. In particular, we have been fortunate to train at an institution where there is close collaboration between internal medicine and dermatology, and we have countless friends, mentors, and colleagues who have contributed to the care of our challenging inpatient dermatology patients, teaching us invaluable tips, tricks, and pearls along the way. We are delighted to share our approach and an up-to-date, evidence-based, and expert opinion-supplemented guide to inpatient dermatology.

In particular, we would like to thank Dr. William James, who is the pinnacle of dermatologic knowledge and a tireless teacher and generous mentor. He has served as a role model and inspiration for all of us, and we would not be where we are without him. Additionally, we are fortunate to have trained just as the hospitalist movement was starting in dermatology. Dr. Lindy Fox helped spark the field of inpatient dermatology, with inspiration from her mentor and legendary clinician, Dr. Marc Grossman, whose career as an inpatient dermatologist helped demonstrate that this career path was possible. Both editors Drs. Rosenbach and Micheletti rotated with Dr. Fox as residents and feel she is the trailblazer of our generation who has launched the entire field of inpatient dermatology; without her, we would not know what we know or do what we do, and we are forever grateful for her mentorship and example. We would like to thank the rest of the other founders of the inpatient dermatology society, Dr. Kanade Shinkai, Dr. Jonathan Cotliar, Dr. Lauren Hughey, and Dr. Daniela Kroshinsky, and the rest of the Society of Dermatology Hospitalists, a close-knit group of like-minded dermatologists who, like us, have chosen to focus their careers on the care and management of hospitalized patients and their dermatologic problems. We also must thank our collaborators in dermatopathology, in particular Drs. Rosalie Elenitsas, David Elder, George Xu, Mary Stone, Vincent Liu, and Brian Swick, without whom we would be unable to confirm many of these challenging diagnoses. Finally, we would like to dedicate this book to our patients, from whom and for whom we are always learning. Thank you for reading.

Dr. Rosenbach would like to dedicate this book to his family, who are endlessly loving and supportive and who never complain that he keeps an unpredictable schedule determined entirely by the number of consults in a given day. His wife, Anna, and children, Lara and Jake, are his loving family and his greatest joy. He thanks all of them for being so patient and understanding and is sorry for the many weekends spent working on this; he thinks they are the absolute best, and they make him thankful each and every day. Dr. Rosenbach would also like to thank his co-editors, who have put up with him for years in all sorts of ways and are the best colleagues one could ask for.

Dr. Wanat would like to dedicate this book to her always supportive, upbeat, and large Wanat family and her incredible husband, Steven, who is unwavering in his support, love, calming presence, and balance. In addition, she feels eternally grateful to her dermatology colleagues including the co-editors for being great to work with, authors of the book who worked so hard on their chapters, near and far mentors for always being there, her co-residents for being the absolute best, and all the residents and patients she has already had the chance to work with—her passion for dermatology is fueled by their presence.

Dr. Micheletti would like to dedicate this book to his wife, Dorothy; son, Andrew; and daughter, Elisa, by whom he is inspired daily and of whom he is endlessly proud. He would also like to thank his mother and father, a dermatologist, for setting him on this path, as well as the countless medical school and residency mentors, students, residents, colleagues, and patients who have helped sustain him along the way. The practice of medicine is an incredible privilege, and the work of a dermatology hospitalist is never boring. May we all continue to learn and strive together daily for the benefit of our patients.

Dr. Taylor would like to dedicate this book to her incredible family and friends. She would like to specifically thank her father who instilled in her a love of learning, travel, and medicine and her mother who taught her to dream big and work hard. She would like to thank Dr. Leeman who is largely responsible for her enthusiasm for and dedication to academic research and to Dr. Louis DePalma for inspiring her to become a pathologist. She would like to thank Drs. Elder, Rosenbach, and Elenitsas for their invaluable support and mentorship and for providing models for the type of clinician she hopes to become. She feels that it has been a fantastic privilege to work on this book alongside such knowledgeable and inspiring colleagues.

Preface

Welcome to inpatient dermatology!

This book aims to fill a novel space in dermatology education: the recognition and appropriate initial management of key dermatologic diseases you will encounter in the inpatient setting. Inpatient dermatology is an exciting, dynamic, and challenging field that may seem overwhelming in the beginning. We hope that this book will help provide the reader with a practical initial approach to the complex patient.

Dermatology is unique in that its organ of study is visible to the naked eye, often providing clues to the etiology of systemic diseases (including autoimmune, infectious, and neoplastic conditions) that otherwise span a variety of disciplines. Therefore, an informed assessment of the skin is an invaluable component of the inpatient workup. As such, this textbook is not geared solely toward dermatologists but also may be used as a resource for anyone who cares for patients in the hospital setting. By providing essential information in a concise, usable package, we hope to provide a systematic approach for evaluating inpatients with cutaneous pathology.

We have attempted to provide concise, bulleted, easy-to-read-and-reference, key material to help physicians diagnose and differentiate the dermatologic diseases that occur in the inpatient setting. Each brief chapter is focused on one specific inpatient dermatologic condition, with carefully curated clinical photographs and corresponding histopathologic images to aid readers in developing clinical-pathologic correlation and pattern recognition for these entities. We have provided a list of essential differential diagnoses which are important to consider and a day-one, initial workup and management plan for each condition. The sections are preceded by diagnostic pearls from the editors, where we share our approach to these often-challenging conditions.

The literature underscores the importance of inpatient dermatology consults by demonstrating that skin findings are often overlooked by non-dermatologists in hospitalized patients, with over three quarters of patients' relevant skin findings not noted by the primary team. One study demonstrated that when dermatologists consult on hospitalized patients, the diagnosis and/or treatment is changed 60% of the time. Other works have demonstrated that involving a dermatologist in the evaluation of common diagnoses such as cellulitis can reduce misdiagnoses (as one large study demonstrated, 75% of cases of "cellulitis" may instead represent pseudocellulitis, stasis dermatitis, contact dermatitis, Lyme, and other entities). Therefore, it is paramount that physicians, regardless of their specialization, are attentive to cutaneous findings so they can request the appropriate consultation or provide the appropriate review.

In this era of cost-conscious care and penalties for readmission, it is important dermatologists are able to identify and mitigate some of the cutaneous risk factors for cellulitis, so that they can guide management and reduce recurrent disease and readmissions. A study in England demonstrated that involving dermatologists in the diagnosis and management of lower limb cellulitis led to alternate diagnoses in 1/3 of cases and dramatically reduced the need for inpatient admission. Finally, emerging data suggest that simply having timely access to inpatient dermatologists can lead to reduced mortality and improved overall survival in patients presenting with Stevens-Johnson syndrome/toxic epidermal necrolysis.

This book is not a comprehensive textbook covering the breadth of dermatology; our focus is to guide point-of-care physicians as they are confronted with skin problems in hospitalized patients. The initial workup that we present is detailed and designed to help clinicians narrow their differential and hone in on a specific diagnosis and treatment plan. Our suggested evaluation is not exhaustive—what we have laid out should help clinicians make the vast majority of correct diagnoses and exclude alternate possibilities in a prompt and economical manner.

As with any text, the pages herein may quickly become outdated as the practice of medicine evolves. Inpatient medicine in particular is a rapidly changing environment: Patients present with novel acute illnesses, new pathogens and patterns of antibiotic resistance emerge, and cutaneous side effects result from clinical trial drugs and cutting-edge chemotherapeutic regimens. When evaluating inpatients, it is always worthwhile to consider searching the primary medical literature. The contents of these pages are designed to give a structured, algorithmic framework for evaluating inpatients, but should not be used in isolation to decide on treatment plans. Instead, each individual patient and case represent a unique combination of comorbidities and problems, requiring a tailored approach.

The practice of inpatient dermatology is humbling, and in many cases a specific final diagnosis is elusive. The approach we advocate is to cast a wide net, considering a broad array of differential diagnoses, and then to supplement the patient's history and clinical exam with a focus on the specific cutaneous morphology, using appropriate diagnostic tests to narrow in on a more focused differential or specific diagnosis. This textbook is designed to help guide that process, with a mind toward cost-conscious care and avoiding unnecessary, extraneous laboratory evaluations whenever possible. We hope readers find the format and content helpful as they care for these challenging conditions and help improve the health and lives of inpatients suffering from skin disease or cutaneous manifestations of systemic illness or treatments.

We hope you find this text helpful in your evaluation and management of inpatients with dermatological issues!

Misha Rosenbach, MD
Karolyn A. Wanat, MD
Robert G. Micheletti, MD
Laura A. Taylor, MD

References

Nahass GT, Meyer AJ, Campbell SF, Heaney RM. Prevalence of cutaneous findings in hospitalized medical patients. J Am Acad Dermatol. 1995;33:207–2011.

Falanga V, Schachner LA, Rae V, et al. Dermatologic consultations in the hospital setting. Arch Dermatol. 1994;130:1022–25.

Hughey LC. Why perform inpatient consultations. Dermatol Ther. 2011;24:149–50.

Strazzula L, Cotliar J, Fox LP, Hughey L, Shinkai K, Gee SN, Kroshinsky D. Inpatient dermatology consultation aids diagnosis of cellulitis among hospitalized patients: a multi-institutional analysis. J Am Acad Dermatol. 2015;73:70–5.

Kroshinsky D, Cotliar J, Hughey LC, Shinkai K, Fox LP. Association of dermatology consultation with accuracy of cutaneous disorder diagnoses in hospitalized patients. JAMA Dermatol. 2016;152(4):477–80.

Levell NJ, Wingfield CG, Garioch JJ. Severe lower limb cellulitis is best diagnosed by dermatologists and managed with shared care between primary and secondary care. Br J Dermatol. 2011;164:1326–8.

Micheletti R. The United States Dermatology Hospitalist Experience with Stevens-Johnson syndrome/toxic epidermal necrolysis: a multicenter retrospective study of 405 patients. Medical Dermatology Society Abstract Session, 2016, Washington, DC.

Contents

Contributors

Jack Abbott, MD Department of Dermatopathology, University of Pennsylvania, Philadelphia, PA, USA

Katherine K. Brown, MD Department of Dermatology, University of Pennsylvania, Philadelphia, PA, USA

Aileen Y. Chang, MD Department of Dermatology, University of California, San Francisco, CA, USA

Pooja Chitgopeker, MD University of Iowa, Iowa City, IA, USA

Juliana K. Choi, MD Department of Dermatology, University of Pennsylvania, Philadelphia, PA, USA

Department of Dermatology, Veteran Affairs Medical Center, Philadelphia, PA, USA

Nkanyezi N. Ferguson, MD University of Iowa Hospital and Clinics, Iowa City, IA, USA

Amy K. Forrestel, MD Department of Dermatology, Perelman School of Medicine, University of Pennsylvania, Philadelphia, PA, USA

Grant Ghahramani, MD Cotton O'Neil Dermatology, Topeka, KS, USA

Rachel Klein, MD Accent Dermatology, Medford, NJ, USA

Reid W. Masters, MD Department of Dermatology, Virginia Mason Medical Center, Seattle, WA, USA

Robert G. Micheletti, MD Department of Dermatology, Perelman School of Medicine, University of Pennsylvania, Philadelphia, PA, USA

Badri Modi, MD Division of Dermatology, City of Hope, Duarte, CA, USA

Molly Moye, MD Forefront Dermatology, Louisville, KY, USA

Krishna A. Mutgi, MD Mercy Health Dermatology, Toledo, OH, USA

Megan H. Noe, MD, MPH Department of Dermatology, University of Pennsylvania, Philadelphia, PA, USA

Lauren Orenstein, MD, FAAD Department of Dermatology, Temple University, Philadelphia, PA, USA

Lisa Pappas-Taffer, MD Department of Dermatology, University of Pennsylvania, Philadelphia, PA, USA

Evan Piette, MD University of Pennsylvania, Philadelphia, PA, USA

Douglas J. Pugliese, MD Department of Dermatology, Penn Presbyterian Medical Center, Perelman School of Medicine, University of Pennsylvania, Philadelphia, PA, USA

Misha Rosenbach, MD Department of Dermatology, Perelman School of Medicine, University of Pennsylvania, Philadelphia, PA, USA

Sara Samimi, MD Department of Dermatology, University of Pennsylvania, Philadelphia, PA, USA

Inbal Sander, MD Johns Hopkins School of Medicine, Baltimore, MD, USA

John C. Selby, MD, PhD University of Iowa Hospitals and Clinics, Iowa City, IA, USA

Natalie Spaccarelli, MD University of Pennsylvania, Philadelphia, PA, USA

Katherine T. Steele, MD Department of Dermatology, Perelman School of Medicine at the University of Pennsylvania, Philadelphia, PA, USA

Sasha Stephen, MD Department of Dermatology, Perelman School of Medicine at the University of Pennsylvania, Philadelphia, PA, USA

Campbell L. Stewart, MD Division of Dermatology, Department of Medicine, University of Washington, Seattle, WA, USA

Laura A. Taylor, MD Department of Pathology and Laboratory Medicine, University of Pennsylvania, Philadelphia, PA, USA

Amanda J. Tschetter, MD University of Minnesota Health, Minneapolis, MN, USA

Elizabeth A. Vanderah, MD Mercy Clinic, Washington, MO, USA

Nahid Y. Vidal, MD Dartmouth-Hitchcock Medical Center, Department of Surgery, Section of Dermatology, Geisel School of Medicine, Hanover, NH, USA

Joy Wan, MD Children's Hospital of Philadelphia, University of Pennsylvania, Philadelphia, PA, USA

Karolyn A. Wanat, MD Department of Dermatology, Medical College of Wisconsin, Milwaukee, WI, USA

Natalie Wright, MD Department of Dermatology, Brigham and Women's Hospital, Harvard University, Boston, MA, USA

Part I

Introduction

General Principles and Approach to Inpatient Dermatology

1

Misha Rosenbach

Introduction

Inpatient dermatology comprises a challenging subset of dermatologic care. As criteria for hospitalization have become more stringent, the inpatient population has become more complex, often requiring interdisciplinary care to manage patients' multiple comorbid problems. The dermatologist plays a crucial role, as many systemic diseases with high morbidity and mortality—from infections to autoimmune diseases to cancer to adverse drug reactions—can primarily present in the skin or involve the skin in isolation. Much of patient disease management, dermatologic and otherwise, has shifted to the outpatient setting, making inpatient treatment highly focused on acute disease management. The dermatologist is often consulted to determine if a patient's cutaneous lesions represent clues to an underlying illness necessitating inpatient treatment, or if the acuity of the lesion itself is such that the patient should be admitted or have their hospital stay prolonged. As most physicians receive only minimal exposure to dermatology in their training and due to the highly variable presentations of cutaneous disease, the dermatologist's insight, guidance, and education in this area can greatly improve patient care.

This text is focused on the initial diagnosis and management of cutaneous findings seen during the practice of inpatient medicine, from the emergency room, through the wards, up to the intensive care unit. In this book we emphasize clinical/pathologic correlation, as inpatients are often acutely ill, and it is important to zero in on a precise diagnosis and rule out alternative explanations as quickly as possible. Doing so often requires a thorough history, detailed cutaneous examination, and frequently a skin biopsy to identify diagnostic features of a particular dis ease.

In order to accurately diagnose and manage skin diseases, a basic framework of dermatologic nomenclature is essential. These terms help to guide the physician during the initial evaluation of the patient, and when interfacing with the descriptions laid out in this text, or during conversations with colleagues across specialties. Most skin findings can be broken down into a description of the primary lesion's most prominent morphology, the color of the lesions, secondary characteristics of the eruption, and distribution. While a comprehensive discussion of which differential diagnoses fall under each morphologic type is beyond the scope of this book, a general framework is essential when discussing inpatients' skin eruptions.

M. Rosenbach, MD
Department of Dermatology, Perelman School of Medicine, University of Pennsylvania, Philadelphia, PA, USA
e-mail: Misha.Rosenbach@uphs.upenn.edu

M. Rosenbach et al. (eds.), *Inpatient Dermatology*,
https://doi.org/10.1007/978-3-319-18449-4_1

Primary Morphologies

Primary morphologic descriptions allow lesions to be broadly characterized based on size, palpability, and contents.

Flat, nonpalpable lesions:	
Macule	Small (<1 cm), flat, non-palpable
Patches	Broad (>1 cm) flat lesions
Raised, solid, palpable lesions:	
Papules	Small (<1 cm) palpable "bumps"
Plaques	Broad (>1 cm) elevated lesions, like a raised patch, or "plateau"
Nodules	Large firm lesions bigger than typical papules; may be subcutaneous, dermal-based, or superficial
Tumors	Infiltrative masses; may be endophytic or exophytic
Raised, fluid filled lesions	
Vesicles	Small fluid-filled papule
Pustules	Small papule filled with purulent fluid
Bullae	Large blisters with clear, serous, or hemorrhagic fluid (Figs. 1.1–1.8)

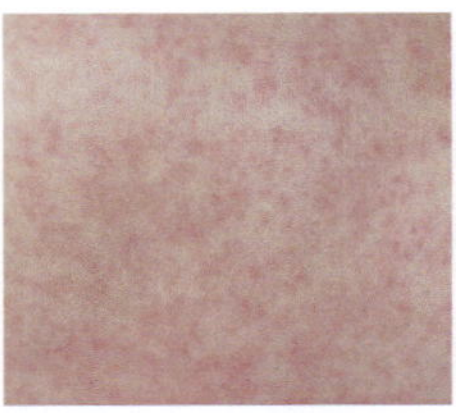

Fig. 1.1 Macules: These lesions are flat and <1 cm; in this case, there are blanchable erythematous macules due to a mild cutaneous adverse drug reaction.

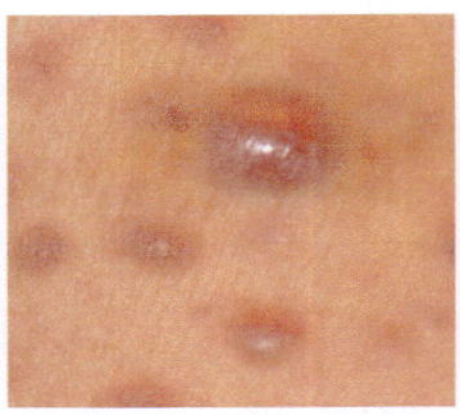

Fig. 1.2 Papules: These lesions are small, <1 cm, raised, palpable bumps, in this case due to leukemic cells infiltrating the dermis.

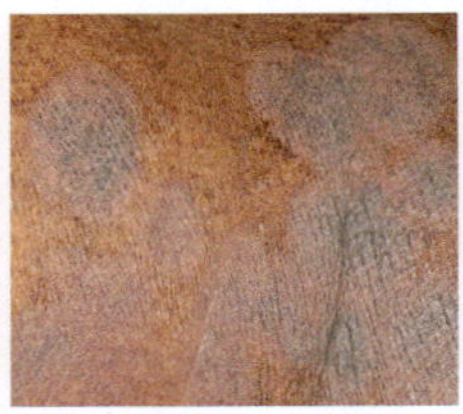

Fig. 1.3 Patches: These are broad, >1 cm, flat areas with minimal surface change or very fine scale, as shown here in a case of mycosis fungoides.

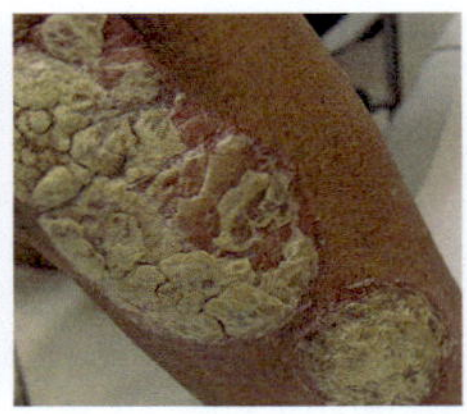

Fig. 1.4 Plaques: These are broad, slightly elevated "plateaus;" this case of psoriasis also had extensive adherent scale.

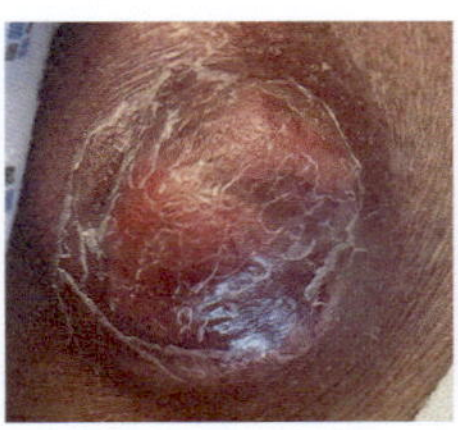

Fig. 1.5 Nodule: This large, 2–3 cm dermal-to-subcutaneous growth is protruding out from the dermis due to metastatic cancer.

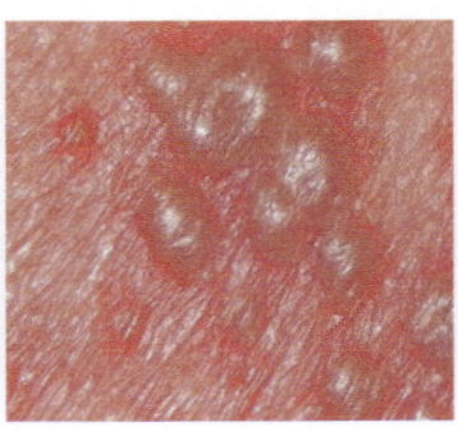

Fig. 1.6 Vesicle: A small <1 cm lesion filled with clear fluid; if filled with pus, may be referred to as a "vesiculopustule".

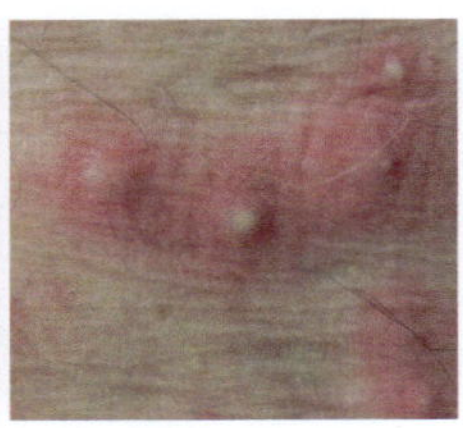

Fig. 1.7 Pustule: A papule or vesicle filled with pus, which may vary in size from near-microscopic to larger, almost bullous lesions.

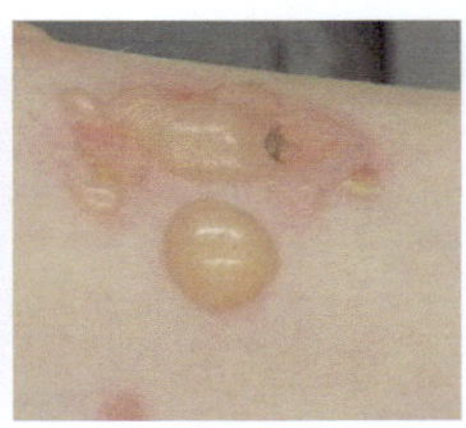

Fig. 1.8 Bullae: These are tense, fluid-filled blisters, as seen in this case of bullous pemphigoid.

Color

When describing the color of a skin eruption, it is best to simply describe what you see, rather than trying to use the "correct" term. Too often lesions are described as "erythematous" by default; one problem with that descriptor is that if it is the only descriptor used, it loses its meaning. The term erythematous should be reserved to refer to lesions that are pink and blanchable, where the color resolves with gentle pressure, signifying inflammation. In general, pink lesions imply inflammation, red lesions imply there has been damage, purple lesions imply there is a concerning infiltrate or ongoing damage, and black lesions imply death or dying (Figs. 1.9–1.13).

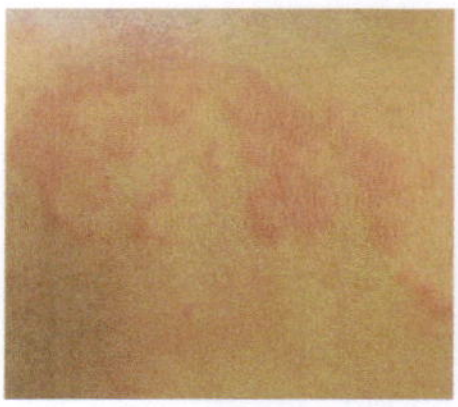

Fig. 1.9 Pink: This very faint erythema is a sign of mild inflammation, as seen in this case of an early urticarial drug reaction.

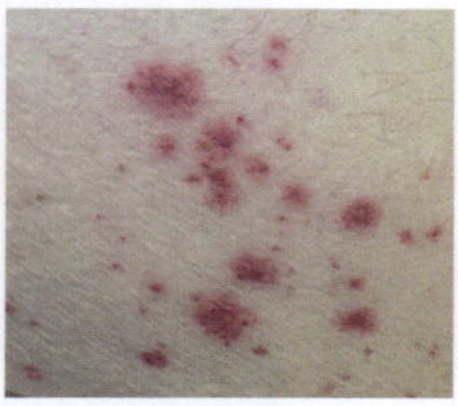

Fig. 1.10 Red: This color is non-blanching, illustrating that there is very intense inflammation or damage, as in this case of small vessel vasculitis.

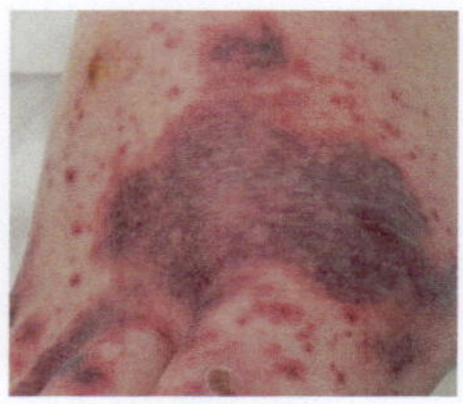

Fig. 1.11 Purple: This color is usually a sign of some form of tissue damage; in this case, confluent red lesions of vasculitis growing together and showing purple due to the amount of vascular injury and extravasated blood.

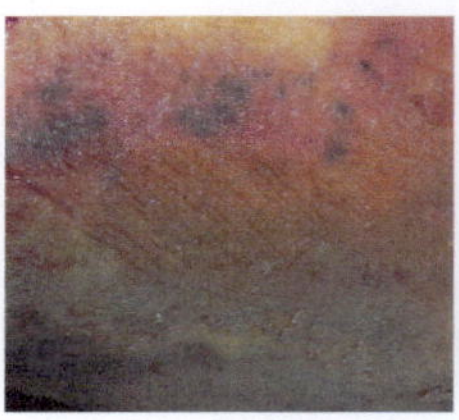

Fig. 1.12 Purple and Black: These colors suggest intense inflammation or damage occurring in the skin. This case of angioinvasive fungal infection is purple due to vascular destruction and extravastated blood, and black at sites of tissue ischemia and early necrosis.

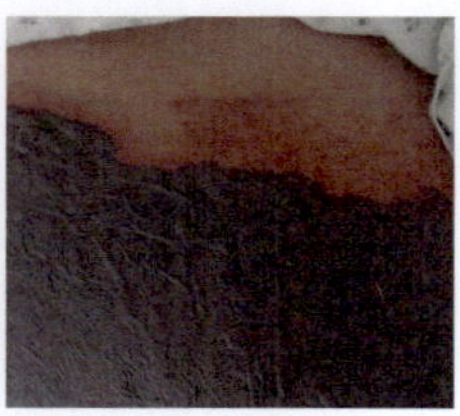

Fig. 1.13 Black: This broad area of necrotic skin has turned black from hypoperfusion, ischemia, and tissue necrosis due to warfarin necrosis.

Secondary Characteristics

Secondary characteristics refer to additional features of the lesions which can be diagnostic clues to their underlying etiology. These are generally extra clinical findings which develop in association with primary lesions, often as a result of change over time. Secondary changes can also include whether there has been ulceration of a lesion, lichenified thickening of the skin, scale build-up on top of a lesion, adherent serous crusts, or malodorous bacterial superinfection, all of which imply some chronicity (Figs. 1.14–1.18).

Secondary change	Description
Crust	Serous fluid which dries on the skin; color may vary depending on the etiology (e.g. honey-colored crust is common in impetigo)
Scale	Adherent fine flakes of skin; thickness may vary depending on the etiology (e.g. thick silvery scale in psoriasis, vs. fine scale in graft-v-host)
Lichenification	Thickening of the skin with accentuation of the normal skin markings (often a result of chronic scratching)
Fissure	A linear erosion or crust (variety of causes, e.g. physical factors (moisture damage in skin creases), infections (herpes), or inflammation (Crohn disease))
Erosion	Superficial damage to the skin involving the epidermis (e.g. ruptured bullae in pemphigus or opened vesicles in varicella)
Ulcer	A deeper injury to the skin resulting in exposed dermis or subcutaneous structures (severity varies by depth, may extend to muscle/bone; multiple causes including physical factors (pressure ulcers), infection, or inflammatory diseases)
Scar	The end result following injury to the skin; occasionally the characteristics of the scar may serve as a diagnostic clue (e.g. cribriform scarring is characteristic of healed ulcers of pyoderma gangrenosum)

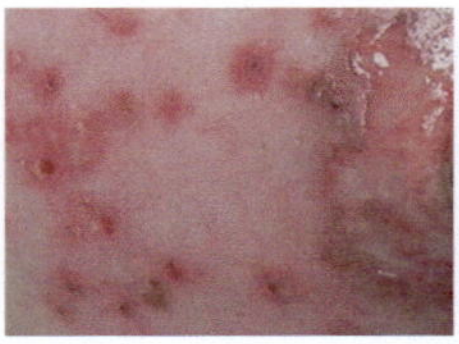

Fig. 1.14 Erosions (with a few vesicles): These flaccid, small vesicles and vesiculo-pustules from herpes simplex are easily ruptured, leaving shallow erosions exposed, which can grow together into a broad, confluent erosion, as shown on the right.

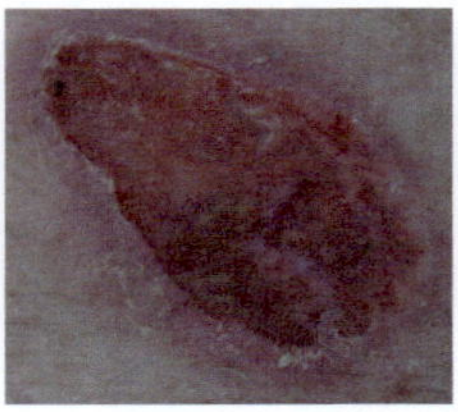

Fig. 1.15 Ulcer: an area of tissue loss through the entire epidermis and into the dermis or deeper layers.

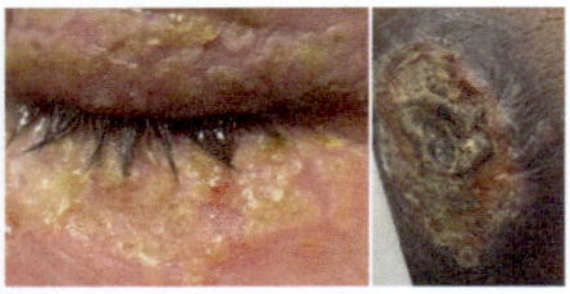

Fig. 1.16 Crust: An adherent layer of dried serous exudate often admixed with surface bacteria. The left image shows orange-yellow, honey colored crust is characteristic of *Staphylococcal* impetigo, as seen here in a patient with superinfected herpes simplex virus infection. The right image is a thicker crust over a deeper wound, with fibrin and dried serous crust overlying a shallow ulcer.

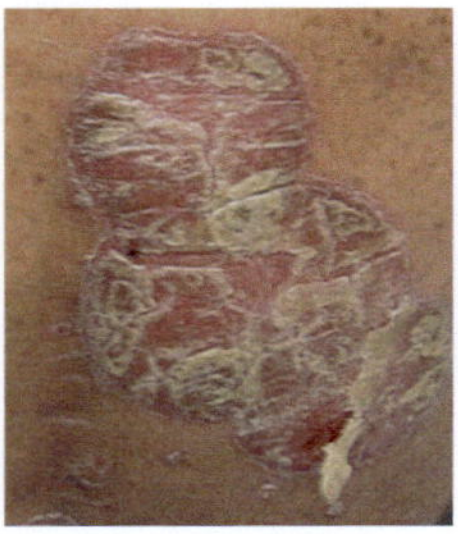

Fig. 1.17 Scale: An area of thickened, hyperkeratotic epidermis which can often be peeled back or picked off.

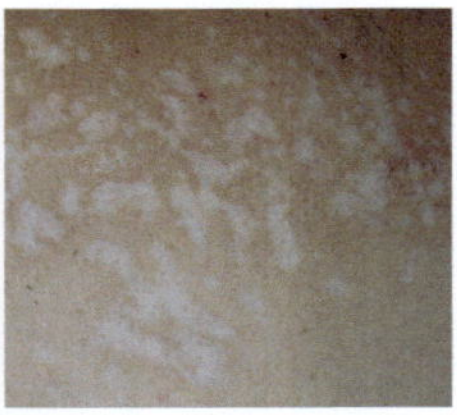

Fig. 1.18 Scar: Sclerotic, damaged skin at a site of prior injury.

Beyond primary lesions and secondary characteristics, another key diagnostic clue is the grouping, pattern, and distribution of skin lesions. Lesional distribution is best thought of in broad categories, such as whether the lesions are localized, diffuse, or limited to specific areas, such as flexural exanthems, dermatomal eruptions, or geometric shapes. Additionally the patterns or groupings of lesions in these areas are important to note, such as whether the lesions are annular, linear, or angulated. More specific localization, such as dermatomal, acral, or intertriginous accentuation, or perifollicular, can be aid in identifying and diagnosing certain diseases.

While appropriately describing a dermatologic eruption can be useful when calling a consult or discussing a case with a remote dermatologist, in the evaluation of complex hospitalized patients, a skin biopsy and histologic assessment coupled with clinical-pathologic correlation is often essential to making accurate, rapid diagnoses. There are two main biopsy techniques: Shave biopsy, which is most commonly used to remove single lesions or intact bullae, and punch biopsy, which allows deeper sampling of the dermis and subcutis and can be closed with sutures. Large lesions may rarely require excisional biopsy, or removal of the entire lesion, while some diagnoses with deeper pathology may require incisional biopsy, or a wedge or ellipse cut into part of the lesion to obtain a broad, deep specimen. In most cases, a punch biopsy of a representative lesion will suffice.

Generally when biopsying inflammatory dermatoses, it is best to biopsy a relatively newer lesion. Most often this means a punch biopsy of the leading edge of inflammation, although there are a number of exceptions and if in doubt it is best to consult with an experienced dermatologist. To exclude infection, sterile tissue culture may be performed by a similar method, i.e., a 4-mm punch biopsy of inflamed skin. This is particularly important when evaluating immunosuppressed patients or when biopsying conditions that are expected to demonstrate substantial neutrophilic infiltrates on pathology (such as Sweet syndrome), in which cases it may be important to correlate the pathology with microbiologic culture data to exclude infection. If evaluating a patient with suspected vasculitis, immunofluorescence studies may be helpful, and it is important to biopsy a fresh lesion for direct immunofluorescence (DIF). When evaluating bullous lesions, a DIF may be helpful as well–however, in that case, the specimen is taken from uninvolved perilesional skin. Immunofluorescence studies allow examination of antibody deposition in the superficial skin. This is often essential in differentiating between certain diagnoses, particularly the autoimmune blistering dermatoses, where the immunofluorescence pattern often defines the disease. Immunohistochemistry is another invaluable tool for dermatopathologists to hone in on a specific diagnosis histologically, with special stains to highlight microorganisms, distinguish specific cell types or highlight deposits of material within the skin.

Bedside Diagnostic Techniques

Additional bedside diagnostic techniques besides may be helpful in narrowing down a differential diagnosis. If a superficial skin fungal infection is suspected, one can wet the skin with an alcohol pad and use a 15-blade to scrape a thin layer of scale onto a glass slide to examine with chlorazol black or potassium hydroxide; the presence of thin branching hyphae can confirm the diagnosis. Similarly, when evaluating a patient with vesicles, simply piercing a vesicle and using a 15-blade to scrape the base onto a slide (Tzanck smear) can allow rapid staining to look for characteristic multinucleated cells and/or nuclear molding suggestive of a herpes-virus-family infection. When evaluating a patient with history and exam findings suggestive of a potential scabies infestation, it is important to know how to scrape and where (and on what magnification) to examine the slide for evidence of the mite, eggs, or feces. Generally, a drop of mineral oil on a 15-blade and a rigorous scraping of scaly web spaces or papular lesions on the hands—to the point of drawing a scant amount of blood—can obtain a sufficient specimen to allow low-power scanning for circular or oval shapes suggestive of mites or eggs. More advanced bedside diagnostic techniques include performing touch preps with the punch biopsy specimen to quickly look for evidence of angioinvasive fungal infections, or India-ink staining to evaluate for Cryptococcus.

Evaluation and Management

Evaluating inpatients using morphology, bedside diagnostic techniques, and skin biopsy can help lead to a narrow, focused differential diagnosis. However, many inpatients are acutely ill—and may be presenting with an early, undifferentiated pattern of a skin disease which will later blossom into a recognizable, diagnosable, and treatable entity. When initially evaluating inpatients, it is often enough to place each patient's eruption into a broad category: Benign (if there is only blanchable erythema, or a localized, minimally symptomatic eruption, or a single banal appearing lesion); dangerous (if there is evidence of skin damage, purpura, necrosis, blisters, or lesions in a suppressed host); or uncertain. If the eruption appears benign, many patients can be reassured and monitored, and may often be treated and supported through their hospitalization despite their rash. If the eruption is concerning or dangerous, it should be managed appropriately. The most challenging case is where there is uncertainty; a widespread morbilliform eruption which spares the face and lacks characteristic features of a systemic hypersensitivity reaction like DRESS, for instance. While mild morbilliform eruptions may be "treated through," and DRESS warrants treatment with systemic steroids, a widespread non-DRESS morbilliform eruption may warrant close monitoring and further workup, to ensure there is no sign of subtle systemic inflammation.

When managing inpatients for dermatological diagnosis, it is important to remember that the inpatient setting is quite different than the outpatient arena. While patients are often sicker and more medically complicated than most outpatients with dermatologic issues, there are a number of advantages to treating inpatients. First and foremost is that patients can be seen on a daily basis. This allows for close clinical follow-up and medical monitoring, thus making it easier to decide to "treat through" certain eruptions and closely monitor patients for progression. For more concerning eruptions, pathology is often rapidly available. It may take a phone call, but most hospital-based pathology labs can turn around a skin biopsy specimen in 24 h, and pathologists are often happy to be contacted with clinical information to help ensure clinical/pathologic correlation—which can help lead to a rapid, accurate diagnosis.

Furthermore, in the inpatient setting other consultants are often readily available. If patients are suspected of having an autoimmune disease, outpatients may wait weeks to see a rheumatologist, yet consultation rarely takes more than 24 h for hospitalized patients. Similarly, if a patient is seen with small-vessel vasculitis and it is unclear whether their urinalysis is concerning, it is quite simple to request a nephrologist evaluate the patient and spin the urine. Additionally, having patients in a monitored setting often makes it easier to initiate certain treatments. At home, recommending a "soak and smear" with topical steroids for a widespread dermatitis may be met with resistance as patients are reluctant to have ointment on their clothing or bedding. Inpatients can easily be wrapped in damp towels, have thick layers of greasy topical steroids applied, and be placed in a sauna suit, for rapid treatment of broad body surface areas with mid-to-high-potency topical steroids twice daily. This can result in rapid improvement in many cases. It is also important to remember that when patients are admitted and being seen on a daily basis, it may be reasonable to use higher potency, stronger medications than one would otherwise prescribe. We frequently recommend a single day of triamcinolone or clobetasol for facial eruptions in the inpatient setting, knowing that, while there are concerns about the long-term safety of high-potency steroids on the face or in skin folds, hospitalized patients' medications can be adjusted on a day-to-day basis and there is no concern for self-administered long-term overuse or misunderstanding of directions. One day of high-potency steroids can often clear an eruption that as an outpatient might take weeks to resolve. This can be helpful in time-sensitive situations, for instance, in vascular surgery patients with inflamed intertriginous eruptions that impair safe transcutaneous vascular access procedures through the inflamed skin.

Perhaps most importantly, in the inpatient setting it is quite easy to assess response to treatment. Through daily assessment of the patient's lesions, the main concept we would emphasize is to ask each day whether the patient requires continued hospitalization on the basis of their skin condition. Patients may be admitted for autoimmune blistering diseases such as bullous pemphigoid, and while it may be important to make a diagnosis during their stay, patients (and their doctors) should realize that even with appropriate therapy, it may take some time for new bullae to cease and old erosions to start to heal. These patients do not need to be admitted for the entire process. More importantly, however, is to recognize when treatments are failing. In such cases, one must always ask whether the wrong treatment is being used, or if the diagnosis needs to be reassessed. Frequently physicians can become fixated on a specific diagnosis, and persist with second, third, and fourth line therapeutic options geared at managing that entity, without going back and questioning the accuracy of the initial diagnosis. When managing inpatient dermatologic diseases, if patients are not responding to what should be appropriate treatment, it is important to keep an open mind and revisit the diagnosis.

One final aspect worth discussing related to inpatient dermatology is the concept of handoffs. While dermatologists are serving as consultants, we encourage physicians to take the time to call and discuss cases directly with the primary team, allowing an opportunity for them to learn about the dermatologic diagnosis and understand the workup, treatment plan, and time course involved. Frequently a simple phone call can ensure that a patient with a full body rash receives an appropriate one-pound jar of ointment instead of a default 15-g tube, which can have a tremendous effect on outcome. Similarly, it is essential to help manage the transition from the inpatient setting through discharge to the outpatient arena. The inpatient dermatology team should ensure that there is written and verbal communication about the inpatient diagnosis, course, and treatment plan, and should ensure there is a follow-up appointment within an appropriate amount of time. If these handoffs are done appropriately, it can help avoid unnecessary readmission or delays in treatment, and can help ensure that patients with dermatologic problems are cared for throughout their hospital stay, during their transition home, and post-hospital course.

Part II

Medication Reactions

Medication reactions are the source of many inpatient dermatology consultations. The dermatologist's job is to screen for serious reactions and provide guidance to the primary medical team. In order to effectively do so, one must balance the risks and benefits associated with continued treatment, specifically, "is the rash or the medication more harmful to the patient?" In this chapter, our purpose is to introduce clues to help distinguish different types of drug eruptions, and strategies for diagnosing and managing patients with medication reactions.

As most common morbilliform eruptions are mild, in the absence of concerning signs patients may be "treating through" the skin rash with topical steroids and antihistamines without altering their therapeutic regimen. However, drug rashes can be life-threatening, as is the case in SJS/TEN or DRESS, necessitating the identification and immediate discontinuation of the culprit medication. The potential lethality of a drug reaction makes the recognition of associated cutaneous findings paramount. The presence of facial involvement, widespread rash, bright red skin lesions, fever, or swelling should raise the possibility of a systemic hypersensitivity reaction (DRESS), while dusky, non-blanching skin lesions, mucosal inflammation or erosions should raise concern for SJS/TEN. Diffuse erythroderma, fine sterile non-folliculocentric pustules, extensive urticaria with facial involvement or associated systemic inflammation should also prompt rapid medication review and consideration for changing the patients' drug regimens.

Some medications can be easily replaced. However, if a patient is on a life-saving medication for which similarly efficacious alternatives do not exist, a medication change should only be suggested in the setting of a severe eruption; in this case one must consider whether it is more harmful to continue or discontinue the medication. It is helpful to keep in mind which medications or classes of medications are frequently associated with drug reactions and which are considered less "reactive," i.e., prone to the induction of cutaneous and systemic manifestations. Antimicrobial agents (particularly sulfa drugs), anti-epileptic agents, allopurinol, minocycline, and nevirapine are frequent offenders that often result in severe reactions, while beta-blockers and calcium channel blockers rarely cause cutaneous sequelae.

Ideally, all patients' medication lists should include only essential agents, and as few PRN medications or overlapping medications as possible (e.g., some order sets include a variety of PRN opiates for pain; it's best when evaluating patients with suspected drug reactions to trim their medication lists to include a single class of drugs for pain control).

Finally, it is important to remember that not everything appears on a medication list. Patients with suspected drug reactions should be queried about home medications, over-the-counter non-prescription medications, and herbal medications or alternative treatments. In the hospital, patients may be exposed to medications in the operating room, to contrast dye during radiographic procedures, or to dialysates if on renal-replacement therapy, all of which can precipitate cutaneous eruptions and may be missed on a cursory review of the medication list.

Morbilliform Drug Eruption

2

Megan H. Noe

Overview

- Morbilliform drug eruptions are the most common type of cutaneous adverse drug eruption comprising 75–90% of all drug reactions
- Frequently implicated medications include: antibiotics (penicillins, sulfonamides, cephalosporins), anticonvulsants, NSAIDs, and calcium channel blockers, although eruptions can occur with any medication
- The underlying mechanism is likely a type IV drug hypersensitivity reaction, caused by the presentation of a drug hapten to T cells, where binding to MHC-II receptors causes the release of cytotoxic proteins

Clinical Presentation

- Erythematous macules and papules coalescing into patches ("morbilliform", or measles-like, eruption) (Fig. 2.1)
  - Typically begin on the trunk, back, flanks, and upper extremities and then can spread to the lower trunk and extremities, becoming confluent in areas
- Generally, more prominent in areas of pressure, such as elastic waistbands or sock bands, or dependent areas in hospitalized patients while typically sparing the face and mucous membranes
  - Facial involvement should prompt consideration of DRESS (see page 33)
- Pruritus and low-grade fever can accompany the rash
- An eruption typically begins 4–14 days after the start of a new medication, but may present sooner if the patient has been previously exposed to the drug and resolves spontaneously in 1–2 weeks

Histopathology

- Overall histology is non-specific but can help rule out other potential causes for the eruption
- Characteristically demonstrates mild perivascular lymphocytic inflammation with or without eosinophils (Fig. 2.2)

M. H. Noe, MD, MPH
Department of Dermatology, University of Pennsylvania,
Philadelphia, PA, USA
e-mail: Megan.Noe@uphs.upenn.edu

M. Rosenbach et al. (eds.), *Inpatient Dermatology*,
https://doi.org/10.1007/978-3-319-18449-4_2

Differential Diagnosis

- Viral Exanthem (EBV, enterovirus, adenovirus, HIV, HHV-6, parvovirus B19): hard to distinguish without exposure history or classic patterned eruption (e.g., slapped cheeks and reticulate erythema in parvovirus)
- Drug reaction with eosinophils and systemic symptoms (DRESS): facial erythema and edema, high fever, lymphadenopathy, and hepatitis
- Acute generalized exanthematous pustulosis (AGEP): minute fine pustules often with fever
- Stevens-Johnson syndrome/toxic epidermal necrolysis (SJS/TEN): mucosal erosions, non-blanching dusky "targetoid" lesions
- Acute GVHD: hard to distinguish in recent transplant patients on multiple medications; aGVH may be more monomorphous, favor the outer arms and upper back, and have fine scale, and may be accompanied by diarrhea or bilirubin elevation

Work-Up

- Evaluation of medication list including new formulations, dose changes, drug-drug interactions, and over the counter medications
- If associated fever, swelling, facial involvement, or other concerning features order a CBC with differential to assess for peripheral eosinophilia and AST/ALT to rule out early DRESS
- Mucosal involvement or dusky, non-blanching macules should prompt consideration of SJS/TEN
- A skin biopsy could be considered if there is concern for other etiologies

Management

- Treatment is based on symptoms and can include topical steroids and/or oral anti-histamines but is mainly supportive
- All unnecessary medications should be discontinued
- If there is a viable alternative medication to the suspected offending agent, substitution should be attempted
- If the triggering medication is medically necessary, stopping the inciting medication is sometimes not necessary, and the morbilliform reaction can be monitored while "treating-through" the rash
- If dusky, non-blanching lesions, bullae, or mucosal involvement develops, or the eruption spreads to involve the face with facial edema, the patient should be reevaluated for progression to more severe drug reaction (SJS, DRESS)

Suggested Readings

1. Gerson D, Sriganeshan V, Alexis JB. Cutaneous drug eruptions: a 5-year experience. J Am Acad Dermatol. 2008;59:995–9.
2. Rawlin M. Exanthems and drug reactions. Aust Fam Physician. 2011;40:486–9.

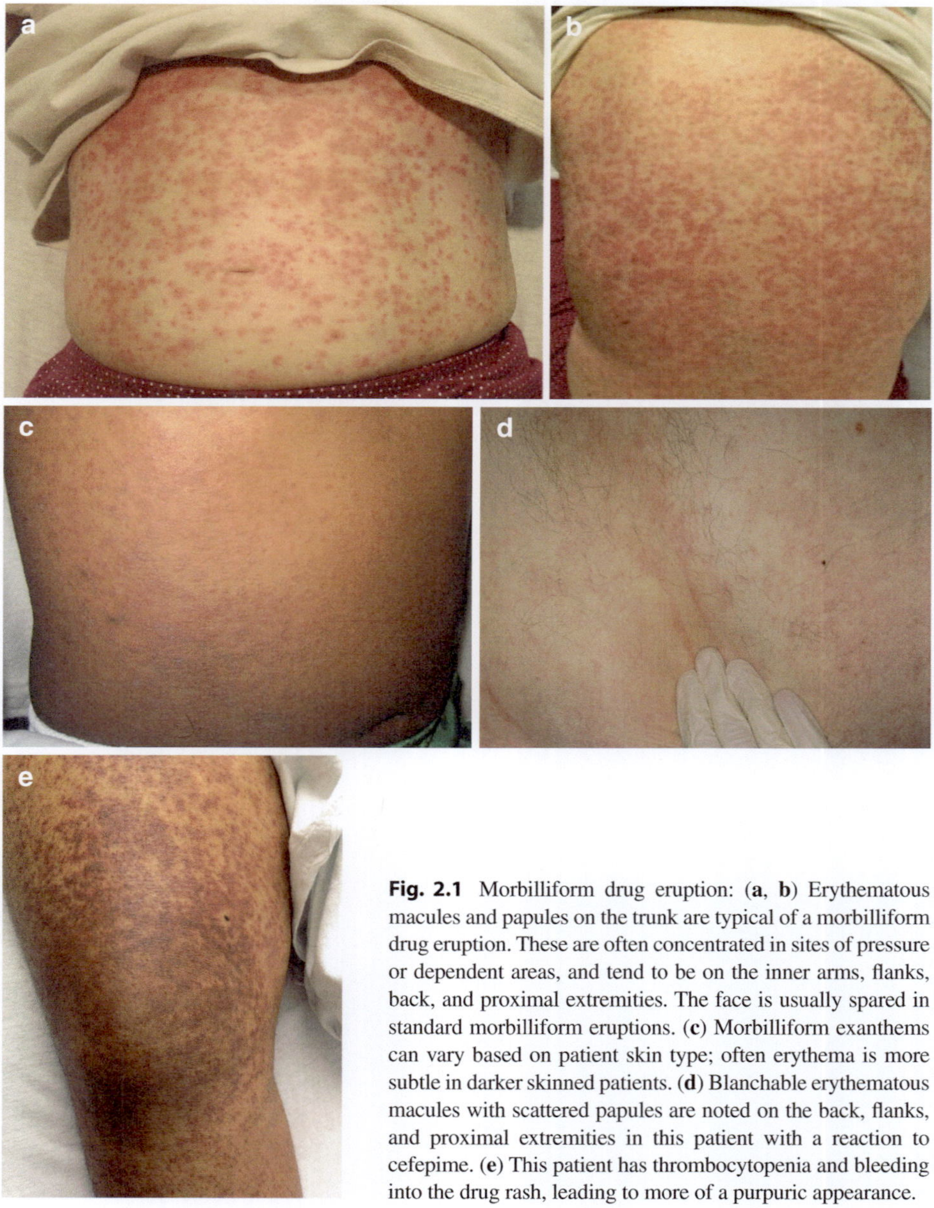

Fig. 2.1 Morbilliform drug eruption: (**a**, **b**) Erythematous macules and papules on the trunk are typical of a morbilliform drug eruption. These are often concentrated in sites of pressure or dependent areas, and tend to be on the inner arms, flanks, back, and proximal extremities. The face is usually spared in standard morbilliform eruptions. (**c**) Morbilliform exanthems can vary based on patient skin type; often erythema is more subtle in darker skinned patients. (**d**) Blanchable erythematous macules with scattered papules are noted on the back, flanks, and proximal extremities in this patient with a reaction to cefepime. (**e**) This patient has thrombocytopenia and bleeding into the drug rash, leading to more of a purpuric appearance.

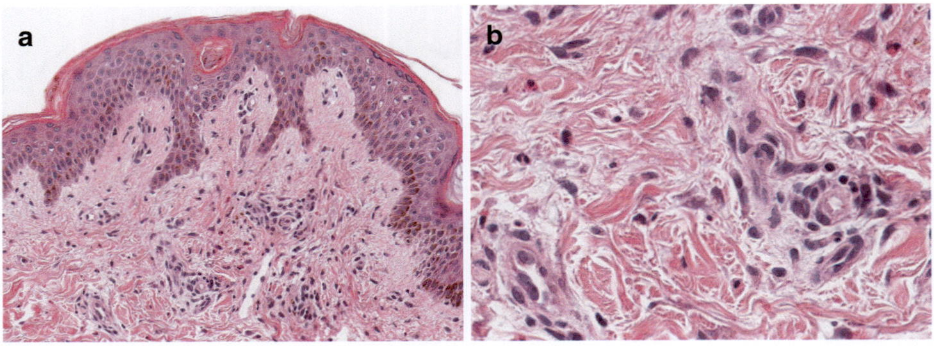

Fig. 2.2 Morbilliform (*10*×, *40*×; *H&E*): The density of the cellular infiltrate is highly variable in morbilliform drug eruptions. (**a**) There is a perivascular lymphocytic infiltrate with eosinophils. (**b**) Higher power demonstrates lymphocytes with occasional eosinophils; eosinophils are typically present but not necessary to make a diagnosis.

Urticaria

3

Aileen Y. Chang

Overview

- Urticaria refers to pink, edematous, pruritic wheals which may be acute (less than 6 weeks of lesions) or chronic (more than 6 weeks); inpatient urticaria is almost always acute
- Acute urticaria is typically due to infections or medications (in the inpatient setting, usually due to recently administered medications)
- IgE-mediated immediate Type I hypersensitivity reaction

Clinical Presentation

- Eruptions tend to arise within minutes to hours of exposure to inciting agent
  - Medications (antibiotics, NSAIDS, opiates) and radiocontrast dye are common triggers; less common causes include viral illnesses, food, and physical triggers (pressure, heat, cold induced urticaria)
- While an urticarial eruption can persist for days, weeks, or sometimes months, the individual lesions should resolve within 24 h (usually within 1–2 h), but patients may have ongoing eruptions with new lesions replacing fading ones at the same anatomic location
- Typical urticarial lesions are generally not painful, and resolve without residua (Fig. 3.1)
  - Urticarial vasculitis presents with wheals that are painful (not pruritic) and persist for hours (often more than 24 h), and resolve with bruising due to the vascular injury; these findings warrant further evaluation as many will have an underlying disease, particularly lupus
  - Urticaria multiforme may occur, particularly in children, as part of a viral exanthema; urticarial wheals can develop central pallor and clear areas
- Angioedema is a form of deep hives with subcutaneous/submucosal swelling, which may be tender, threaten the airway, and last up to 2–3 days
  - Patients with extensive facial urticaria, lip or tongue swelling, or stridor, wheezing, or drooling, should be monitored closely, ideally in an ICU

A. Y. Chang, MD
Department of Dermatology, University of California, San Francisco, CA, USA
e-mail: aileen.chang@ucsf.edu

M. Rosenbach et al. (eds.), *Inpatient Dermatology*,
https://doi.org/10.1007/978-3-319-18449-4_3

Histopathology

- Interstitial dermal edema, dilated venules with endothelial swelling, with a paucity of mixed inflammatory cells although occasional neutrophils and eosinophils may be seen (Fig. 3.2)

Differential Diagnosis

- Urticarial vasculitis: wheals last >24 h, burn rather than itch, fade with bruising
- Erythema multiforme: urticaria may develop central clearing and appear "multiform"—erythema multiforme lesions exhibit central duskiness
- Serum sickness: urticaria tend to be distal and over joints, and patients are systemically ill with joint pain and fever
- Bullous pemphigoid (BP), urticarial phase: the presence of bullae suggests BP, but very early disease may lack blisters; biopsy and immunofluorescence may be necessary
- Auto-inflammatory or autoimmune syndromes (Familial Mediterranean Fever, Muckle-Wells, Stills, Schnitzler, EGPA): family history and disease-specific manifestations from each entity may be necessary
- Parasitic infections, arthropod assault: puncta or bite sites, grouped lesions ("breakfast, lunch, dinner"), or clusters at exposed sites/clothing folds can be helpful clues

Work-Up

- A thorough history and review of systems should screen for concerning "red flag" systemic symptoms such as fever, joint pain, lesions lasting longer than 24 h which burn and fade with bruising
- New medications, recent infection, and other potential triggers should be noted
- Consider physical urticarias: pressure, heat, cold, sun, stress
- Biopsy should be performed in those with red flags or refractory disease in order to rule out other entities and guide treatment
- Extensive laboratory evaluation is not warranted in the absence of specific features prompting further investigation; a trigger is rarely identified in chronic urticaria
- A work-up for specific urticaria mimics should proceed if concerning features are present

Management

- Patients with perioral or airway involvement should be monitored closely; if airway involvement is present patients may warrant ICU level care
- First-line: combination long-acting non-sedating antihistamine therapy for at least 4–8 weeks (H1 and H2 blockers twice daily or more), with breakthrough short acting antihistamines as needed
- Second-line:
  - Consider dapsone or colchicine, particularly if neutrophilic infiltrate on biopsy
  - Consider prednisone for severe cases
  - Consider omalizumab (monoclonal anti-IgE antibody) or immunosuppressive therapies (e.g. mycophenolate) in rare cases

Suggested Readings

1. Tarbox JA, Gutta RC, Radojicic C, et al. Utility of routine laboratory testing in management of chronic urticaria/angioedema. Ann Allergy Asthma Immunol. 2011;107(3):239–43.
2. Kozel MM, Mekkes JR, Bossuyt PM, et al. The effectiveness of a history-based diagnostic approach in chronic urticaria and angioedema. Arch Dermatol. 1998;134(12):1575–80.
3. Kaplan AP. Clinical practice. Chronic urticaria and angioedema. N Engl J Med. 2002;346(3):175–9.

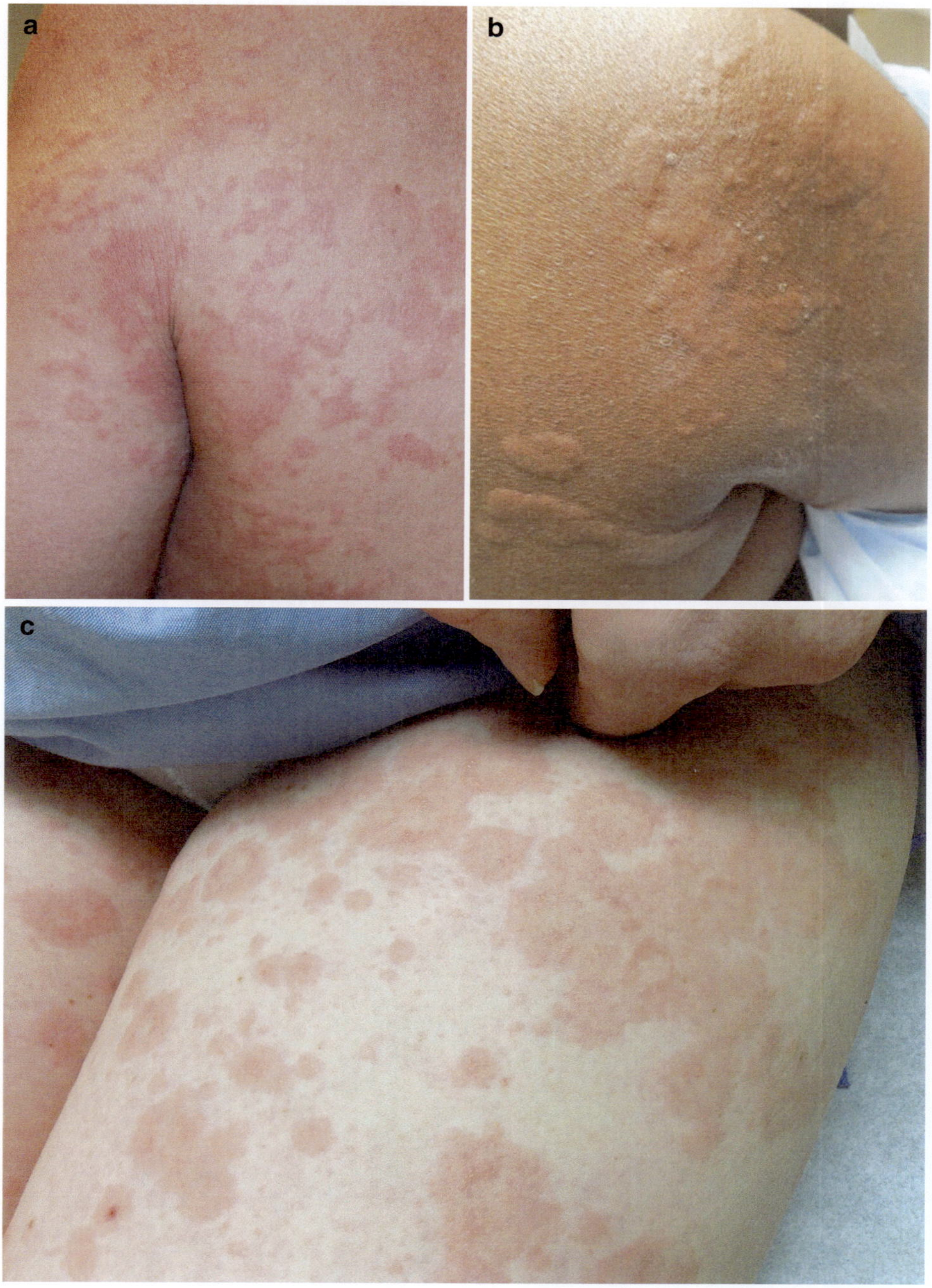

Fig. 3.1 Urticaria: (**a**) Pink, edematous wheals of typical urticaria. (**b**) In dark-skinned patients, urticaria may appear flesh-colored. (**c**) Localized edema may cause the lesions to blanch, resulting in an annular or polycyclic appearance as in this case of urticaria multiforme. The centers are often clear, helping to distinguish these lesions from those of erythema multiforme.

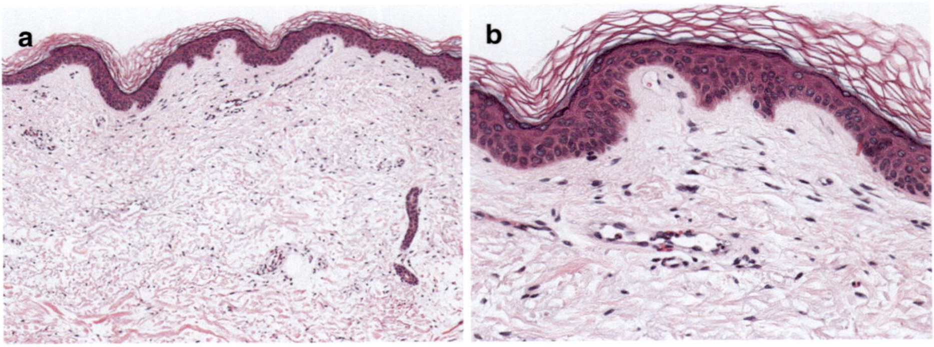

Fig. 3.2 Urticaria (*5×, 10×; H&E*): (**a**) There is interstitial dermal edema with dilated vessels and mixed inflammatory infiltrate. (**b**) Higher power demonstrates eosinophils, neutrophils, and lymphocytes in variable amounts depending on the age of the lesion, with increased spaces between collagen fibers secondary to dermal edema.

Stevens-Johnson Syndrome/Toxic Epidermal Necrolysis

4

Nkanyezi N. Ferguson

Overview

- Stevens-Johnson syndrome (SJS) and Toxic epidermal necrolysis (TEN) are life-threatening mucocutaneous diseases where the epidermal barrier is lost and patients experience pain, fluid and electrolyte shifts, and are at high risk for secondary infection, scarring, and long-term morbidity
- SJS and TEN exist on a spectrum and are defined by the percentage of the patient's body surface area with epidermal detachment (measured when the disease is at its worst)
  - <10% for SJS; 10–30% for SJS/TEN overlap >30% for TEN
  - Characterized by severe mucous membrane inflammation and full-thickness epidermal necrosis leading to wide spread mucocutaneous sloughing and denudation
- Affects all age groups, with an increased incidence noted in individuals with HIV, autoimmune diseases, immunosuppression, and underlying malignancy
- In adults, almost always drug associated
  - Antibiotics (particularly sulfonamides), anticonvulsants, allopurinol, NSAIDs, nevirapine, are common offenders but can be seen with several other medications
  - Infectious causes are uncommon in adults but maybe seen in children (HSV or *M. pneumoniae*; some consider mycoplasma-induced mucositis a separate entity)
- May represent an immune mediated drug reaction with higher rates in certain genetically at-risk populations
  - For example, carbamazepine-associated SJS/TEN among Han Chinese and other Asian groups has been associated with HLA-B*1502
- Type IV hypersensitivity reaction: CD8+ cytotoxic T-cell mediated apoptosis of keratinocytes via granulysin, Fas ligand (FasL), TNF-alpha, perforin/granzyme B, and nitric oxide

Clinical Presentation

- Mucocutaneous symptoms often accompanied by fever, rhinorrhea, cough, malaise and anorexia
- Mucosal inflammation often shortly precedes the cutaneous eruption and typically involves at least two mucosal surfaces
  - Dysphasia, photophobia, "gritty" eyes, rectal/vaginal pain, and dysuria may be symptoms of mucosal involvement

N. N. Ferguson, MD
University of Iowa Hospital and Clinics, Iowa City, IA, USA
e-mail: nkanyezi-ferguson@uiowa.edu

M. Rosenbach et al. (eds.), *Inpatient Dermatology*,
https://doi.org/10.1007/978-3-319-18449-4_4

- Cutaneous involvement is characterized by a tender, painful macular eruption with non-blanching "targetoid lesions" (central red spots surrounded by minimal erythema) which classically develop symmetrically on the face and trunk and spread to the extremities (Fig. 4.1)
- The dusky, non-blanching lesions represent sites of epidermal damage; as the disease progresses the dusky lesions can blister and form bullae or widespread sheets of epidermal sloughing
  - Positive Nikolsky sign: separation of epidermis at the sub-basilar plane with gentle lateral pressure
- Symptoms most commonly develop within 1–2 weeks of initial drug exposure, but can occur 1–2 months out, or following dose change, formulation change, or alteration in drug metabolism; more rapid reactions can occur with subsequent repeated exposure
  - Worst offenders: lamotrigine, carbamazepine, phenytoin, phenobarbital, allopurinol, trimethoprim-sulfamethoxazole, cephalosporins, aminopenicillins, quinolones, oxicam non-steroidal anti-inflammatory drugs, nevirapine; can occur with any agent
- Mucositis involving ocular, oral and genital locations is seen in the majority of patients; a lack of mucosal inflammation should prompt consideration of alternate etiologies
- Patients with TEN can develop multiorgan involvement resulting in renal, gastrointestinal, respiratory and cardiovascular damage
- High risk for secondary infection potentially resulting in sepsis and increased risk for thromboembolic disease significantly contribute to morbidity and mortality

Histopathology

- Early SJS/TEN resembles erythema multiforme and is marked by the presence of necrotic keratinocytes and interface dermatitis with lymphocytes tagging the epidermal-dermal junction; can be pauci-inflammatory (Fig. 4.2)
- Late SJS/TEN is characterized by full-thickness epidermal necrosis, which may be accompanied by subepidermal clefting and bullae formation at the dermoepidermal junction and an accompanying inflammatory infiltrate within the superficial dermis

Differential Diagnosis

- Erythema multiforme (EM): often HSV-associated, and thus recurrent, with one mucous-membrane mildly inflamed and symmetric (typically central lip and bilateral palms or soles), true "target" lesions with three distinct zones of inflammation
- Staphylococcal scalded skin syndrome (SSSS): Diffuse superficial desquamation sparing the mucosa
- Morbilliform drug eruption: fully blanching erythema with no dusky/targetoid lesions, spares the mucosa
- Acute graft versus host disease (GVHD): severe acute GVHD can be impossible to distinguish
- Drug induced linear immunoglobulin (IgA) dermatosis: blisters in clusters, with mucosal involvement less common; pathology and immunofluorescence can be definitive
- Drug reaction with eosinophilia and systemic symptoms (DRESS): patients can have overlapping features of both DRESS and SJS; in pure DRESS blistering and mucositis is rare
- Acute generalized exanthematous pustulosis (AGEP): fine pustules with rare mucositis; as the pustules of AGEP run together, lakes of pus can resemble widespread TEN-like peeling
- Bullous dermatoses (e.g pemphigus vulgaris, bullous pemphigoid, paraneoplastic pemphigus bullous lupus erythematosus): biopsy and DIF can help distinguish

Work-Up

- A thorough medication history and complete physical exam including all mucosal sites is imperative
- Frozen sections allow for rapid evaluation for full thickness epidermal necrosis (high sensitivity and low specificity for TEN); "jelly roll" method (peeling off already detached epidermis for evaluation of full thickness necrosis) can be helpful

- Severity of Illness Score for Toxic Epidermal Necrolysis (SCORTEN) is a tool to predict severity and mortality in patients with acute TEN
  - One point is allotted to each of the following variables:
    Age > 40 years, heart rate > 120 beats per minute, epidermal detachment >10% body surface area on day one, comorbid malignancy, blood urea nitrogen >28 mg/dL, glucose >252 mg/dL, and bicarbonate <20 mEq/L
  - Total score and corresponding mortality rate (%):
    0–1 (3.2%), 2 (12.2%), 3 (35.5%), 4 (58.3%), ≥5 (90.0%)
  - The algorithm of drug causality for epidermal necrolysis (ALDEN) score has been proposed to help evaluate likelihood that suspected offending agents are responsible
- Blood cultures and occasional skin bacterial sampling to evaluate for systemic and local infection can be important
- CBC for evaluation of leukocytosis and other abnormalities
- CMP for evaluation of electrolyte abnormalities, liver dysfunction, and renal involvement is important
- Patients should be monitored for DVT
- Consultation to ophthalmology, urology, gynecology, and/or otolaryngology depending on mucosal involvement is important in co-management; even if overt clinical disease is not apparent, ophthalmology should be consulted as the rate of permanent ocular scarring is very high

Management

- Rapid, early intervention is critical
- Identification and discontinuation of the suspected etiologic agent—must be done within the first 24 h
  - All unnecessary medications and any potential culprit agents must be stopped
  - Patients should avoid cross-reacting agents
- Supportive management in a specialty intensive care unit or burn unit for control of fluid and electrolyte balance, hemodynamics, temperature monitoring for infection, and wound care
- Early, aggressive fluid resuscitation (2/3 the volume required as calculated by the Parkland formula for burn victims with similar BSA)
- Early, aggressive nutritional repletion (sometimes requiring parenteral nutrition or tube feedings)
- Management of mucocutaneous detachment
  - Keratinocytes heal best in moist environments:
    Thick layers of hydrophobic ointment can aide in wound healing
    Coverage of denuded skin with lubricated non-adherent dressing (options range from Vaseline TM® to silver-impregnated dressings)
    Ocular lubrication and emergent involvement of ophthalmology (occasional aggressive intervention with amniotic membranes may be indicated)
  - Urethral involvement should be assessed by urology
  - Vaginal involvement should be evaluated by gynecology; moist non-adherent dressings are essential to minimize long-term sequelae
  - Unnecessary catheters, tape, adhesives, or other invasive devices should be minimized in order to prevent infection
- Use of adjuvant systemic therapy has shown conflicting results:
  - Intravenous immune globulin (IVIG) has been utilized to prevent Fas-FasL directed keratinocyte apoptosis
    Using higher doses earlier in the disease process has demonstrated improvement in SCORTEN predicted mortality
  - Corticosteroids have been used historically as an adjuvant treatment with mixed results; some advocate for early, high dose, pulse steroids
    Prolonged steroid use can raise the risk of infection and impair wound healing and is generally not recommended
  - Cyclosporine has shown benefit in limited studies and is now the treatment of choice across much of Europe
  - Recent studies have demonstrated efficacy with the TNF-alpha inhibitor etanercept

Suggested Readings

1. Schwartz RA, McDonough PH, Lee BW. Toxic epidermal necrolysis. Part I. Introduction, history, classification, clinical features, systemic manifestations, etiology, and immunopathogenesis. J Am Acad Dermatol. 2013;69(2):173.e1–13.
2. Schwartz RA, McDonough PH, Lee BW. Toxic epidermal necrolysis. Part II. Prognosis, sequelae, diagnosis, differential diagnosis, prevention, and treatment. J Am Acad Dermatol. 2013;69(2):187.e1–16.
3. Downey A, Jackson C, Harun N, Cooper A. Toxic epidermal necrolysis: review of pathogenesis and management. J Am Acad Dermatol. 2012;66(6):995–1003.
4. Wang CW, Yang LY, Chen BC, et al. Randomized, controlled trial of TNF-alpha antagonist in CTL-mediated severe cutaneous adverse reactions. J Clin Invest. 2018;128(3):985–96.

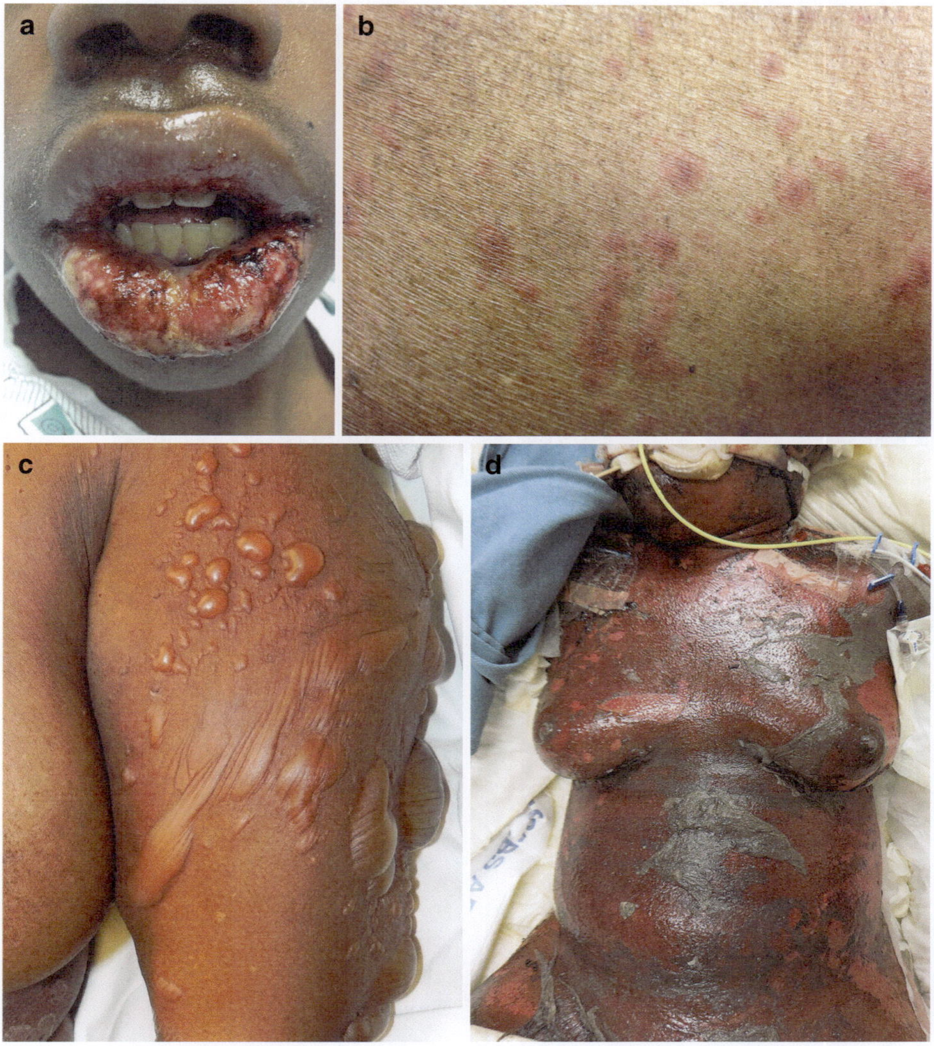

Fig. 4.1 Stevens-Johnson syndrome/toxic epidermal necrolysis: (**a**) Eroded, crusted lips typical of the oral mucosal involvement seen in SJS/TEN. (**b**) Atypical target with a dusky center and rim of erythema (two zone, "targetoid" lesion) is characteristic of SJS. (**c**) Numerous bullae superimposed on dusky skin in a patient with SJS/TEN, Nikolsky (induction of blister with firm twisting pressure) and Asboe-Hansen (expansion of blister with pressure on the bulla) sign positive. (**d**) Dusky, necrotic skin of SJS/TEN with sloughing resulting in erosions with moist skin revealed, demonstrating the full thickness necrosis and exposed underlying dermis.

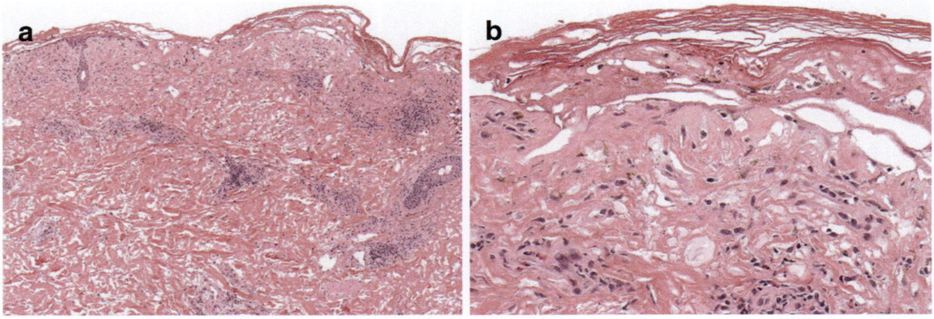

Fig. 4.2 Stevens Johnson syndrome/toxic epidermal necrolysis (SJS/TEN) (*5×, 10×; H&E*): (**a**) There is full thickness epidermal necrosis with overlying intact basket weave stratum corneum demonstrating the acuity of the process. (**b**) Underlying the full thickness necrosis is mild-to-moderate dermal lymphocytic perivascular infiltrate. Classically these lesions exhibit minimal inflammation.

Erythema Multiforme

5

Lauren Orenstein

Overview

- Erythema multiforme (EM) is an acute, immune mediated mucocutaneous eruption that is most often caused by infection (~90%) and less commonly by medications. Current knowledge suggests that EM occurs as a type IV hypersensitivity reaction in predisposed individuals
  - Eruption composed of “true target” lesions with three concentric zones of coloration
  - Mucosal involvement is variable with typically only one mucosal surface involved
- HSV-1 is the most commonly associated infection
  - Less common examples include: HSV-2, *Mycoplasma pneumonia* (especially in children), and much less likely HCV, CMV, HIV, or VZV
- Commonly implicated medications include: sulfonamides, NSAIDs, antiepileptics, and other antibiotics
- Classification of EM/SJS/TEN is controversial; some view them as distinct entities while others view them as a spectrum
  - “Classic EM” was historically referred to as “erythema multiforme minor”, with symmetric acral target lesions and variable mucosal involvement
  - “EM major” is a more severe disease which most agree is simply SJS. This distinction is a source of confusion and not a clinically relevant subtype characterized by more extensive mucosal involvement—typically of multiple sites, systemic symptoms (fevers/arthralgias); <10% of total body surface area with epidermal sloughing
- Rare subtypes include:
  - Recurrent EM: defined as >6 episodes per year
  - Persistent EM: may be linked to underlying autoimmune disease (IBD), persistent infection, or malignancy; if all other etiologies excluded can be classified as idiopathic

L. Orenstein, MD, FAAD
Department of Dermatology, Temple University, Philadelphia, PA, USA

M. Rosenbach et al. (eds.), *Inpatient Dermatology*,
https://doi.org/10.1007/978-3-319-18449-4_5

Clinical Presentation

- Typical target lesions are characteristic of EM and distinguish it from SJS/TEN. Typical targets contain three concentric zones (Fig. 5.1)
  - Central epidermal necrosis causes the dusky or bullous centers, which are surrounded by an area of lighter erythema and finally a third darker erythematous ring
  - In contrast to atypical targetoid papules, with only two zones of erythema present, which are more characteristic of SJS/TEN
- Lesions usually arise over 3–5 days and resolve within 1–2 weeks
  - Lesions do not scar but may heal with residual post-inflammatory hyperpigmentation
- Distribution: Symmetric, on the acral extremities, particularly palms and soles, and with a predilection for extensor surfaces
  - Trunk is relatively spared, unlike SJS/TEN
- May be accompanied by oral, genital, upper respiratory, pharyngeal and/or ocular erosions, but generally only 1 mucous membrane is involved
- Skin lesions are usually asymptomatic; occasionally itchy or painful
- Negative Nikolsky sign

Histopathology

- Vacuolar interface change and a dermal inflammatory infiltrate, predominantly mononuclear lymphocytes at the dermal/epidermal junction, with varying degrees of apoptotic keratinocytes; eosinophils are frequently present (Fig. 5.2)
- The stratum corneum maintains its basket-weave pattern signifying the acute nature of this process
- Epidermal necrosis is present but its extent depends on the biopsy location and age of the lesion
  - More prominent necrosis will be seen in biopsies taken from the center of the target lesion
  - Histopathologic findings are often insufficient to distinguish EM from SJS/TEN (or other interface reactions, such as GVHD)

Differential Diagnosis

- SJS/TEN: Usually starts on the trunk and then progresses distally, more likely to be painful, have atypical targetoid macules (not true three layer targets), patient systemically ill, more likely associated with medication, positive Nikolsky sign
- Ecthyma gangrenosum: Fewer larger lesions, signs of sepsis, more frequently in perineal/gluteal areas
- Autoimmune blistering diseases (bullous pemphigoid, pemphigus vulgaris, paraneoplastic pemphigus, and linear IGA bullous dermatosis): patients will have syndrome-specific findings
- Rowell Syndrome: Lupus presenting with EM-like lesions; patients will have history of lupus, chilblains, ANA and/or SS-A/SS-B antibody positive
- Fixed drug eruption: Large flat oval lesion with 1–2 zones of violaceous erythema and a darker center which may blister; consider in cases of recurrent EM (the patient could be misdiagnosed)
- Acute annular urticaria: lesions resolve within 24 h
  - In the pediatric community "urticarial multiforme" refers to polycyclic urticaria with dusky centers which can be confused clinically with EM

Work-Up

- Complete a detailed review of medications started in the preceding month
  - Drug-related EM usually starts within 7–21 days of medication initiation
- Biopsy for H&E and direct immunofluorescence (DIF)
  - Findings of EM are often non-specific, but biopsy can rule other disorders
  - DIF may be helpful to distinguish from other bullous lesions (DIF in EM will be negative)
- To detect HSV, perform a Tzanck smear or swab an unroofed vesicle and send it for viral culture, polymerase chain reaction, or direct fluorescent antigen testing
  - Serologic HSV IgM and IgG antibodies are low yield
  - Negative titers can rule out HSV, but positive titers can't rule in HSV as the cause
- If the patient is a child or has respiratory symptoms, consider Mycoplasma serology, polymerase chain reaction of a throat swab, and/or chest X-ray
- In extensive cases can perform laboratory testing for white blood cell count, liver function enzymes, electrolytes
- Positive serum ANA (speckled), SS-A, or SS-B may be helpful if Rowell Syndrome is suspected
- In a patient with recurrent or persistent idiopathic EM, consider further systemic workup

Treatment

- Stop the instigating drug if applicable
- If there is evidence of Mycoplasma or other non-HSV infection, treat the infection
- Antivirals for HSV do not appear to reduce the severity or shorten the acute episode of EM, but are low risk and may offer patients some relief
  - In a patient with recurrent HSV-related EM, consider suppressive treatment with antivirals
- Treatment is mostly supportive:
  - Antihistamines and topical corticosteroids may relieve pruritus
  - Mouth wash with local anesthetic and mild antiseptic may alleviate oromucosal symptoms
  - Wound care should be initiated for skin breakdown
- Severe cases may benefit from a short (2–3 week) course of oral corticosteroids
- If ocular mucosal involvement is present, consult ophthalmology
- Hospitalization may be warranted in cases of severe skin involvement or poor oral intake secondary to severe mucosal involvement

Suggested Readings

1. Hughey L. Approach to the hospitalized patient with targetoid lesions. Dermatol Ther. 2011;24: 196–206.
2. Sokumbi O, Wetter D. Clinical features, diagnosis, and treatment of erythema multiforme: a review for the practicing dermatologist. Int J Dermatol. 2012;51:889–902.

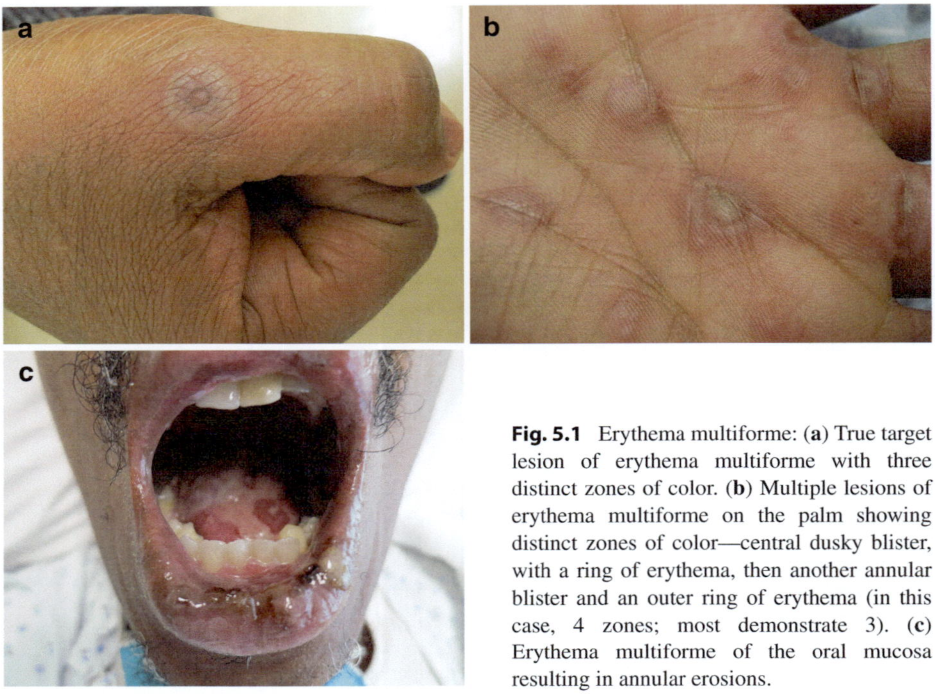

Fig. 5.1 Erythema multiforme: (**a**) True target lesion of erythema multiforme with three distinct zones of color. (**b**) Multiple lesions of erythema multiforme on the palm showing distinct zones of color—central dusky blister, with a ring of erythema, then another annular blister and an outer ring of erythema (in this case, 4 zones; most demonstrate 3). (**c**) Erythema multiforme of the oral mucosa resulting in annular erosions.

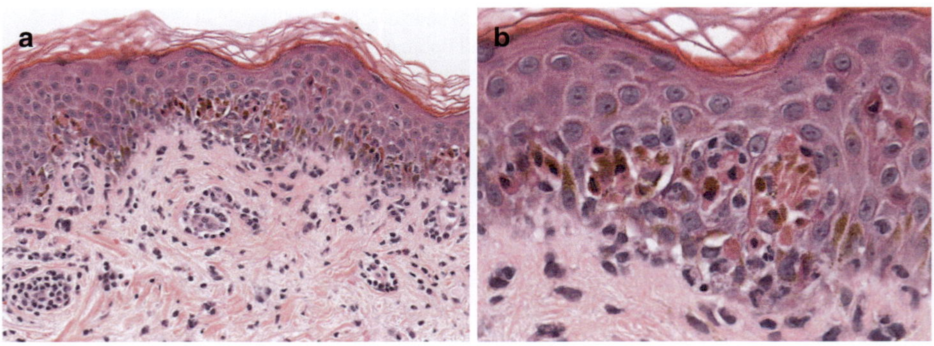

Fig. 5.2 Erythema multiforme (EM) (*10×, 20×; H&E*): (**a**) Characterized by a brisk interface dermatitis with scattered necrotic keratinocytes and mild vacuolar change. There is overlying basket weave stratum corneum secondary to the acute nature of the process. (**b**) The necrotic keratinocytes are deeply eosinophilic. Although there are overlapping histologic features between EM and SJS, EM will often have less extensive epidermal necrosis and more dermal inflammation.

Drug Rash with Eosinophilia and Systemic Symptoms

6

Aileen Y. Chang

Overview

- Drug rash with eosinophilia and systemic symptoms (DRESS) is a systemic drug hypersensitivity reaction ranging in clinical presentation from more mild (rash, transient eosinophilia, lymphadenopathy) to severe (multi-organ dysfunction)
  - Encompassing term including: Anti-convulsant hypersensitivity syndrome, drug-induced hypersensitivity syndrome, drug-induced delayed multiorgan hypersensitivity syndrome
- Mortality rate is 10%, with most patients dying from fulminant liver failure or cardiac complications
- Most common offending agents: Antiepileptic drugs (carbamazepine, phenytoin, lamotrigine), Sulfa-based antimicrobials (trimethoprim/sulfamethoxazole, sulfasalazine), NSAIDs, minocycline, allopurinol, abacavir, and nevirapine
- Latency period: 2–6 weeks from drug exposure to disease onset
- Symptoms may persist for weeks following discontinuation of the inciting medication
- The exact mechanism of pathogenesis is unknown but leading theories include:
  - Drug-induced transient host lymphocyte suppression, allowing latent virus reactivation
  - EBV, CMV, HHV7, and particularly HHV6 reactivation can be seen in as many as 75% of cases
  - Another possible contributor to disease is a deficiency in detoxifying enzymes (such as epoxide hydrolase) which prevents proper clearing of drug metabolites with their accumulation resulting in an immunologic response

Clinical Presentation

- Extensive deep red-erythematous morbilliform eruption involving the face with facial and sometimes acral swelling (Fig. 6.1)
  - The facial edema is a prominent and an essential diagnostic feature as most morbilliform drug eruptions spare the face
  - There is typically periorbital sparing (relative pallor), and occasionally impetigo-like crusting around the chin

A. Y. Chang, MD
Department of Dermatology, University of California,
San Francisco, CA, USA
e-mail: aileen.chang@ucsf.edu

M. Rosenbach et al. (eds.), *Inpatient Dermatology*,
https://doi.org/10.1007/978-3-319-18449-4_6

- Rarely there is isolated mucous membrane inflammation, and vesicles/bullae, pustules, target lesions, and purpura have been reported
- There are no validated, internationally agreed upon diagnostic criteria, but suggested criteria include:
  - Drug rash
  - Fever >38 °C
  - Lymphadenopathy
  - Peripheral eosinophilia (>1000–1500 absolute eosinophilia), or atypical lymphocytosis
  - Internal organ involvement (liver, kidneys, lungs, heart)
  - HHV6 PCR may be elevated but testing is not widely available
- Despite its name, eosinophilia is not always present and is not a requirement for diagnosis
  - 90% of DRESS cases will have associated eosinophilia
  - Atypical lymphocytosis may be seen as in a viral syndrome

Histopathology

- Histology for DRESS is nonspecific and can include the following (Fig. 6.2):
  - Lymphocytic infiltrate of the papillary dermis may be band-like or perivesicular and may contain eosinophils
  - Dyskeratotic keratinocytes, vacuolar change in basilar keratinocytes, "activated" lymphocytes, and eosinophils may be seen at the dermal/epidermal junction and around follicles
  - May see papillary dermal edema and epidermal spongiosis with subcorneal pustules
  - Variable parakeratosis

Differential Diagnosis

- Morbilliform drug eruption: spares the face, less deep-red, no systemic inflammation
- Viral exanthem: varied depending on the virus, but facial involvement is less common
- Stevens-Johnson syndrome/toxic epidermal necrolysis (SJS/TEN): DRESS-SJS overlap can occur; in SJS, mucositis is prominent, and cutaneous lesions have dusky targetoid macules
- Acute generalized exanthematous pustulosis (AGEP): DRESS-AGEP overlap can occur; in AGEP, fine pustules are present
- Staphylococcal scalded skin syndrome: diffuse and flexural superficial desquamation
- Kawasaki disease: red tongue, acral and intertriginous peeling, conjunctivitis
- Graft-versus-host disease: bilirubinemia and diarrhea can help distinguish; cutaneous GVHD often displays a fine scale and may be folliculocentric, often involves the ears

Work-Up

- Complete blood cell count with differential, liver function tests, serum creatinine level, urinalysis to evaluate for extracutaneous involvement
- Organ specific indications depending on symptomatology and presentation:
  - Low threshold to consider cardiac evaluation (EKG, echocardiogram) and pulmonary imaging
  - Small case series suggest specific drugs may be more likely to lead to specific organ dysfunction (allopurinol-renal, minocycline-pulmonary, etc.)
- Patients are at risk for delayed autoimmunity, including thyroid disease and diabetes, and should have thyroid function and glucose testing regularly for 3–6 months post-DRESS onset

Management

- Removal of offending agent and labeling patients allergic; re-exposure may be fatal
  - DRESS may have a genetic component, and ideally patients' first degree relatives will avoid similar agents
  - Avoid cross-reacting drugs, which is a particular issue with anti-epileptic agents
- Systemic corticosteroids at moderately high to high doses (e.g. prednisone 1-2mg/kg per day)
  - Median duration of systemic corticosteroids is 50 days
  - Patients often require close follow-up for delayed autoimmunity, flares of DRESS with steroid taper, and steroid-related adverse effects
- Supportive care

Suggested Readings

1. Cacoub P, Musette P, Descamps V, et al. The DRESS syndrome: a literature review. Am J Med. 2011;124(7):588–97.
2. Walsh SA, Creamer D. Drug reaction with eosinophilia and systemic symptoms (DRESS): a clinical update and review of current thinking. Clin Exp Dermatol. 2011;36(1):6–11.

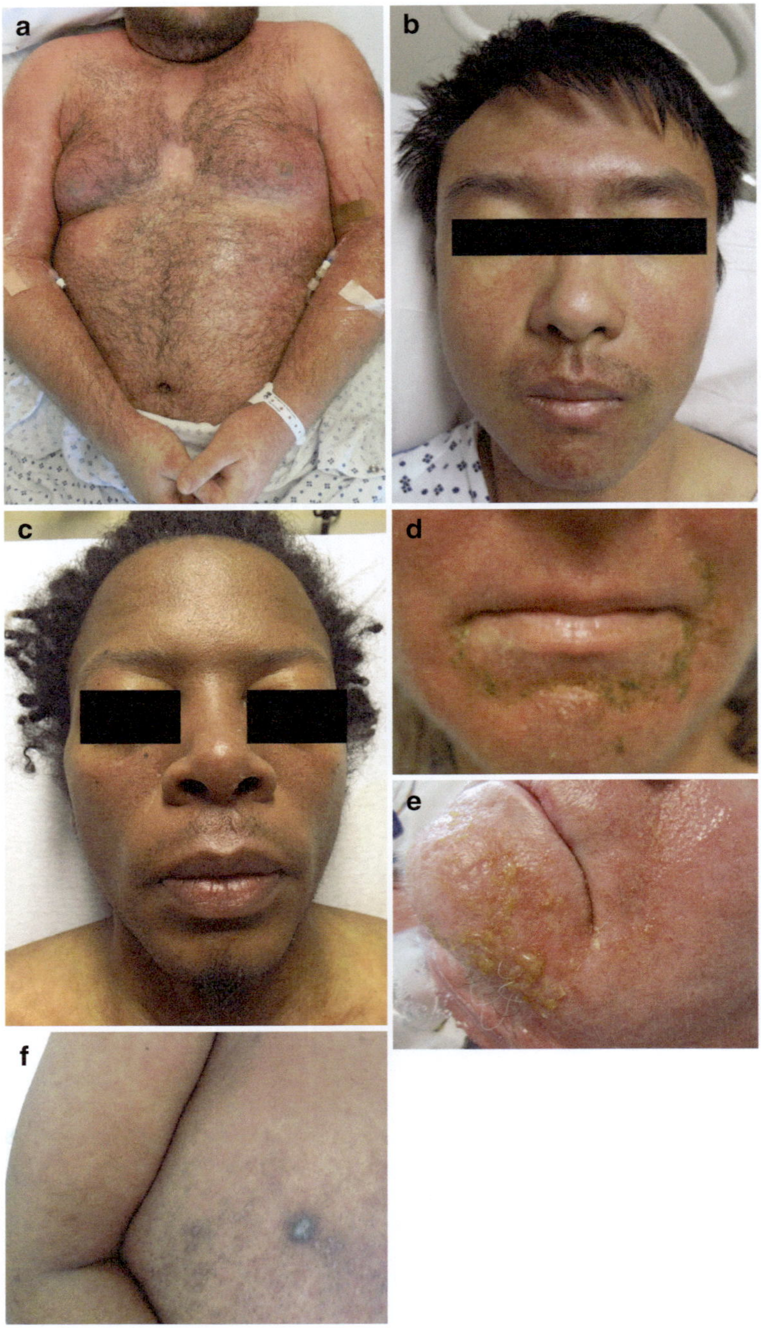

Fig. 6.1 Drug reaction with eosinophilia and systemic symptoms (DRESS): (**a**) A full-body morbilliform eruption, often deeply erythematous, is typical of DRESS syndrome. (**b**, **c**) Erythema and swelling of the face are typical findings in DRESS but may be subtle in those with darker skin (**c**). (**d**) Patients may develop impetigo-like crusting, as is seen here on the chin of a patient with DRESS syndrome. (**e**) This patient with DRESS from phenytoin exhibits extensive impetigo-like crusting of the chin. (**f**) Erythematous macules and papules coalescing into larger patches and plaques can occur in DRESS.

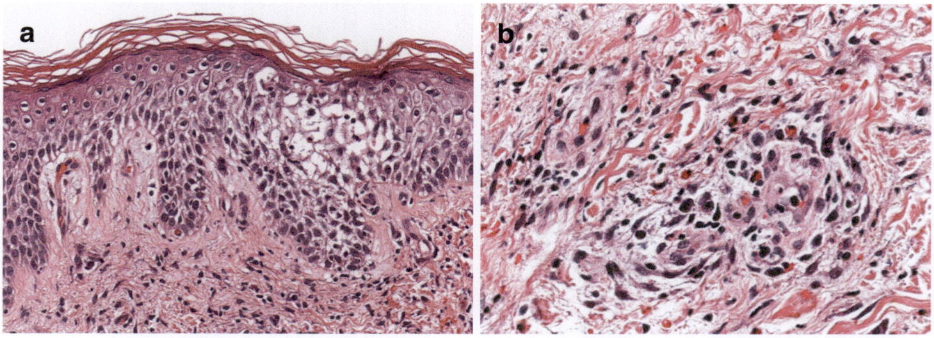

Fig. 6.2 Drug reaction with eosinophilia and systemic symptoms (DRESS) (*20×*, *40×*; *H&E*): (**a**) The histologic presentation of DRESS is variable. Features can include epidermal spongiosis, interface dermatitis with vacuolar change, perivascular lymphocytic infiltration, and eosinophils. (**b**) The perivascular lymphocytes may appear large and atypical.

Acute Generalized Exanthematous Pustulosis

7

Sara Samimi

Overview

- Acute generalized exanthematous pustulosis (AGEP) is a rapidly progressing erythroderma with studded pustules which typically occurs within 24–48 h of medication exposure and resolves quickly with its cessation
  - May recur with drug re-exposure
- AGEP can occur at any age, but is uncommon in children; when AGEP occurs in children it is typically in the setting of a viral infection
- Most common inciting medications include antibiotics (penicillin and derivatives, macrolides, others), calcium channel blockers, antimalarials, radiocontrast dye, dialysate
  - Rarely other causes (viruses, bacteria, spider bites, radiation therapy)
- Typically, a type IV hypersensitivity reaction caused by medication induced recruitment and activation of neutrophils via IL-8

Clinical Findings

- A rapidly expanding morbilliform eruption develops initially and often progresses to erythroderma
- Within 1–2 days of rash onset, there is acute evolution of innumerable pinpoint fragile non-follicular sterile pustules, favoring intertriginous areas (Fig. 7.1)
- Fever and leukocytosis with a neutrophil predominance are often present
- Resolution occurs within 4–10 days, resulting in superficial desquamation
- Other findings:
  - Pruritus
  - Fever (>38 °C)
  - Leukocytosis +/– eosinophilia
  - Lymphadenopathy
  - Rare mucous membrane involvement
- Rarely patients may present with an overlap of both DRESS and AGEP, with characteristic multiorgan inflammation (fever, lymphadenopathy, hepatitis, CBC abnormalities) in addition to the cutaneous pustules of AGEP

S. Samimi, MD
Department of Dermatology, University of Pennsylvania, Philadelphia, PA, USA
e-mail: sara.samimi@uphs.upenn.edu

M. Rosenbach et al. (eds.), *Inpatient Dermatology*,
https://doi.org/10.1007/978-3-319-18449-4_7

Histopathology

- Spongiform pustules are subcorneal or superficially intraepidermal and often contain admixed neutrophils and eosinophils; apoptotic keratinocytes may be seen (Fig. 7.2)
- Papillary dermal edema is present with a perivascular leukocytosis (mostly neutrophils with some eosinophils); rarely with associated leukocytoclastic vasculitis

Differential Diagnosis

- Pustular psoriasis: patients may have a history of psoriasis and triggers (strep, steroids, medication cessation), nail pitting, or other findings of chronic/plaque psoriasis
- Bullous impetigo: more localized, with characteristic honey-colored crusting
- Drug rash with eosinophilia and systemic symptoms (DRESS): DRESS-AGEP overlap can occur; pure DRESS should have facial edema and lack pustules
- Stevens Johnson Syndrome (SJS) and Toxic Epidermal Necrolysis (TEN): should have prominent mucositis and dusky targetoid lesions; notably in AGEP the superficial pustules can run together to form lakes of pus which can resemble bulla of SJS—though the epidermal split in AGEP is higher, and when the lesions rupture there is not raw, exposed dermis in AGEP, unlike in SJS
- Sweet syndrome: usually "juicy" edematous bright red plaques and nodules, but Sweet syndrome can develop pustules and pustulonodules, usually larger than AGEP
- Candidiasis: can have fine pustules; culture and/or biopsy can help distinguish

Diagnostic Work-Up

- Vital signs—To evaluate for fever and hemodynamic instability
- Complete blood count (CBC) with differential—To evaluate for leukocytosis, neutrophilia (in 90%; $> 7 \times 10^9$/L), and eosinophilia (30%)
- Complete metabolic profile (CMP)—To assess renal function (decreased creatinine clearance in 30%), liver function (usually normal, but may have mild elevation of aminotransferases), and calcium (rarely develop hypocalcemia)
- Urinalysis (UA)—To assess renal function
- Punch biopsy—Perform biopsies if necessary to make a definitive diagnosis and exclude entities on the differential diagnosis

Management

- Drugs are the most common triggers for AGEP; once the offending agent is removed, the cutaneous eruption will resolve with supportive care
- Patients can be given systemic anti-pyretics and anti-histamines for symptomatic relief
- Topical corticosteroids may help alleviate pruritus; emollients are important to manage the commonly seen post-AGEP desquamation
- Corticosteroids may be given, but are generally only necessary in severe cases

Suggested Readings

1. Goh TK, Pang SM, Thirumoorthy T, Goh SGN. Acute generalised exanthematous pustulosis and toxic epidermal necrolysis induced by carbamazepine. Singap Med J. 2008;49(6):507–10.
2. Peermohamed S, Haber RM. Acute generalized exanthematous pustulosis simulating toxic epidermal necrolysis: a case report and review of the literature. Arch Dermatol. 2011;147(6):697–701.
3. Speeckaert MM, Speeckaert R, Lambert J, Borchez L. Acute generalized exanthematous pustulosis: an overview of the clinical, immunological and diagnostic concepts. Eur J Dermatol. 2010;20(4):425–33.

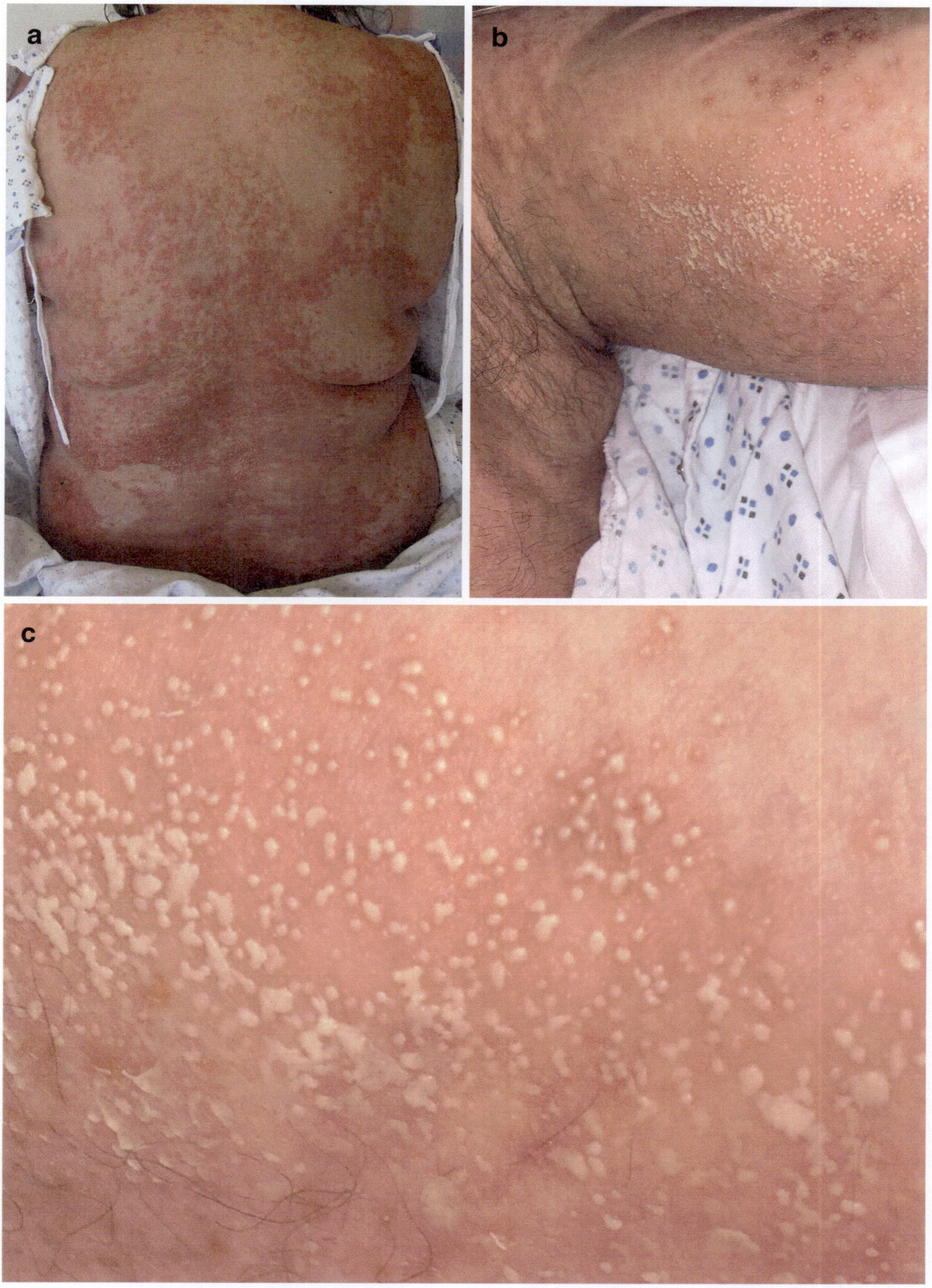

Fig. 7.1 Acute generalized exanthematous pustulosis (AGEP): (**a**) Widespread erythema/erythroderma with pinpoint pustules, which may not be readily visible except on close examination. (**b**, **c**) Pustules in AGEP favor body fold areas and, due to their superficial nature, are easily ruptured. They can become confluent “lakes of pus” resembling large bullae.

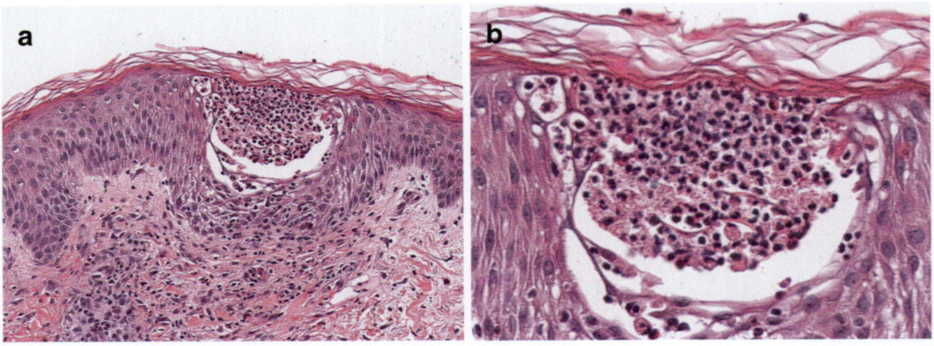

Fig. 7.2 Acute generalized exanthematous pustulosis (AGEP) (*10×*; *40×*; *H&E*): (**a**) There is a psoriasiform epidermis with subcorneal or intraepidermal pustules. (**b**) The intraepidermal pustules may have dyskeratotic keratinocytes and eosinophils. This can sometimes differentiate from pustular psoriasis.

Fixed Drug Eruption

8

Aileen Y. Chang

Overview

- Fixed drug eruption (FDE) is a distinctive drug reaction characterized by oval dusky macules/patches which develop soon after medication exposure and will recur in the same anatomical site with drug re-exposure
  - Continued, repeated exposure can worsen the eruption at specific anatomic sites and can lead to progressive involvement of new sites with each exposure
- FDE usually occurs due to medications taken intermittently with common inciting agents including NSAIDs, tetracycline antibiotics, trimethoprim-sulfamethoxazole, pseudoephedrine, laxatives
- Pathogenesis likely involves interaction of a portion of the offending medication acting as a hapten trigging an immune response that involves skin-resident memory T cells

Clinical Presentation

- Sharply demarcated oval, dusky, violaceous patches which appear on average 2 h after medication exposure (but can occur as quickly as within 30 min) (Fig. 8.1)
  - May itch or burn and severe cases (often after repeated re-exposure) can develop central bullae/blisters
- Distribution typically includes: lips, tongue, perioral region, face, acral areas, and/or genitalia
  - Erosive oral and genital mucosal involvement is common
- Re-exposure to the offending medication will result in recurrence of lesions at the same anatomical site; may develop additional multifocal lesions
- Generalized bullous fixed drug eruption (GBFDE) can present with widespread ovals with dusky centers that blister and may be mistaken for SJS/TEN
  - Widespread GBFDE with epidermal sloughing can have a course similar to SJS/TEN with sloughing, morbidity, and risk for secondary infection; it is markedly more severe than typical FDE and requires early recognition, supportive care, and intervention
- Resolution will occur with drug cessation and often results in post-inflammatory hyperpigmentation which maybe permanent
  - Nonpigmenting FDE is less common

A. Y. Chang, MD
Department of Dermatology, University of California,
San Francisco, CA, USA
e-mail: aileen.chang@ucsf.edu

M. Rosenbach et al. (eds.), *Inpatient Dermatology*,
https://doi.org/10.1007/978-3-319-18449-4_8

Histopathology

- The normal appearing basket weaved stratum corneum signifies an acute process while the underlying dermis shows evidence of prior damage, notably pigment incontinence
  - Lymphocytic interface dermatitis results in degeneration of the basal keratinocytes and pigment incontinence leading to melanin filled macrophages in an edematous upper dermis with an associated mixed inflammatory infiltrate (Fig. 8.2)
- Variable amounts of keratinocyte apoptosis can be present; may be confluent and lead to epidermal detachment

Differential Diagnosis

- Erythema multiforme: usually accompanied by mucositis and smaller true target lesions symmetrically on acral sites
- Stevens-Johnson syndrome/toxic epidermal necrolysis: challenging to distinguish from GBFDE; SJS will have conjunctival and wider mucosal involvement
- Bullous pemphigoid: urticarial plaques and tense bullae without characteristic oval shaped lesions
- Contact dermatitis: eczematous, more pruritic, more often linear/geometric (as opposed to the oval lesions of FDE)
- Cellulitis: large patches of FDE may be mistaken for cellulitis; cellulitis should have fever, an elevated white count, and lack the violaceous color and oval shape
- Erythema migrans: the expanding lesion of Lyme may have a dark red center and be hard to distinguish, a bite site or tick can help

Diagnostic Work-Up

- Usually a clinical diagnosis; can be confirmed with biopsy
- A thorough medication history can help identify a potential trigger; if the trigger is unclear, a topical provocation test (using increasing concentrations of drug applied to the skin) or an oral provocation test can confirm the clinical suspicion, but are rarely necessary and should be avoided in cases of GBFDE
  - Provocation tests should be done >2 weeks after the rash's resolution

Treatment

- Avoid offending agent
- Topical steroids and oral antihistamines for symptomatic relief
- Systemic steroids can be considered in severe cases

Suggested Readings

1. Gendernalik SB, Galeckas KJ. Fixed drug eruptions: a case report and review of the literature. Cutis. 2009;84(4):215–9.

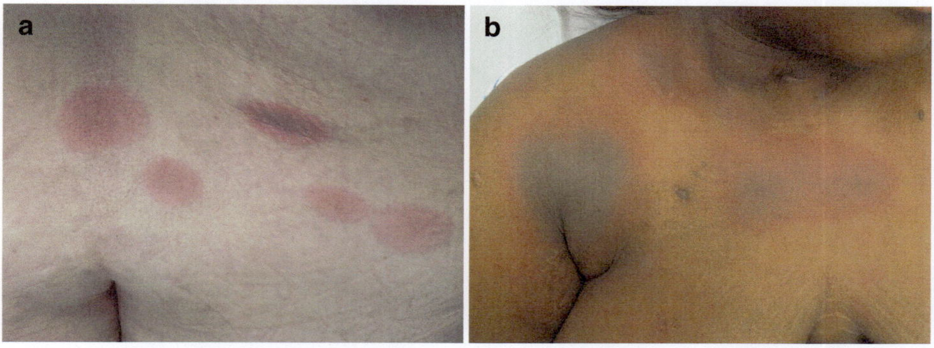

Fig. 8.1 Fixed drug eruption: (**a**) Round and oval dusky patches typical of fixed drug eruption. (**b**) Large patches of fixed drug eruption with central dusky areas eventuating in bullae.

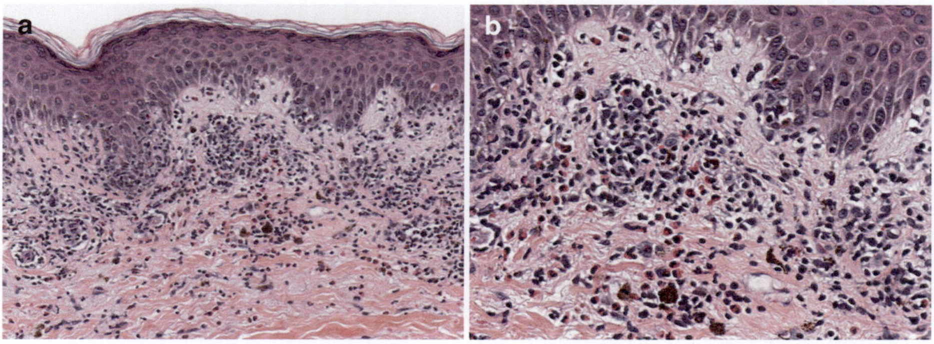

Fig. 8.2 Fixed drug reaction: (**a**) There is a lichenoid lymphocytic infiltrate with an associated acute interface dermatitis characterized by vacuolar change with apoptotic keratinocytes in the epidermis. (**b**) The superficial dermis often contains eosinophils, neutrophils, and melanophages (which suggest repeated injury and pigment incontinence).

Serum Sickness-Like Reaction

9

Elizabeth A. Vanderah

Overview

- Rare, multi-system reaction seen mostly in children, clinically resembling serum sickness with fevers, arthralgias, and urticarial rash typically developing 1–3 weeks after medication exposure
  - Internal organ involvement (renal, hepatic) is less common in serum-sickness-like reaction (SSLR) than in true serum sickness
- Common inciting agents:
  - Frequently secondary to medication exposure:
    Cefaclor is the most classic precipitant
    Other medications include anti-seizure medications, penicillin, amoxicillin, trimethoprim-sulfamethoxazole, and more
  - May also be secondary to infections (streptococcal, hepatitis or non-protein containing vaccines
- True serum sickness (SSR) is classically caused by the combination of antibodies and serum or foreign proteins to create circulating immune complexes (Type III hypersensitivity reaction which can be seen with anti-toxin treatments), whereas SSLR have a similar clinical presentation but may result from direct cytotoxic effects from medications or inflammatory reaction to drug metabolites in some cases

Clinical Presentation

- Urticarial lesions, particularly distally over joints and the lateral hands or feet; associated hand and foot edema often present (Fig. 9.1)
  - May start as a flexural presentation that then generalizes
  - Erythematous macules or multiforme lesions resembling targets
  - May have non-specific morbilliform or scarlatiniform eruptions
  - Mucosa are spared
- Patients often experience fever and polyarticular joint swelling with pain
  - Patients may have lymphadenopathy and rarely gastrointestinal, renal, or neurological involvement

E. A. Vanderah, MD
Mercy Clinic, Washington, MO, USA
e-mail: Elizabeth.Vanderah@Mercy.Net

M. Rosenbach et al. (eds.), *Inpatient Dermatology*,
https://doi.org/10.1007/978-3-319-18449-4_9

Histopathology

- Pathology is non-specific, and often utilized to primarily rule out other potential diagnoses
- Mild perivascular infiltrates consisting of lymphocytes and histiocytes, in the absence of vasculitis

Differential Diagnosis

- Serum sickness: clinically indistinguishable, depends on history of exposure (antitoxin, ATG, monoclonal antibodies, animal-derived therapies)
- Urticaria/urticaria multiforme: lacks the joint involvement and edema, less localized to joints/distal sites
- Erythema multiforme: often HSV eruption present, true targets on palms, recurrent
- Kawasaki's disease: strawberry tongue, intertriginous/acral peeling, high fever, conjunctivitis
- Viral exanthem: varies depending on the specific virus
- Acute hemorrhagic edema of infancy: purpura in florets/circular arrangements

Work-Up

- Often diagnosis can be made clinically with history and physical examination
- Skin biopsy may be indicated primarily to rule out alternative diagnoses
- Laboratory evaluation in patients who are moderately to severely ill to rule out other causes, especially if patient does not have strong clinical history of medication or viral exposure
  - CBC/Differential
  - ESR/CRP: Nonspecific inflammatory markers that may track with disease activity
  - CMP: liver and renal sequelae rare in SSLR compared to SSR
  - Complement studies: SSLR typically has normal to mildly decreased complement levels while C3/C4, CH50 levels are significantly decreased in SSR
  - Urinalysis: Typically, normal in SSLR; in SSR proteinuria is common

Treatment

- Discontinue culprit medication, reaction spontaneously resolves in 1–2 weeks
- Avoid future use of offending medication
- Short course of oral corticosteroids if symptoms are severe
- NSAIDs/analgesics
- Antihistamines

Suggested Readings

1. Dodiuk-Gad RP, et al. Epidemiology of severe drug hypersensitivity. Semin Cutan Med Surg. 2014;33:2–9.
2. Mathur AN, et al. Urticaria mimickers in children. Dermatol Ther. 2013;26:467–75.
3. Zhang Z, Xiang Y, Wang B, et al. Intestinal mucosal permeability of children with cefaclor-associated serum sickness-like reactions. Eur J Pediatr. 2013;172:537–43.

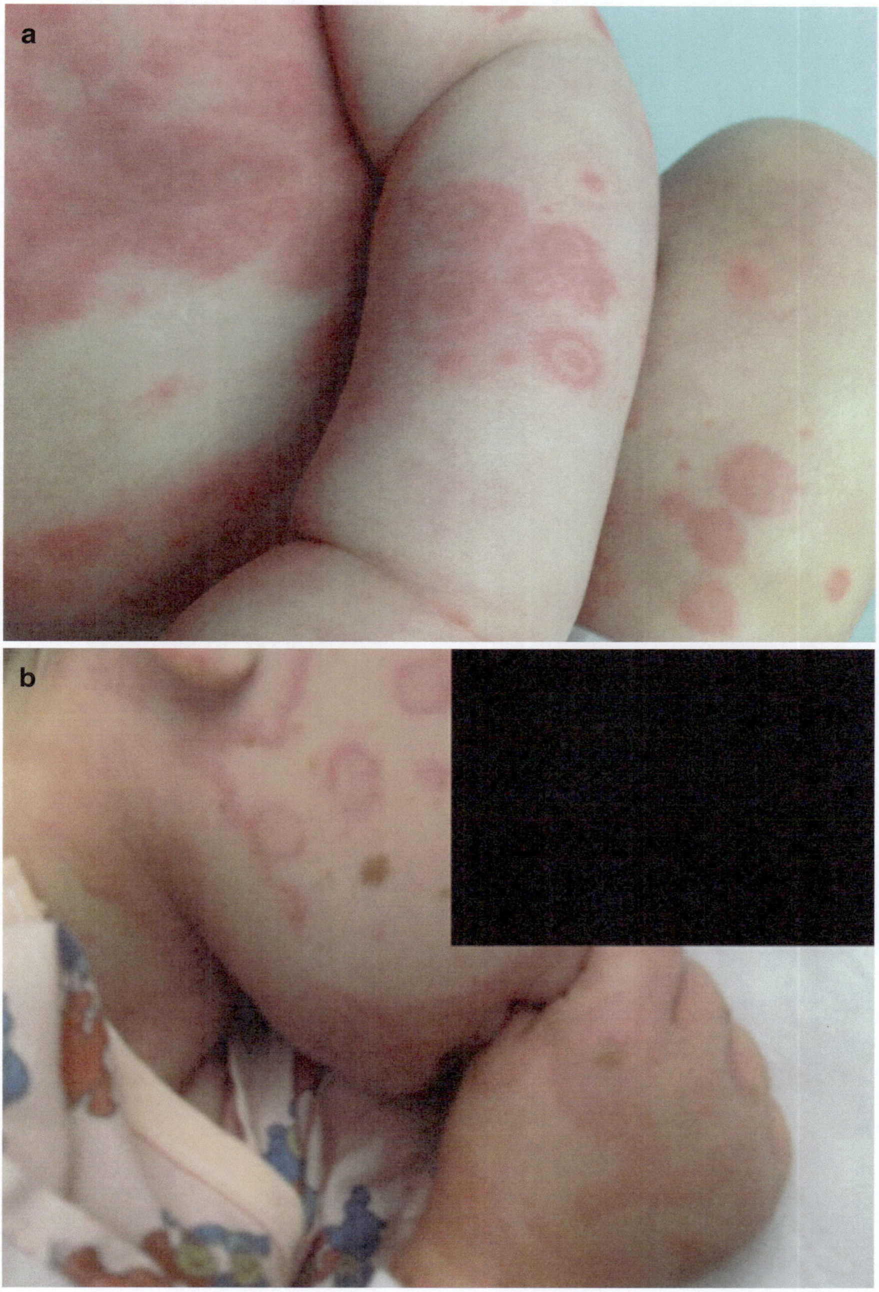

Fig. 9.1 Serum sickness: Annular and edematous urticarial lesions of serum sickness. These are often more prominent over joints (**a**, **b**), which may also be swollen; lesions on the distal feet and over the ankles are also common presentations.

Part III

Oncodermatology: Cancer- and Treatment-Related Skin Issues

The management of skin issues in patients battling cancer can be challenging. Patients can develop rashes directly due to their malignancy (cutaneous metastases or direct extension to the skin), paraneoplastic phenomena (Sweet syndrome and other skin eruptions), chemotherapy toxicities (direct cytotoxic effect or immune-mediated phenomena), cutaneous manifestations of infection (particularly in patients with hematologic malignancy and neutropenia), and rashes from the supportive medications and antibiotics required to carry patients through their disease treatment. Those who receive transplants are at risk of graft-versus-host disease as well, which involves the skin in the majority of cases. The main philosophic point to keep in mind is treatment of the cancer is of paramount importance.

Consultants evaluating the skin should consider the theory of "supportive oncodermatology:" that is, the goal of evaluating the skin is to help minimize and manage cutaneous side effects of cancer treatment in such a way as to allow patients to continue on the optimal treatment for their malignancy. Whenever possible, supportive measures should be used to alleviate skin toxicities to improve patient comfort, reduce symptoms, and allow patients to continue on their therapeutic regimen.

Patients with hematologic malignancies are a special challenge, as patients are often severely immunosuppressed due to their disease and chemotherapy. Any skin finding in neutropenic hosts can be quite significant – a red papule or violaceous nodule may be the "tip of the iceberg," as it is important to remember that without an intact immune system, these patients cannot mount a normal host response to infection. Often a red nodule which appears otherwise innocuous can be the only sign of a rapidly spreading, angioinvasive fungal organism—timely diagnosis (with frozen section or touch prep) can help make a potentially life-saving diagnosis in these cases. It is essential to thoroughly evaluate all neutropenic patients, including examination of the mucosa, skin folds, and tape sites, as life threatening infections can display subtle cutaneous findings which may be missed on cursory inspection.

Evaluating patients in the peri-transplant period represents a special challenge. 'Morbilliform' eruptions can be challenging to identify as viral exanthem, drug reaction, or graft-versus-host (GvH). Technologically, widespread testing for specific viruses is an emerging field, and there is limited data regarding diagnosis or treatment of most viruses in this setting (excluding HSV and VZV, which are frequent pathogens, but do not typically cause morbilliform eruptions). Clues to distinguish drug eruptions from acute GvH include the following: eruptions on the ears, upper back, outer arms, hands and feet, which are folliculocentric and may have fine scale favor GvH. Eruptions on the inner arms/flanks, lower back, and more pruritus favors drug. GvH may be accompanied by diarrhea more frequently. Histopathologically, GvH is more likely to display a lichenoid reaction with lymphocytes at the dermal/epidermal junction, often extending down follicles; morbilliform drug eruptions are more often perivascular lymphocytes and eosinophils. While it may be impossible to completely exclude one or the other, generally astute clinicians can lean heavily in one direction using clinical/pathologic correlation.

10 Sweet Syndrome

Aileen Y. Chang

Overview

- Sweet syndrome (acute febrile neutrophilic dermatosis) is a rare inflammatory disorder characterized by sudden onset variably tender brightly erythematous-to-violaceous papules, plaques, or nodules
- Three subtypes:
  - *Classical:* majority of cases worldwide but less common in inpatients; most frequently associated with recent upper respiratory and gastrointestinal infections, inflammatory bowel disease, or sometimes pregnancy
  - *Malignancy-associated*: usually seen with hematologic malignancies (AML and MDS most common), rarely seen with solid tumors
  - *Drug-associated*: typically 1–2 weeks after exposure to offending agent

    Common offenders: granulocyte-colony stimulating factors, all-trans retinoic acid, emerging cases with azacitadine, targeted chemotherapeutics (such as BRAF, multikinase, and FLT3-inhibitors)

    Less commonly seen with azathioprine, trimethoprim-sulfamethoxazole, minocycline, nitrofurantoin, carbamazepine, diazepam, hydralazine, furosemide, abacavir, propylthiouracil

    Rarely reported after radiation therapy or other atypical triggers
- Exact pathogenesis is unknown; likely a neutrophil-mediated reactive process due to hypersensitivity, cytokine dysregulation, and genetic susceptibility

Clinical Presentation

- Red tender lesions most commonly present on the head, neck, upper back, and upper extremities; may be associated with substantial dermal edema leading to a swollen, "juicy" appearance which may resemble pseudo-vesicles (Fig. 10.1)
  - In leukemia patients lesions may also be necrotic or bullous
  - May be associated with pathergy (lesions occur or worsen at site of prior injury)

A. Y. Chang, MD
Department of Dermatology, University of California,
San Francisco, CA, USA
e-mail: aileen.chang@ucsf.edu

M. Rosenbach et al. (eds.), *Inpatient Dermatology*,
https://doi.org/10.1007/978-3-319-18449-4_10

- Fever, malaise, and joint/muscle pain are often present; fever may be less common in drug-induced cases
  - Lesions are typically preceded by fever with many patients experiencing febrile illnesses (such as upper respiratory tract infections) 1–3 weeks prior to cutaneous findings
  - Can be associated with ocular findings with approximately 30% of patients having conjunctivitis or episcleritis
- Pulmonary and renal involvement can rarely occur

Histopathology

- Dense neutrophilic infiltrate with papillary dermal edema (Fig. 10.2)
- Leukocytoclasis without associated vasculitis is common

Differential Diagnosis

- Cutaneous infection: challenging to distinguish; biopsy and tissue culture are necessary
- Leukemia cutis (LC): clinically similar, though LC lesions may be smaller, more violaceous, less edematous, and less tender
- Drug eruption: widespread eruption of small papules in Sweet syndrome can resemble morbilliform reactions, but Sweet syndrome is usually redder, and histopathology will be different
- Leukocytoclastic vasculitis: often smaller, more numerous, and localized to legs; most Sweet syndrome cases lack extensive vasculitis on biopsy
- Erythema nodosum: Duller color, symmetrical, mostly on legs
- Pyoderma gangrenosum (PG): Bullous/ulcerative Sweet syndrome can be identical to ulcerative PG (lesions like this in a patient with myelodysplastic syndrome (MDS) are called Sweet syndrome, while if the patient had inflammatory bowel disease would likely be called PG)
- Neutrophilic eccrine hidradenitis: usually concentrated on areas with many eccrine coils (palms/soles/axilla)

Work-Up

- Biopsy for histology and tissue culture; infection must be ruled out to make a diagnosis of Sweet syndrome
- CBC, LFTs, BMP, UA to evaluate for signs of extracutaneous involvement
- ESR and CRP are typically elevated but nonspecific
- Age-appropriate cancer screening
- Most patients warrant a bone marrow biopsy in the absence of a clear explanation for Sweet syndrome
- Diagnostic criteria for classical subtype: two major and two out of four minor criteria
  - *Major:*
    Abrupt onset of painful erythematous plaques or nodules
    Dense neutrophilic infiltrate without vasculitis evident on pathology
  - *Minor:*
    Fever >38 °C
    Underlying malignancy
    Inflammatory disorder
    Pregnancy
    Preceded by upper respiratory/gastrointestinal infection, or vaccination
    Excellent response to steroids
    The presence of three of four lab findings: ESR >20 mm/h, positive CRP, >8000 leukocytes, >70% neutrophils

Treatment

- Oral prednisone is highly effective and will need to be tapered over 4–6 weeks
  - With prednisone, fevers stop quickly and lesions start to fade within 24–48 h with complete resolution over 1–2 weeks; lesions resolve without scarring
  - Intralesional or topical steroids may be effective for some lesions
- Colchicine, dapsone, or potassium iodide may be effective steroid-sparing agents

Suggested Readings

1. von den Driesch P. Sweet's syndrome (acute febrile neutrophilic dermatosis). J Am Acad Dermatol. 1994;31(4):535–56. quiz 557–60.
2. Alavi A, Sajic D, Cerci FB, Ghazarian D, Rosenbach M, Jorizzo J. Neutrophilic dermatoses: an update. Am J Clin Dermatol. 2014;15(5):413–23.
3. Nelson CA, Stephen S, Ashchyan HJ, James WD, Micheletti RG, Rosenbach M. Neutrophilic dermatoses. J Am Acad Dermatol. 2018;Epub ahead of print.

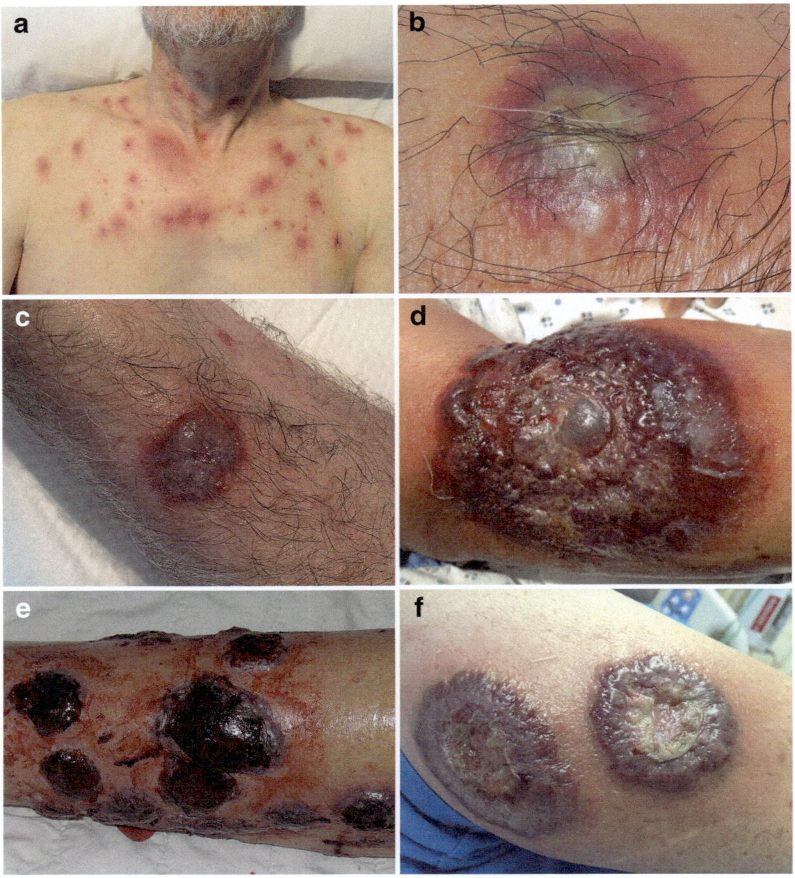

Fig. 10.1 Sweet syndrome: (**a**) Multiple juicy, purple-red nodules on the head and neck and upper trunk, typical of Sweet syndrome. (**b**) Early lesion of Sweet syndrome developing at a site of venipuncture, demonstrating pathergy. (**c**) Erythematous plaque with intense edema leading to a pseudo-bullae in a patient with myelodyspastic syndrome. (**d**) Massive violaceous and necrotic plaque of AML-associated bullous Sweet syndrome demonstrating pathergy following punch biopsy of a smaller lesion. (**e**) Indurated violaceous plaques with "juicy" edematous appearance from subepidermal edema. (**f**) These two lesions have an annular morphology (which can be seen in neutrophilic eruptions) and occurred at sites of trauma (pathergy phenomenon).

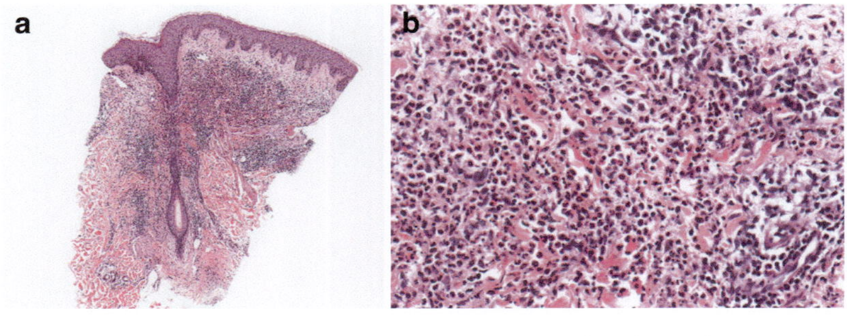

Fig. 10.2 Sweet syndrome (*2.5×, 20×; H&E*): (**a**) On low power, there is prominent papillary dermal edema, occasionally leading to pseudovesicles, and a diffuse dermal infiltrate of neutrophils. (**b**) At higher power sheets of neutrophils can be appreciated. Although not present in the current images, occasional eosinophils and secondary vasculitis can be observed.

11 Leukemia Cutis

Aileen Y. Chang

Overview

- Leukemia cutis (LC) refers to cutaneous infiltration by neoplastic leukocytes
  - Most commonly associated with acute myeloid leukemia (AML) with monocytic differentiation (historically referred to as FAB types M4 and M5), or *NPM1* mutated leukemias
  - LC can occur prior to overt leukemia
- LC arising in patients with AML may confer a poorer prognosis and is typically associated with multiple sites of extramedullary disease; these patients commonly have CSF involvement (40%)
- LC in patients with chronic leukemias (CML/CLL) may coincide with blast transformation
- Exact pathogenesis of leukemia cutis is not known
  - Likely related to the expression of skin-homing receptors and surface molecules facilitating cutaneous leukemic migration, with neoplastic cells ultimately gaining the ability to proliferate locally in the skin

Clinical Presentation

- Patient presents with papule, nodules or plaques, ranging in color from red-brown to violaceous, sometimes hemorrhagic; "plum colored papules" are most common (Fig. 11.1)
- Legs are the most common site, followed by the arms, trunk, scalp, face
- Systemic disease usually precedes the development of skin lesions
- Rarely cutaneous involvement occurs prior to bone marrow involvement, systemic symptoms, or lab abnormalities and in these situations is referred to as aleukemic leukemia cutis or primary extramedullary leukemia

A. Y. Chang, MD
Department of Dermatology, University of California,
San Francisco, CA, USA
e-mail: aileen.chang@ucsf.edu

M. Rosenbach et al. (eds.), *Inpatient Dermatology*,
https://doi.org/10.1007/978-3-319-18449-4_11

Histopathology

- Dermal infiltrate of leukemic cells, often perivascular or periadnexal; can be diffuse/sheet-like, often extending into the subcutis; typically mitotic figures are present (Fig. 11.2)
- As the leukemic cells do not exhibit epidermotropism there is a distinct separation of the lymphocytic infiltrate from the epidermis known as the Grenz zone
- Cytology and immunohistochemical profile of neoplastic cells depends on subtype of original disease

Differential Diagnosis

- Sweet syndrome: can be hard to distinguish; Sweet syndrome lesions are normally redder, larger, and more edematous with a "juicy" appearance
- Cutaneous lymphoma: can be identical and require pathology and ancillary testing to distinguish
- Graft-versus-host disease: usually thin, pink, scaly, and not as indurated as LC
- Drug eruption: usually flatter, pinker lesions compared to the violaceous papules of LC
- Erythema nodosum: usually symmetrical and with ill-defined edges compared to the indurated, more superficial dermal papules of LC
- Sarcoidosis: usually on the face, around the nares, eyes, mouth, and/or around scars/tattoos
- Metastatic carcinoma of the skin: history is key, but pathology evaluation can distinguish
- Neutrophilic eccrine hidradenitis: usually localized to palms, soles, axilla and/or face

Important Work-Up

- CBC with differential to asses for cytopenias and degree of peripheral blood involvement
- Biopsy for histology and potential molecular workup:
  - If the patient has a previous diagnosis, it is important to know the immunohistochemical profile of the original tumor cells so targeted staining can be performed
  - If LC is diagnosed in the absence of known leukemia, referral to hematology/oncology for urgent bone marrow biopsy is indicated
- Lumbar puncture if concerned for leukemic meningitis
- Cultures and/or radiologic imaging if concern for infection

Treatment

- Systemic chemotherapy aimed at treating the underlying leukemia subtype
- Palliative radiation therapy or localized corticosteroids for symptomatic relief of pain or pruritis in patients who are not candidates for systemic chemotherapy

Suggested Readings

1. Cho-Vega JH, Medeiros LJ, Prieto VG, Vega F. Leukemia cutis. Am J Clin Pathol. 2008;129(1):130–42.
2. Luskin MR, Huen AO, Brooks SA, Stewart C, Watt CD, Morrissette JJ, Lieberman DB, Bagg A, Rosenbach M, Perl AE. NPM1 mutation is associated with leukemia cutis in acute myeloid leukemia with monocytic features. Haematologica. 2015;100(10):e412–4.

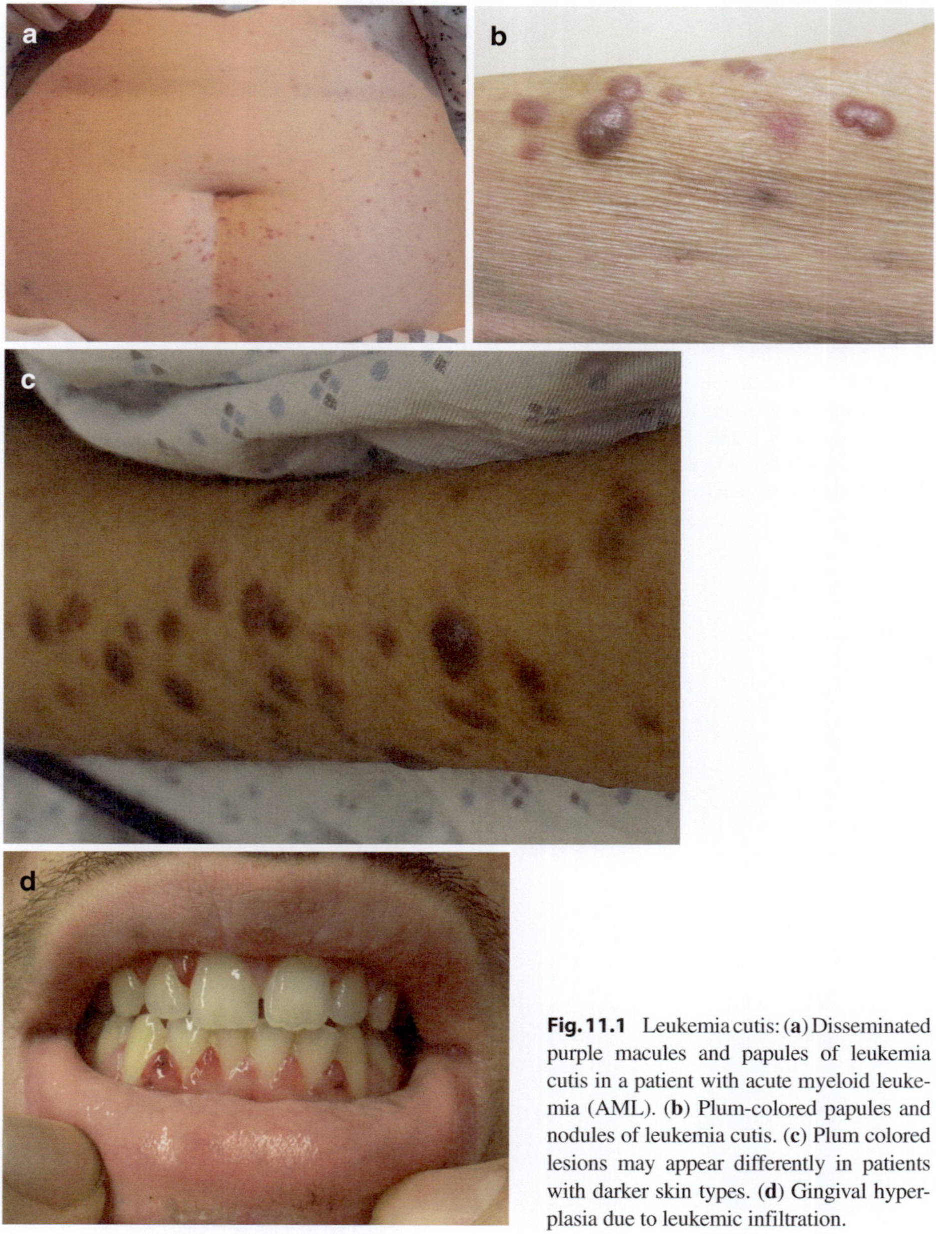

Fig. 11.1 Leukemia cutis: (**a**) Disseminated purple macules and papules of leukemia cutis in a patient with acute myeloid leukemia (AML). (**b**) Plum-colored papules and nodules of leukemia cutis. (**c**) Plum colored lesions may appear differently in patients with darker skin types. (**d**) Gingival hyperplasia due to leukemic infiltration.

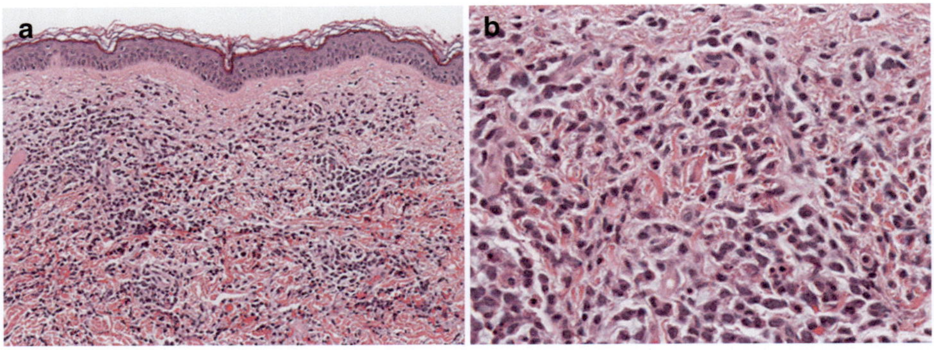

Fig. 11.2 Leukemia cutis *(10×, 40×; H&E):* (**a**) There is a dense dermal infiltrate of large atypical lymphocytes representing the patient's leukemic cells (which can be confirmed with immunohistochemistry and ancillary studies). The leukemic cells do not exhibit epidermitropism but instead there is a Grenz zone, which is a separation of the lymphocytic infiltrate from the epidermis. (**b**) In the dermis, the leukemic cells spread between and splay collagen fibers (as demonstrated in the image on the right).

Toxic Erythema of Chemotherapy

12

Lisa Pappas-Taffer

Overview

- Toxic erythema of chemotherapy (TEC) is an umbrella category of overlapping cutaneous reactions to cytotoxic chemotherapy agents, including: hand-foot syndrome (HFS), eccrine squamous syringometaplasia (ESS); some include neutrophilic eccrine hidradenitis (NEH) under this overarching term (the authors feel that NEH has some distinguishing features and is discussed separately)
- TEC is characterized by painful erythema and peeling favoring hands, feet, and intertriginous areas occurring most commonly 2–3 weeks after chemotherapy initiation
  - It is thought to be caused by damage associated with the concentration of cytotoxic agents in sweat ducts
- Risk factors include higher doses, greater cumulative doses, increased half-life, increased frequency of administration
- *Subclassifications*:
  - **HFS:** Historically referred to as palmar-plantar erythrodysesthesia and acral erythema
    Most common causes: pyrimidine analogs (cytarabine, 5-FU, capecitabine), anthracyclines (pegylated liposomal doxorubicine > doxorubicine), and taxanes (doxetaxel)
    Less common causes: paclitaxel, hydroxyurea, methotrexate, 6-mercaptopurine, cyclophosphamide, and more
  - **ESS:** Considered to be a non-inflammatory version of NEH, and is largely a histopathologic descriptor of what is seen in patients with HFS clinically
  - **NEH:** Some consider NEH to be a reactive process akin to Sweet syndrome, however, the concentration around eccrine coils and temporal association with cytotoxic chemotherapy suggests it is pathophysiologically related to TEC though the clinical manifestations are often distinctive
    Most common causes: cytarabine and daunorubicin
- Hand foot skin reaction (**HFSR**) is not generally grouped as a form of traditional TEC:
  - HFSR is caused by targeted kinase inhibitors and may be associated with friction or pressure-induced injury
  - Patients develop focal, localized reactions concentrated in the creases of the hands or feet or on pressure points

L. Pappas-Taffer, MD
Department of Dermatology, University of Pennsylvania, Philadelphia, PA, USA
e-mail: lisa.pappas-taffer@uphs.upenn.edu

M. Rosenbach et al. (eds.), *Inpatient Dermatology*,
https://doi.org/10.1007/978-3-319-18449-4_12

Clinical Presentation

- **HFS**
  - Prodrome of tingling or pain of palmoplantar skin that progresses to confluent, painful, well-demarcated diffuse symmetric erythema within days typically notable on the distal palmar aspect of the fingers (Fig. 12.1)
    - With time the erythema will fade and turn darker with superficial denuded skin and superficial desquamation
  - Severity can range from asymptomatic finger peeling to severe, extremely painful widespread bullae
  - The intertriginous involvement is often a red-brown erythema which can display fine superficial peeling desquamation
- **NEH**
  - Tender violaceous dermal-based papules, nodules, or plaques
  - Most commonly affects the palms, axilla, and face

Histopathology

- All forms of TEC may display epidermal dysmaturation and focal keratinocyte cell necrosis (Fig. 12.2)
- Squamitization of the eccrine coils may be seen (squamous syringometaplasia)
- In NEH, neutrophils will infiltrate and surround the glands (may see a paucity of neutrophils in neutropenic patients which is consistent with ESS); associated glandular epithelial necrosis is often seen

Differential Diagnosis

- Hand-foot skin reaction: History is essential; HFSR will display targeted involvement of acral flexural creases and pressure points versus the widespread diffuse acral involvement of HFS/TEC
- Acute Graft-versus-Host Disease: may also affect palms and soles, but typically involves ears, upper back, outer arms, and is accompanied by bilirubin elevations and diarrhea
- Sweet syndrome: can closely resemble NEH, but will rarely involve palms/soles and rarely be desquamative
- Leukemia cutis: usually scattered plum-colored papules, not palmar/intertriginous red-brown superficial peeling
- Drug hypersensitivity reaction (DRESS): usually more diffuse and just blanchable erythematous macules, lacking the characteristic localization of TEC
- Candida/intertrigo: intertriginous TEC can be mistaken for candida, but candida should have a rim of fine papules or small pustules and satellite lesions, and lack the peeling of TEC

Work-Up

- Generally the diagnosis is made clinically and based on the timing and history of chemotherapy administration
- A skin biopsy may be indicated in select cases; primarily to help rule out other entities in the differential diagnosis

Treatment

- Drug interruption or dose modification is the most well-documented intervention, but it is important to balance the severity of the skin with the overall management of the malignancy—treating the cancer is usually paramount
- General: wound care to prevent infection, elevation to reduce edema, symptomatic treatment, routine topical emollients
- Reported symptom alleviation in small studies with: oral corticosteroids, vitamin E, celecoxib, and topical 99% dimethylsulfoxide (DMSO); anecdotally many have utilized topical steroids with some improvement
- Prevention:
  - Cooling the extremities during chemotherapy administration may help limit chemotherapeutic deposition and sweating and resultant cutaneous toxicities
  - Statins, Cox-2 inhibitors, pyridoxine, oral vitamin E, and systemic steroids have been utilized with varying degrees of efficacy

Suggested Readings

1. Bolognia JL, Cooper DL, Glusac EJ. Toxic erythema of chemotherapy: a useful clinical term. J Am Acad Dermatol. 2008;59(3):524–9.
2. Huang V, Anadkat M. Dermatologic manifestations of cytotoxic therapy. Dermatol Ther. 2011;24(4):401–10.
3. Balagula Y, Rosen ST, Lacouture ME. The emergence of supportive oncodermatology. J Am Acad Dermatol. 2011;65(3):624–35.

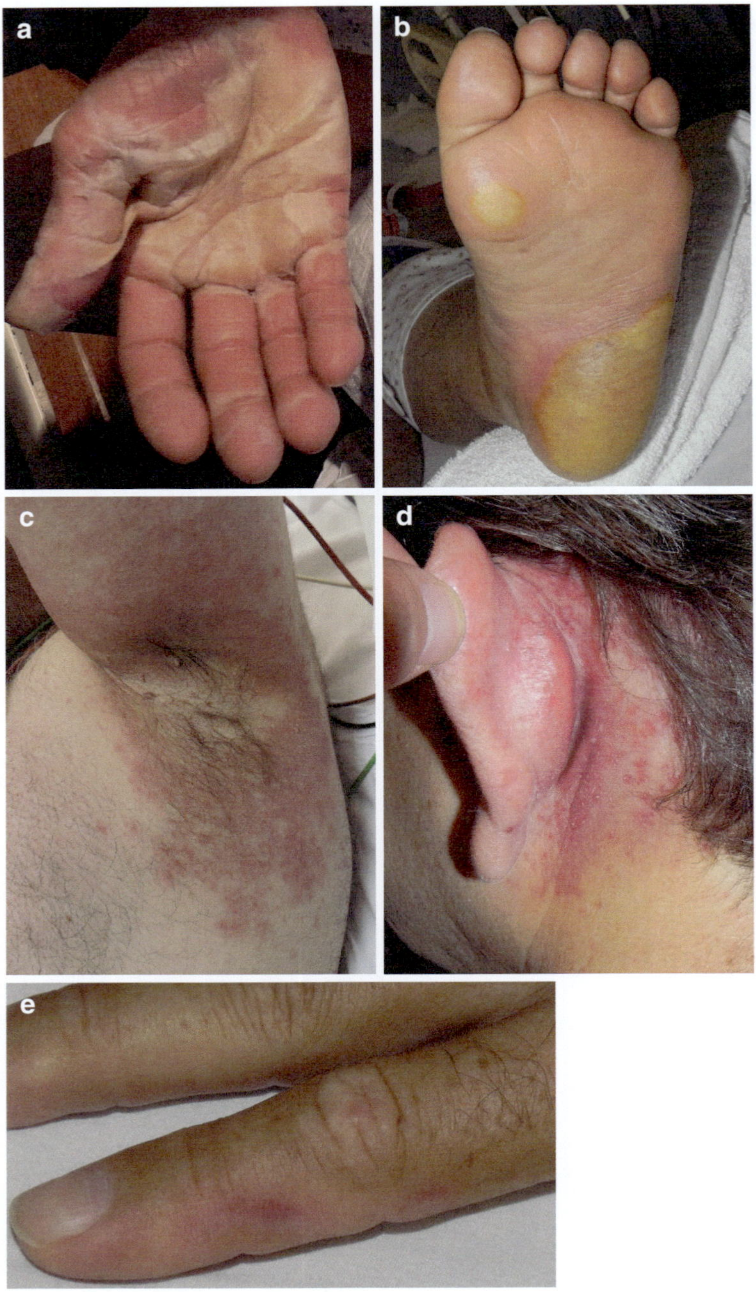

Fig. 12.1 Toxic erythema of chemotherapy (TEC): (**a**) TEC involving areas with increased eccrine sweat gland concentration, shown here on the palms (hand-foot syndrome). (**b**) Sole involvement accentuated here at sites of pressure. Broad areas of involvement are commonly seen with cytotoxic chemotherapy; newer, more targeted therapies such as multikinase inhibitors may lead to smaller lesions, over folds or sites of pressure, termed "hand foot skin reaction." (**c**) TEC commonly leads to red-brown erythema with some scaling in the axilla and groin. (**d**) Involvement of the skin behind the ear is also commonly seen ("Ara-C ears"). (**e**) Targeted involvement of the creases or isolated orange-pink inflammation at sites of pressure may be seen with kinase inhibitors (hand foot skin reaction).

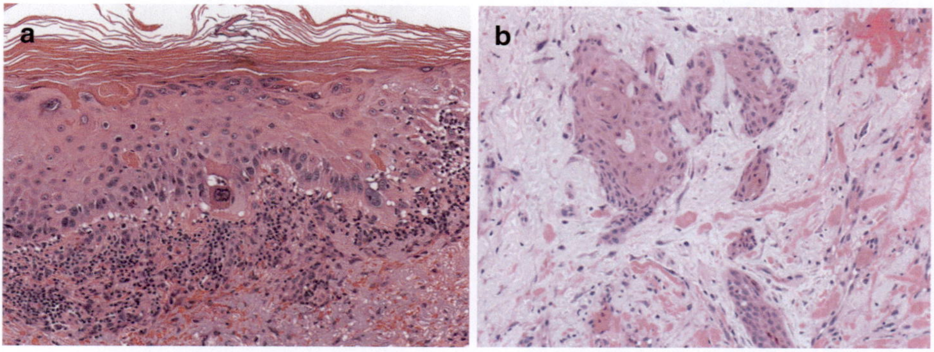

Fig. 12.2 Toxic erythema of chemotherapy (*10×, 20×; H&E*): Histopathologic features can vary depending on the severity of the reaction. (**a**) Features include keratinocyte necrosis and dysmaturation with underlying interface dermatitis, and a variable superficial perivascular predominantly lymphocytic infiltrate. (**b**) Eccrine coil syringosquamous metaplasia can be seen in some sections.

Neutrophilic Eccrine Hidradenitis

13

Molly Moye

Overview

- Neutrophilic eccrine hidradenitis (NEH) is a cutaneous eruption associated with chemotherapy, particularly cytarabine and anthracyclines, in patients with AML
  - Other drugs reported to cause NEH include granulocyte colony stimulating factor (G-CSF), anti-retroviral agents
  - Also been reported in patients with other hematologic malignancies (e.g. Hodgkin's lymphoma, non-Hodgkin's lymphoma, chronic lymphocytic leukemia), solid tumors, and HIV
- Pathogenesis is unknown and is hypothesized to be related to direct cytotoxicity of drugs that are secreted into sweat versus similar pathogenesis to neutrophilic dermatoses
- Rare reports of infections causing NEH exist including Staphylococcus, Streptococcus, Enterobacter, Serratia and Nocardia
- Children may rarely develop localized NEH on the soles from rigorous exercise

Clinical Presentation

- Erythematous to violaceous papules and plaques without overlying epidermal changes, typically on the face (peri-orbital), in the axilla, on the palms, and rarely on the arms and upper torso that develop 1–2 weeks after exposure to culprit drug (Fig. 13.1)
- Patients may be febrile, and are frequently neutropenic due to disease or chemotherapy

Histopathology

- Neutrophilic infiltrate surrounding and involving eccrine glands with degenerative vacuolar change with/without associated necrosis typically primarily involves the secretory portion of the eccrine epithelium, usually with sparing of the acrosyringium (Fig. 13.2)
  - Occasionally, necrosis of eccrine glands exists without accumulation of neutrophils
  - Eccrine squamous syringometaplasia may develop

M. Moye, MD
Forefront Dermatology, Louisville, KY, USA
e-mail: mollymoye@me.com

M. Rosenbach et al. (eds.), *Inpatient Dermatology*,
https://doi.org/10.1007/978-3-319-18449-4_13

Differential Diagnosis

- Infection (bacterial, fungal, mycobacterial): distribution of eruption may suggest NEH (palms, axilla), but ultimately tissue culture and special stains are required to rule out infection
- Other neutrophilic dermatoses, particularly Sweet syndrome: challenging to distinguish as there is substantial history, clinical, and pathologic overlap (location in axilla, palms, face may favor NEH)
- Leukemia cutis: lesions are often firmer, and are more often on the extremities than the palms and soles as with NEH; histology can be used to distinguish

Work-Up

- Skin biopsy and tissue culture (along with blood cultures) are necessary to establish correct diagnosis and rule out infectious etiology
- Complete blood count with differential and peripheral smear should be obtained in an otherwise healthy individual as NEH can be the presenting sign of hematologic malignancies

Treatment

- NEH improves spontaneously as neutropenia resolves, so no treatment is necessary if eruption is asymptomatic
- Systemic corticosteroids lead to resolution of eruption, but are generally not necessary (and may be contraindicated)
- Topical steroids can be utilized by often are typically ineffective due to the location of the inflammation in the deep dermis
- Pain associated with NEH can be treated with NSAIDs or narcotic pain medications, depending upon severity

Suggested Readings

1. Bachmeyer C, Aractingi S. Neutrophilic eccrine hidradenitis. Clin Dermatol. 2000;18:319–30.
2. Srivastava M, et al. Neutrophilic eccrine hidradenitis masquerading as facial cellulitis. J Am Acad Dermatol. 2007;56:693–6.

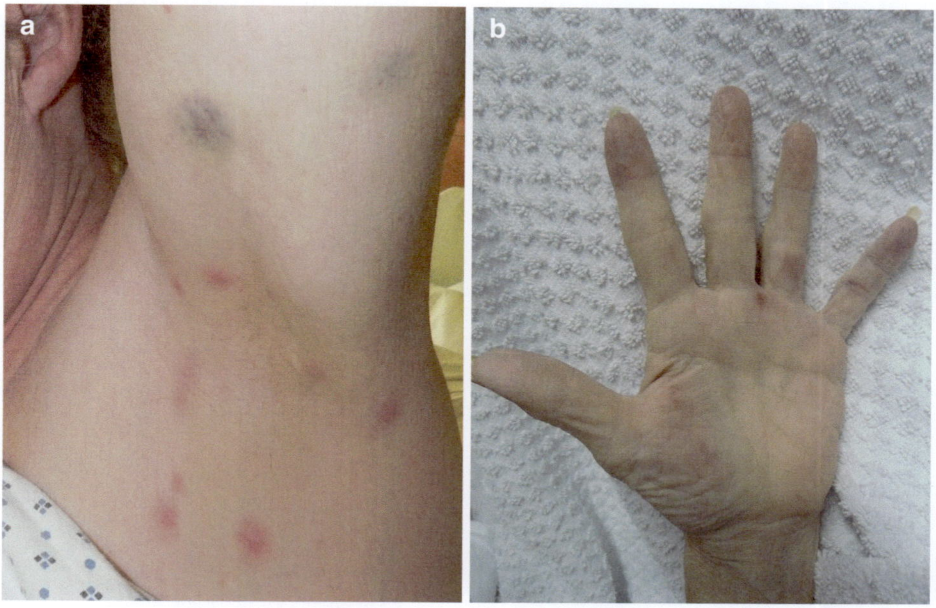

Fig. 13.1 Neutrophilic eccrine hidradenitis of the axilla: (**a**) Juicy pink papules favoring areas with increased eccrine sweat glands. Axilla, palms, and soles are the most common sites of involvement, but facial lesions are not seen infrequently. (**b**) Subtle erythematous macules with slight substance on palpation involving the palms of a patient with recent cytarabine exposure.

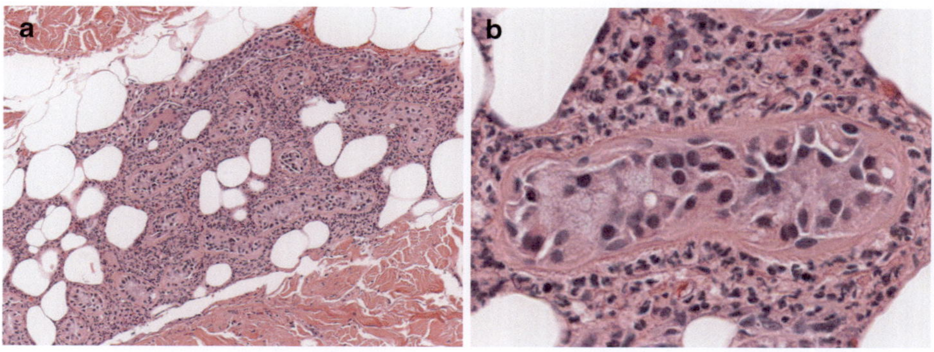

Fig. 13.2 Neutrophilic eccrine hidriadenitis *(10×, 40×; H&E):* (**a**) There is a dense neutrophilic infiltrate involving eccrine glands and the peri-eccrine adipose tissue with associated lymphocytes. (**b**) Eccrine necrosis is evidenced by the deeply eosinophilic cytoplasm and pyknotic nuclei of affected cells.

Transient Acantholytic Dermatosis of Chemotherapy

14

Megan H. Noe

Overview

- Transient acantholytic dermatosis of chemotherapy (TAD) is an eruption of mildly pruritic crusted, eroded, and pseudovesicular erythematous papules most commonly on the chest and back, though can involve the extremities and rarely the scalp
- The eruption is self-limited and not an indication to stop or adjust chemotherapy
- Typically seen in the setting of polychemotherapy, with no particular drug or class of chemotherapeutic agents consistently responsible; Cytarabine may be a more common inciting culprit than others
  - Also has also been reported in association with a hematological malignancy before chemotherapy is administered
  - May be related to excessive heat (fever, sweating, occlusion) and the elimination or accumulation of chemotherapy agents in the eccrine glands

Clinical Presentation

- Self-limited eruption of pruritic, crusted erythematous papules and vesicles typically on the chest, back and thighs following chemotherapy use (Fig. 14.1)
  - Classic transient acantholytic dermatosis (Grover's disease) is a similar eruption on the chest, flanks, and abdomen which tends to occur in the setting of irritated skin, either with sweating, or from hot showers drying out the skin in the winter

Histopathology

- Histopathology shows multifocal hypergranulosis with acantholytic dyskeratosis with epidermal spongiosis and suprabasilar clefting (Fig. 14.2)
- Corps ronds and grains are features of acantholysis
  - Corps ronds: round dyskeratotic keratinocytes with pyknotic nuclei surrounded by a clear or blue halo
  - Grains: basophilic keratinocytes with stretched nuclei
- Direct immunofluorescence is negative

M. H. Noe, MD, MPH
Department of Dermatology,
University of Pennsylvania, Philadelphia, PA, USA
e-mail: Megan.Noe@uphs.upenn.edu

M. Rosenbach et al. (eds.), *Inpatient Dermatology*,
https://doi.org/10.1007/978-3-319-18449-4_14

Differential Diagnosis

- Disseminated HSV or VZV infection: while vesicles are often present, later lesions or excoriated lesions can closely resemble TAD
- Folliculitis: usually more localized to hair follicles and often accompanied by small pustules
- Graft vs. Host Disease: usually involves the ears and upper back, hands/feet, and accompanied by diarrhea/liver abnormalities
- Miliaria: This common heat- and sweat-induced rash on the back, termed "prickly heat," can be hard to distinguish from TAD; while pathology can help, the management is often similar
- Morbilliform drug eruption: less crusted and eroded, more pink macules and usually more widespread
- Viral exanthem: often less crusted/eroded, and more discrete pink macules

Important Work-Up

- Diagnosis can be made clinically; however, as patients are typically immunosuppressed and undergoing chemotherapy, further work-up is often performed to exclude alternate etiologies
- Skin biopsy can confirm the diagnosis
- Skin scrapings are useful to help rule out a potential infestation as a cause of pruritus (example: scabies or mites)
- Appropriate workup to rule out a potential infectious etiology may be necessary
  - Bacterial culture of a pustule
  - Laboratory evaluation for HSV or VZV

Treatment

- Typically benign and self-limited, resolving without treatment in several months without the need to alter or discontinue the patient's chemotherapy regimen
- Mid to high potency topical steroids and antihistamines can be used for symptomatic pruritus
- If bacterial folliculitis is in the differential diagnosis it is reasonable to treat with topical antimicrobials in the morning and topical corticosteroids in the evening to cover for both

Suggested Readings

1. Guana AL, Cohen PR. Transient acantholytic dermatosis in oncology patient. J Clin Oncol. 1994;12:1703–9.
2. Harvell JD, Hashem C, Williford PL, While WL. Grover's-like disease in the setting of bone marrow transplantation and autologous peripheral blood stem cell infusion. Am J Dermatopathol. 1998;20:179–84.
3. Horn TD, Groleau GE. Transient acantholytic dermatosis in immunocompromised febrile patients with cancer. Arch Dermatol. 1987;123:238–40.
4. Villalon G, Martin JM, Monteagudo C, Alonso V, Ramon D, Jorda E. Clinicopathological spectrum of chemotherapy induced Grover's disease. J Eur Acad Dermatol Venereol. 2007;21(8):1145–7.

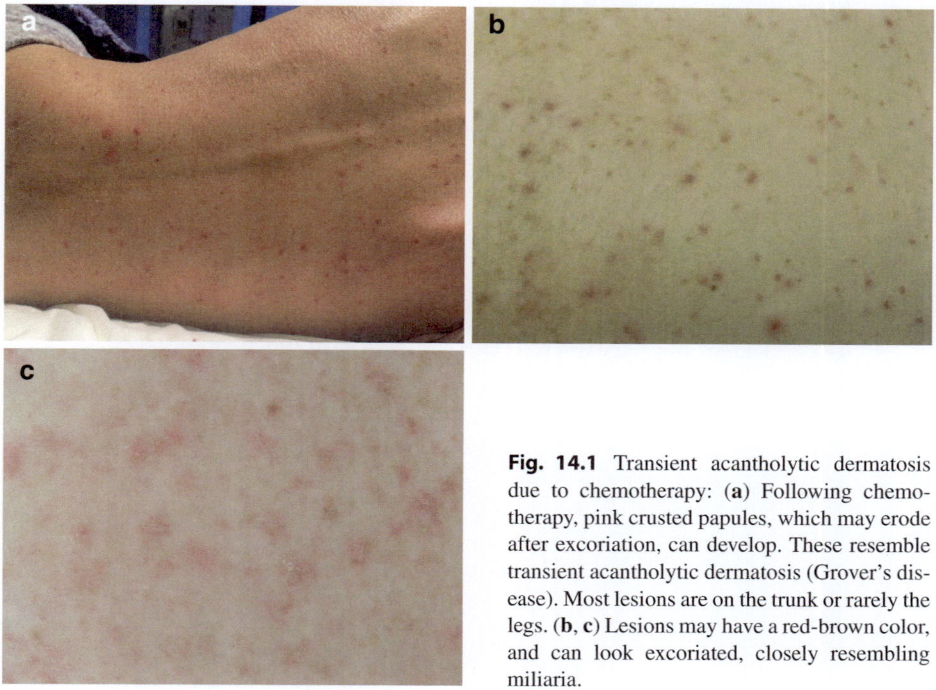

Fig. 14.1 Transient acantholytic dermatosis due to chemotherapy: (**a**) Following chemotherapy, pink crusted papules, which may erode after excoriation, can develop. These resemble transient acantholytic dermatosis (Grover's disease). Most lesions are on the trunk or rarely the legs. (**b**, **c**) Lesions may have a red-brown color, and can look excoriated, closely resembling miliaria.

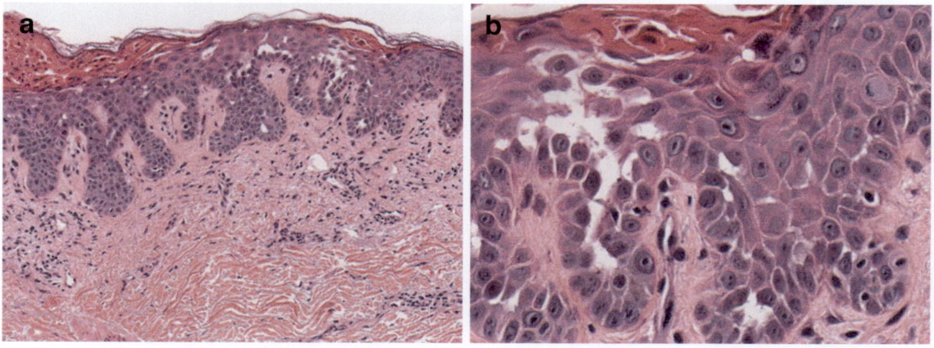

Fig. 14.2 Transient acantholytic dermatosis of chemotherapy *(10×, 40×; H&E)*: (**a**) There is multifocal acantholysis and dyskeratosis as seen in classic Grover's disease. (**b**) In addition to the acantholysis, the cytotoxic effects in the epidermis including dysmaturation and mitotic figures.

Serpentine Supravenous Hyperpigmentation

15

Megan H. Noe

Overview

- Typically seen following chemotherapeutic infusions, patients develop hyperpigmentation in the skin overlying the venous path through which the medication traveled creating a characteristic serpentine and branching rash
- 5-fluoruracil is the most commonly reported medication
  - Less commonly seen secondary to docetaxel, actinomycin, fotemustine, bromodeoxyuridine, vinorelbine, and vincristine
- The exact mechanism of pathogenesis is unclear
  - Proposed theories include hyperpigmentation resulting from a direct cytotoxic effect of the chemotherapy causing endothelial damage, epidermal basal hyperpigmentation and melanin incontinence versus local tissue extravasation injury

Clinical Presentation

- Distinctive clinical appearance with faintly erythematous-to-hyperpigmented streaks which may develop blisters and superficial desquamation (Fig. 15.1)
- The eruption follows the superficial venous network, most often seen on the forearms (streaking proximally from sites of peripheral IVs) but can be observed at any site
  - Deeper pigmentation is noted closest to the infusion site with lightening of the rash as it spreads

Histopathology

- Cytotoxic epithelial changes including keratinocyte dysmaturation and marked cellular pleomorphism are present (Fig. 15.2)
- Hyperplasia of basal melanocytes and melanophages in the upper dermis is consistent with post-inflammatory hyperpigmentation
  - Sparse perivascular inflammation and basilar vacuolization can be seen

M. H. Noe, MD, MPH
Department of Dermatology,
University of Pennsylvania, Philadelphia, PA, USA
e-mail: Megan.Noe@uphs.upenn.edu

M. Rosenbach et al. (eds.), *Inpatient Dermatology*,
https://doi.org/10.1007/978-3-319-18449-4_15

Differential Diagnosis

- Superficial thrombophlebitis: usually red, tender, and less visible branching out into smaller vessels
- Deep vein thrombosis: usually accompanied by swelling and pain
- Linear lichen planus: can be distinguished by history (chemo administration); lichen planus is also very pruritic
- Phytophotodermatitis: history is important, as if patient was drinking lime juice out in the sun, that can help distinguish this from someone receiving IV chemotherapy
- Allergic contact dermatitis: recent history of outdoor plant exposure, but clinically ACD will be more erythematous and spongiotic, with less deep-red-brown color, and won't closely follow vascular patterns

Important Work-Up

- Typically a clinical diagnosis requiring a thorough medication review
- A biopsy can aid in diagnostic confirmation if necessary
- In some cases, ultrasound may help rule out thrombosis or thrombophlebitis

Treatment

- No treatment necessary
- If secondary to chemotherapy, changing from peripheral administration to a central line (if appropriate for the agent in question) can help to resolve the pigmentation
  - Venous washing after chemotherapy may prevent the development of the hyperpigmentation
- The eruption may rarely recur with subsequent chemotherapy infusions, even in some cases when administered at a contralateral site, as a recall-reaction

Suggested Readings

1. Survirya A, Argrawl A, Parihar A. 5-Fluoracil-induced bilateral persistent serpentine supravenous hyperpigmented eruption, bilateral mottling of palms and diffuse hyperpigmentation of the soles. BMJ Case Rep. 2014. https://doi.org/10.1136/bcr-2014-206793.
2. Payne AS, James WD, Weiss RB. Dermatologic toxicity of chemotherapeutic agents. Semin Oncol. 2006;33(1):86–97.

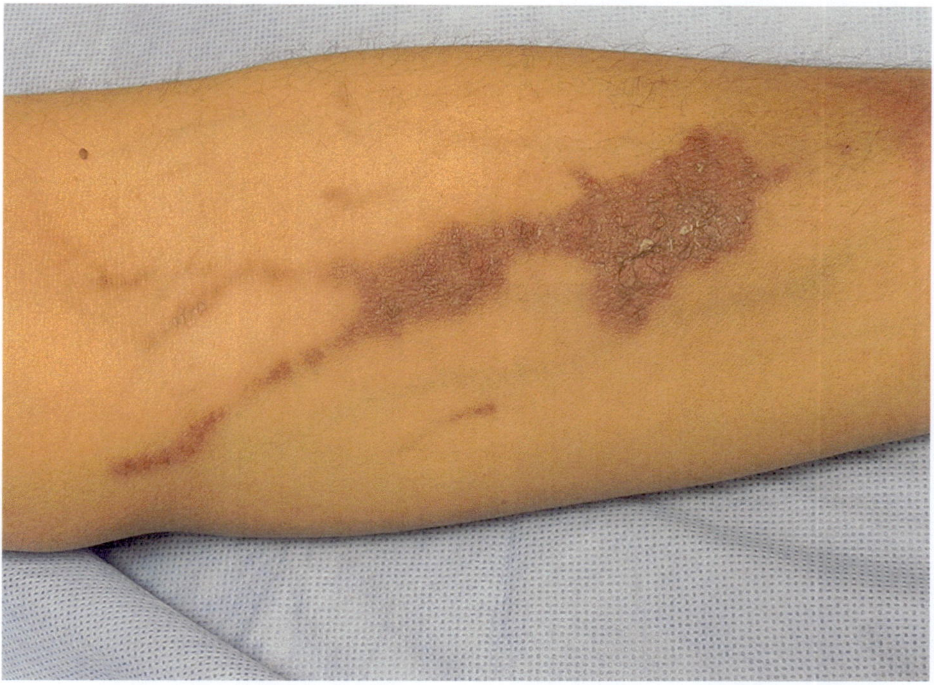

Fig. 15.1 Serpentine reaction: Supravenous serpentine chemotherapy reaction following infusion of docetaxel; 5-fluoruracil is a classic culprit of this patterned chemotherapeutic eruption.

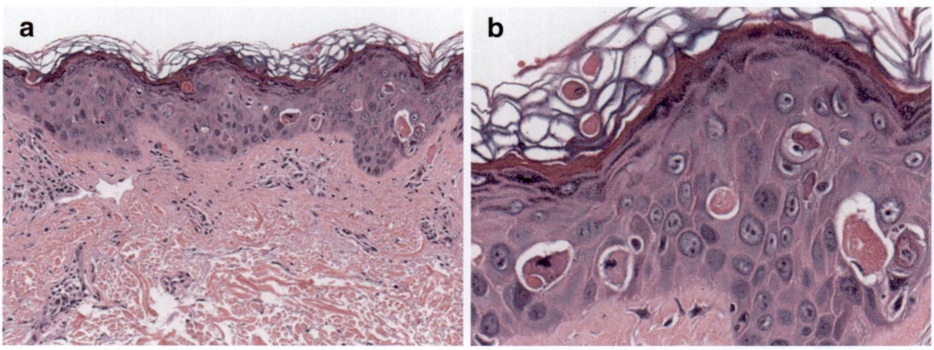

Fig. 15.2 Cytotoxic reaction to chemotherapy *(10×, 20×; H&E)*: (**a**) Cytotoxic changes in the epidermis are characterized by epidermal dysmaturation with similar size and shape of keratinocytes in basal layer and superficial layers of the epidermis and dyskeratosis. (**b**) Large, dyskeratotic and atypical cells can be seen, and mitotic figures may be evident.

Epidermal Growth Factor Inhibitors

16

Nahid Y. Vidal

Overview

- Epidermal growth factor receptors (EGFR) are involved in cell growth, differentiation, and proliferation with overexpression/dysregulation seen in many solid malignancies (including pulmonary and most GI cancers) making epidermal growth factor receptor inhibitors (EGFRI) a common treatment choice
- Two classes exist:
  - Tyrosine kinase inhibitors (TKIs—erlotinib and gefitinib)
  - Monoclonal antibodies (mAbs—panitumumab and cetuximab)
- EGFR is a trans-membrane glycoprotein preferentially expressed in the epidermis explaining why cutaneous side effects are common; although the exact mechanism is unclear
  - Thought that EGFRIs cause follicular occlusion/rupture secondary to increased apoptosis and its pro-inflammatory effects while also altering the local microflora environment leading to cutaneous damage and increased risk for bacterial overgrowth
- Skin manifestations are self-limited and typically resolve without scarring but the associated discomfort and displeasing aesthetics can lead to poor compliance with 1/3 of patients requiring intervention with EGFRI discontinuation in up to 40%
- Appearance and severity of rash correlates with objective tumor response and overall survival—it may be a surrogate marker for degree of receptor saturation by the EGFRI

Clinical Presentation

- Inflamed papules and pustules; often described as acneiform or rosaceaform but are not actually acne (Fig. 16.1)
- Face, neck, shoulders, upper trunk, scalp, and generally sun-exposed areas are most commonly affected with associated burning/stinging pain and pruritus with higher incidence and more severe rash seen with monoclonal anti-EGFR antibodies or Fitzpatrick skin types I/II
- Typical Course:
  - Week 1: Sensory changes, erythema, and edema
  - Weeks 2–3: Papulopustular eruption
  - Week 4: Crusting
  - Erythema and xerosis may persist for weeks after
  - Initially pustules are sterile but secondary infection with Staphylococcus aureus may occur
- Other findings with EGFR inhibitors include: paronychia, pyogenic granuloma, painful fissures on distal digits, palmoplantar hyperkeratosis, mucositis, scalp alopecia, trichomegaly of eyelashes

N. Y. Vidal, MD
Section of Dermatology, Department of Surgery, Dartmouth-Hitchcock Medical Center, Geisel School of Medicine, Hanover, NH, USA
e-mail: nahid.y.vidal@hitchcock.org

M. Rosenbach et al. (eds.), *Inpatient Dermatology*,
https://doi.org/10.1007/978-3-319-18449-4_16

Histopathology

- Acneiform eruption(Fig. 16.2):
  - Superficial perifolliculitis (neutrophils surrounding hyperkeratotic and/or ectatic follicular infundibula)
  - Neutrophilic suppurative folliculitis with rupture of epithelial lining +/– dyskeratosis or acantholysis
  - Hypoplastic sebaceous glands may be seen

Differential Diagnosis

- Drug-induced acne (steroids): clinically very similar to the EFGR-I acneiform eruption, though steroid acne will usually be monomorphic papules
- Pityrosporum folliculitis: usually monomorphic small papules on face, chest, shoulders only
- Eosinophilic folliculitis: this pruritic papular eruption centered on follicles of the face and chest often in HIV+ patients can be hard to distinguish; history is important
- Other anticancer acneiform eruption that can be seen (mTOR inhibitors, MEK inhibitors, BRAF-inhibitors, Multikinase inhibitors): different targeted chemotherapies will display divergent cutaneous phenotypes depending on their particular target, and as the literature is rapidly changing physicians should consult the primary literature in trying to distinguish these eruptions

Treatment

- Prior to EGFRI initiation patients should be instructed to limit/avoid sun exposure as it can worsen cutaneous manifestations
  - Use sun screen and avoid direct sunlight
  - Avoid products/activities which dry out the skin such as hot showers, OTC acne medication, alcohol containing products
- Prophylaxis with minocycline, doxycycline or tetracycline: may lead to overall fewer lesions, less severe, and improved symptoms of pain and itch
  - However, patients must be even more cautious with sun exposure since tetracyclines can increase sun sensitivity
- Treatments: Treating rash and symptoms can allow continuation of EGFRI
  - Oral tetracycline-class antibiotics are the first line treatment for moderate or severe disease (doxycycline, minocycline, tetracycline)
  - Topical antibiotics: 2% topical clindamycin or 1% nadifloxacin
  - Class II or III topical corticosteroids, or topical tacrolimus for anti-inflammatory effects
  - Metronidazole 0.75% cream
  - Recalcitrant: oral isotretinoin 10–20 mg per day during anti-EGFR treatment
  - Topical retinoids do not offer benefit and may cause irritation
  - Symptomatic relief:
    - Moisturize with chilled alcohol-free emollients
    - Oatmeal baths
    - Mild cleansers may be used
- Dose-reduction or discontinuation if failed other treatments and intolerable rash (patient-dependent)

Suggested Readings

1. Melosky B, Burkes R, Rayson D, et al. Management of skin rash during EGFR-targeted monoclonal antibody treatment for gastrointestinal malignancies: Canadian recommendations. Curr Oncol. 2009;16(1):16–26.
2. Wehler TC, Graf C, Mohler M, et al. Cetuximab-induced skin exanthema: prophylactic and reactive skin therapy are equally effective. J Cancer Res Clin Oncol. 2013;139(10):1667–72.
3. Guttman-Yassky E, Mita A, De Jonge M, et al. Characterization of the cutaneous pathology in NSCLC patients treated with EGFR tyrosine kinase inhibitor erlotinib. Eur J Cancer. 2010;46:2010–9.

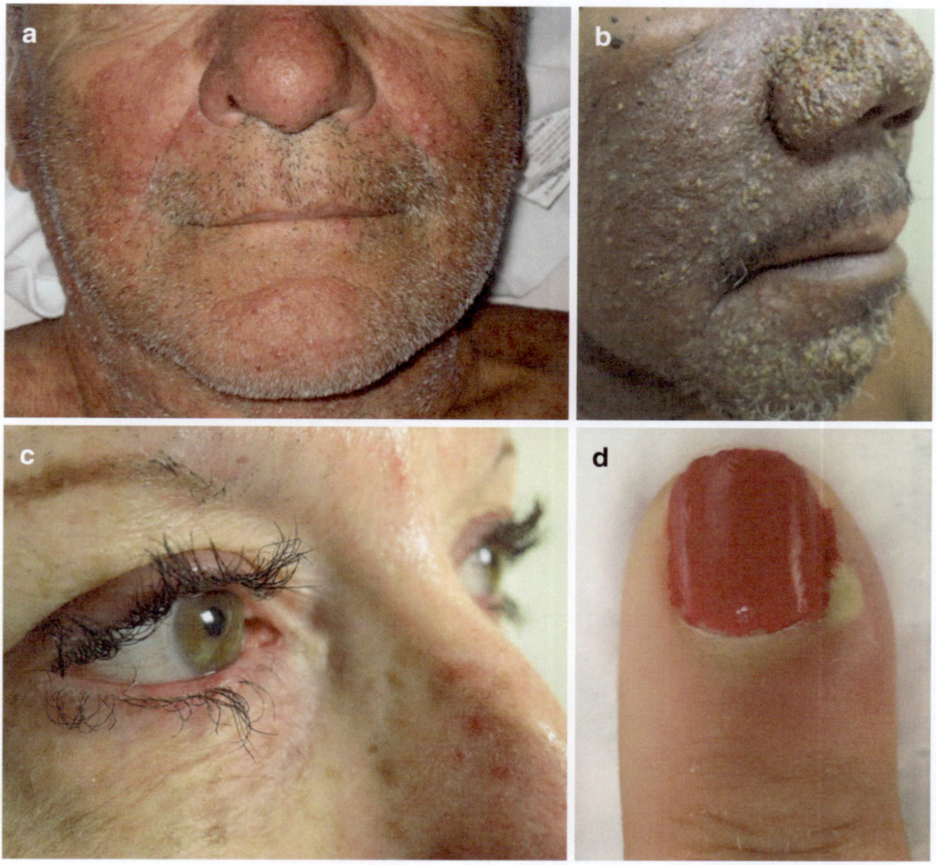

Fig. 16.1 Epidermal growth factor inhibitor eruptions: (**a**) Monomorphic acneiform eruption due to epidermal growth factor receptor (EGFR) inhibitor. (**b**) Severe EGFR inhibitor-induced acneiform eruption, which was dose-limiting. (**c**) Trichomegaly of the eyelashes due to EGFR inhibition. (**d**) Acute paronychia induced by exposure to an EGFR inhibitor.

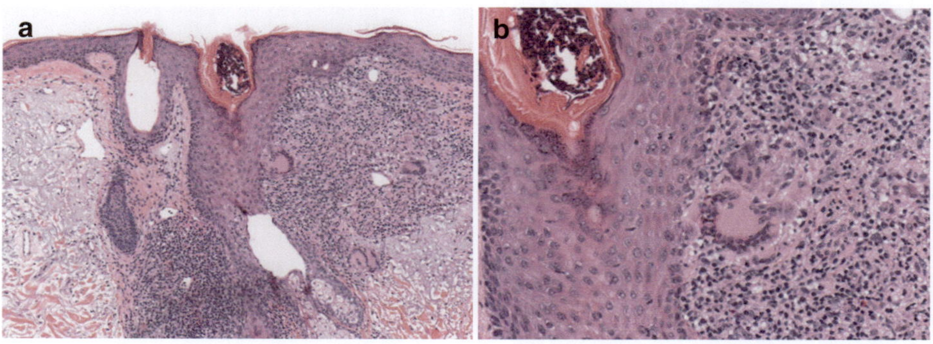

Fig. 16.2 Epidermal growth factor inhibitor eruptions: (*H&E; 10x, 40x*): (**a**, **b**) There is a focus of peri-follicular inflammation consisting of a mixed inflammatory infiltrate with scattered multinucleated giant cells.

Bleomycin-Induced Flagellate Erythema

17

Nkanyezi N. Ferguson

Overview

- Bleomcyin is a *Streptomyces* derived antibiotic/cytotoxic glycopeptide commonly used as an antitumor agent in combination chemotherapy regimens
  - Used to treat a variety of malignancies including Hodgkin and non-Hodgkin lymphomas, squamous cell carcinomas, malignant pleural effusions, and germ cell tumors
  - It is sometimes used to treat recalcitrant warts or keloids with local injection
- Flagellate erythema and persistent hyperpigmentation may result from exposure to bleomycin (systemic or intralesional); occurs in approximatley 10–20% of patients on Bleomycin
  - Other common mucocutaneous side effects include alopecia, stomatitis/mucositis
- Symptom onset after bleomycin exposure can range from 12 to 24 h to 6 months
- Usually resolve within 3–4 months after discontinuation of bleomycin
  - Some patients may have persistent hyperpigmentation for years or decades
- The skin's deficit of inactivating bleomycin hydrolase enzyme leads to cutaneous toxicity
  - It is postulated that the classic flagellate pattern is caused by localized bleomycin accumulation secondary to increased blood flow to regions of trauma from pressure or scratching

Clinical Presentation

- Erythematous to hyperpigmented linear streaks distributed in a flagellate pattern (flagellate meaning "whip-like" in appearance) (Fig. 17.1)
- Pruritus may precede or accompany cutaneous manifestations
- Primarily affects the trunk however can also involve the extremities

N. N. Ferguson, MD
University of Iowa Hospital and Clinics, Iowa City, IA, USA
e-mail: nkanyezi-ferguson@uiowa.edu

M. Rosenbach et al. (eds.), *Inpatient Dermatology*,
https://doi.org/10.1007/978-3-319-18449-4_17

Histopathology

- Hypermelanosis along the epidermal basal layer is prominent feature (Fig. 17.2)
- A range of histopathological features have been described including hyperkeratosis, parakeratosis, spongiosis, dermal edema, melanin incontinence and perivascular lymphocytic infiltration

Differential Diagnosis

- Shiitake dermatitis-associated flagellate erythema: this is more of an acute erythema rather than the hyperpigmentation seen with bleomycin
- Dermatomyositis-associated flagellate erythema: fewer than 5% of patients with dermatomyositis will demonstrate flagellate erythema, which is more acute erythema than hyperpigmentation
- Docetaxel-associated flagellate erythema: this is uncommon, but history can help distinguish these

Work-Up

- A thorough history and review of systems to screen for potential underlying etiologies is warranted; including a thorough medication review
- Skin biopsy of representative skin changes can be performed if unusual clinical presentation, but is rarely necessary

Treatment

- Self-limited with resolution on cessation of bleomycin; hyperpigmentation may persist after therapy
- Pruritus can be managed with topical corticosteroids and antihistamines
- Cutaneous symptoms recur with bleomycin re-challenge

Suggested Readings

1. Reyes-Habito CM, Roh EK. Cutaneous reactions to chemotherapeutic drugs and targeted therapies for cancer: part I conventional chemotherapeutic drugs. J Am Acad Dermatol. 2014;71(2):203.e1–203.e12.
2. Yamamoto T, Nishioka K. Flagellate erythema. Int J Dermatol. 2006;45(5):627–31.
3. Grynszpan R, Niemeyer-Corbellini JP, Lopes MS, Ramos-e-Silva M. Bleomycin-induced flagellate dermatitis. BMJ Case Rep. 2013;27:1–3.

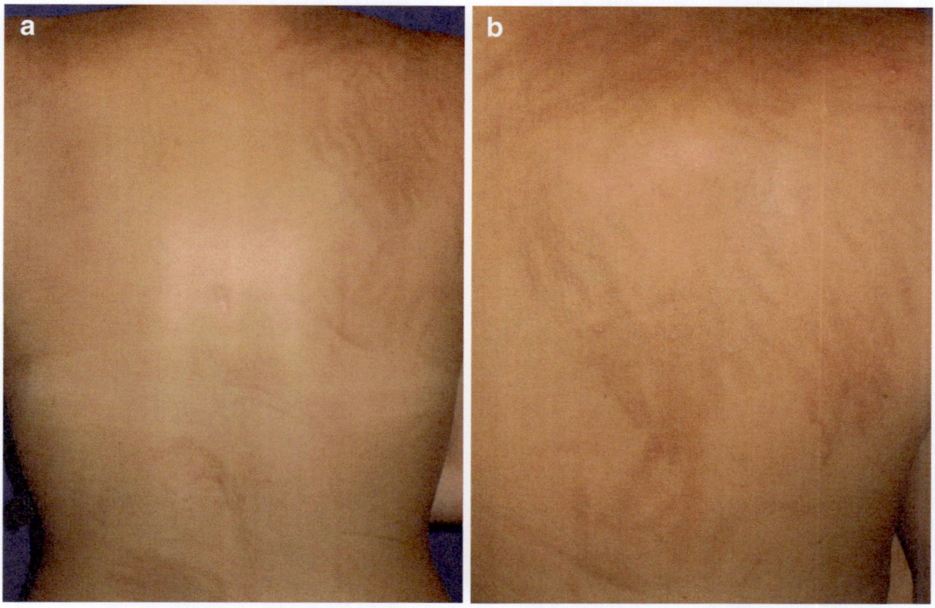

Fig. 17.1 Bleomycin hyperpigmentation: Numerous grouped linear hyperpigmented streaks, resembling stigmata of self-flagellation, on the back following exposure to bleomycin.

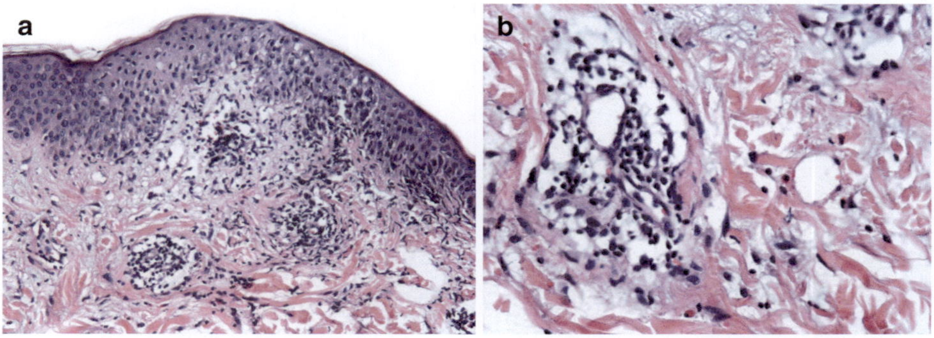

Fig. 17.2 Bleomyocin exposure (*5×*, *20×*; *H&E*): (**a**) Biopsies demonstrate hyperkeratosis, focal parakeratosis, irregular acanthosis and spongiosis. Interface dermatitis and a superficial perivascular lymphocytic infiltrate with eosinophils is seen. (**b**) The dermis has a lymphocytic infiltrate, scattered eosinophils, and variable edema. Superficial dermal melanin pigment can be seen in older lesions.

18 Acute Graft Versus Host Disease

Natalie Spaccarelli

Overview

- Graft versus host disease (GVHD) is caused by the introduction of immunologically competent donor cells into a recipient whose tissues display antigens that the donor cells view as foreign causing the donor cells to attack the host
- GVHD most commonly occurs following allogeneic hematopoietic stem cell transplant (SCT)
  - Can also occur following the transfusion of non-irradiated blood products into an immunocompromised host or after solid organ transplant (particularly liver, where more donor lymphocytes may be transported into the host and can engraft)
- Pre-transplantation chemotherapy and radiation aid in both the destruction of neoplastic cells and the down-regulation of the recipient's immune system (to prevent rejection of the donor cells)
  - Chemotherapy and radiation target cells with rapid turnover (skin, gut, and liver) leading to increased activation/antigen expression by dendritic cells in these areas, increasing their susceptibility to attack by donor cells; this is why much of the sequela of GVHD is associated with cutaneous, gastrointestinal and hepatic damage
- Although classically acute graft versus host disease (aGVHD) was defined as reactions occurring less than 100 days following SCT, and chronic graft versus host disease (cGVHD) occurring after 100 days, these entities are better distinguished by their clinical presentations than by their timing
- Skin is the most commonly affected organ in aGVHD and is usually the first organ involved

Clinical Presentation

- Cutaneous aGVHD usually presents as a morbilliform eruption which is typically symmetric and diffuse, and may be variably pruritic (Fig. 18.1)
- Monomorphic erythematous macules, often with fine scale, are present, sometimes clustered around hair follicles or over stretched/taught areas of skin (dorsal hands/feet, ears, posterior neck, upper back, outer arms, outer legs, scalp)
- Severe cases may cause extensive skin peeling, blister formation, and erosions of the mucosa
- Cutaneous aGVHD is graded (I-IV) based on extent of skin involvement (Table 18.1)
- Cutaneous aGVHD may be accompanied by other manifestations of aGVHD
  - Gastrointestinal GVHD is usually characterized by abdominal pain, diarrhea, vomiting, and/or appetite loss
  - Hepatic GVHD is usually characterized by abnormal LFTs (cholestatic hyperbilirubinemia), hepatomegaly, jaundice, pale stool, and/or dark urine

N. Spaccarelli, MD
University of Pennsylvania, Philadelphia, PA, USA
e-mail: natalie.spaccarelli2@uphs.upenn.edu

M. Rosenbach et al. (eds.), *Inpatient Dermatology*,
https://doi.org/10.1007/978-3-319-18449-4_18

Table 18.1 Clinical and histologic grading of aGVHD: each is graded separately [5]

Grade	Clinical grade of aGVHD	Histologic grade of aGVHD
1	Rash involves 1–18% BSA	Basal vacuolar change (not specific for GVHD)
2	Rash involves 19–50% BSA	Vacuolar interface dermatitis: basal vacuolar change, keratinocyte apoptosis, lymphocyte epidermotropism
3	Rash involves >50% BSA to generalized erythroderma	Focal dermal-epithelial junctional separation/clefting
4	Generalized erythroderma with bullae/blistering	Extensive epidermal necrosis with epidermolysis

Histopathology

- Cutaneous aGVHD is graded (0–IV) based on the extent of epidermis alteration (Table 18.1)
- Classically shows vacuolar interface dermatitis: basal vacuolar alteration, exocytosis of lymphocytes into the basal layer, and necrotic keratinocytes usually in the basal layer (Fig. 18.2)
  - Lymphocytic infiltrates are often scant given the level of immunosuppression in the patient but tend to occur in perivascular, hair follicle, and/or eccrine regions
  - Eosinophilia is rare, but the presence of scattered eosinophils does not exclude GVHD (more than 10–15 eosinophils/hpf may make GVHD less likely)
- Other findings can include:
  - Satellite cell necrosis: epidermal and adnexal epithelial lymphocytes surrounding dying keratinocytes
  - Pigment incontinence in long-standing cases
  - More severe cases can show aggregated necrotic keratinoctyes forming clefts and microvesicles at the dermal-epidermal junction and most severe cases can show detachment of epidermis with epidermolysis
- Full thickness keratinocyte necrosis can occur

Differential Diagnosis

- Viral exanthem: hard to distinguish; presence of a viral prodrome may help, and subtle cutaneous exam differences can help learn towards GVHD (fine scale, folliculocentric, localization to ears)
- Morbilliform drug eruption: hard to distinguish; morbilliform eruptions should not have a fine scale, and histology with an interface reaction can help lean towards GVHD; diarrhea, bilirubinemia, and less pruritus also favor GVHD
- Engraftment syndrome/eruption of lymphocyte recovery: many view this as a form of hyperacute GVHD and the cutaneous signs are very similar; these will often self-resolve rapidly
- Stevens-Johnson syndrome/Toxic epidermal necrolysis: severe aGVHD with widespread blistering can be clinically and histologically identical to TEN; sometimes chimerism studies may be helpful but generally these are challenging to distinguish

Work-up

- Diagnosis is usually based on clinical criteria, but histological confirmation with biopsy should be sought when possible and is ideally obtained prior to starting treatment
- CBC with differential, CMP should be performed; if diarrhea is present, quantification of volume of stool can assist in staging the severity of GI disease
- A thorough analysis of concomitant medications and potential infections to exclude potential alternate etiology (such as a drug eruption) is recommended

Treatment

- High potency topical corticosteroids may provide relief in mild cases, but escalation of systemic immunosuppressive regimen (usually in the form of starting or increasing systemic corticosteroids) is typically necessary
  - High dose corticosteroids are typically given for the first 7–14 days (in addition to the existing GVHD prophylactic therapy)
  - Second line therapy should be closely coordinated with the transplant team, and can include immunosuppressants (mycophenolate mofetil, tacrolimus, or sirolimus), anti-thymocyte globulin, pentostatin, antibodies (anti-TNF alpha, anti-CD52, or anti-IL2 receptor (CD25)), or mesenchymal stem cells
- PUVA phototherapy, UVA1 phototherapy, and extracorporeal photopheresis have shown some efficacy, but are more typically used for cGVHD

Suggested Readings

1. Ferrara J, Levine JE, Reddy P, et al. Graft-versus-host disease. Lancet. 2009;373:1550–61.
2. Peñas PF, Zaman S. Many faces of graft-versus-host disease. Australas J Dermatol. 2010;51:1–10.
3. Sundram U. A review of important skin disorders occurring in the posttransplantation patient. Adv Anat Pathol. 2014;21:321–9.
4. Ziemer M. Graft-versus-host disease of the skin and adjacent mucous membranes. J German Soc Dermatol. 2013;11:477–95.
5. Jagasia MH, Greinix HT, Arora M, et al. National Institute of Health consensus development project on criteria for clinical trials in chronic graft-versus-host disease: 1. The 2014 diagnosis and staging working group report. Biol Blood Marrow Transplant. 2015;21(3):389–401.

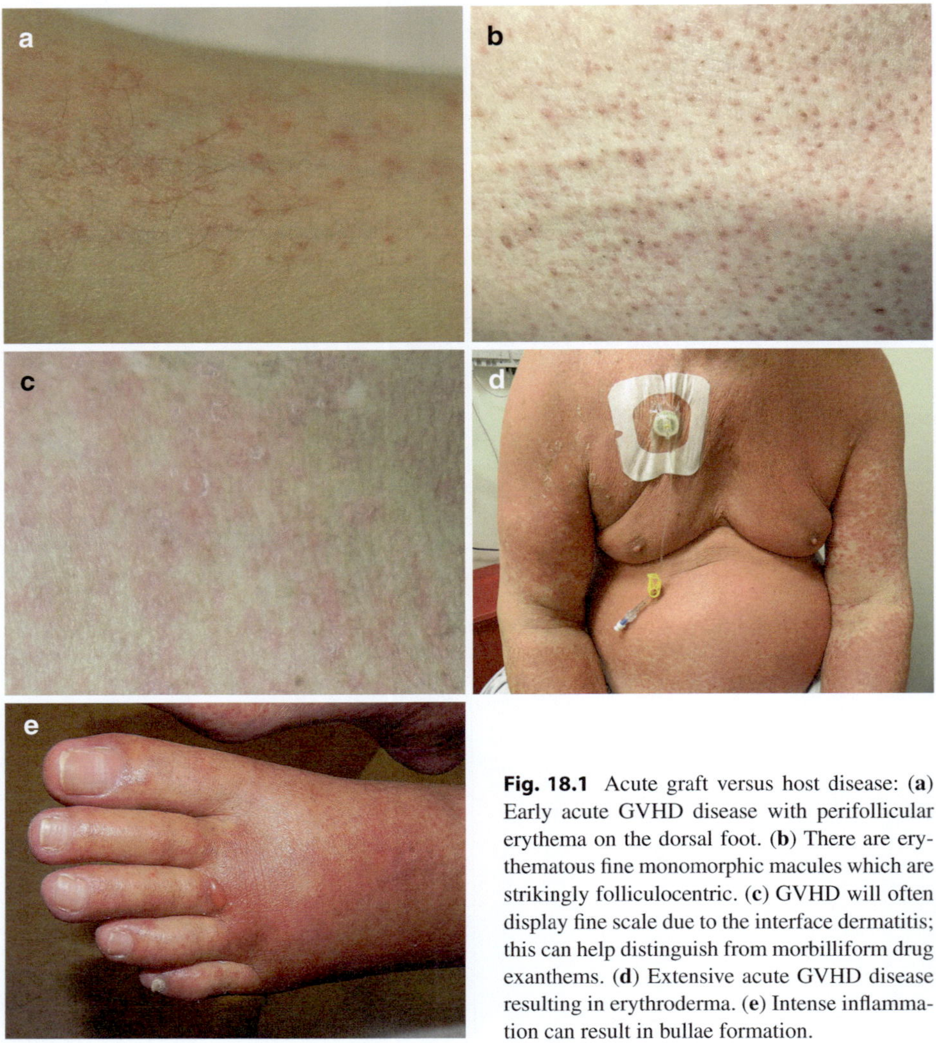

Fig. 18.1 Acute graft versus host disease: (**a**) Early acute GVHD disease with perifollicular erythema on the dorsal foot. (**b**) There are erythematous fine monomorphic macules which are strikingly folliculocentric. (**c**) GVHD will often display fine scale due to the interface dermatitis; this can help distinguish from morbilliform drug exanthems. (**d**) Extensive acute GVHD disease resulting in erythroderma. (**e**) Intense inflammation can result in bullae formation.

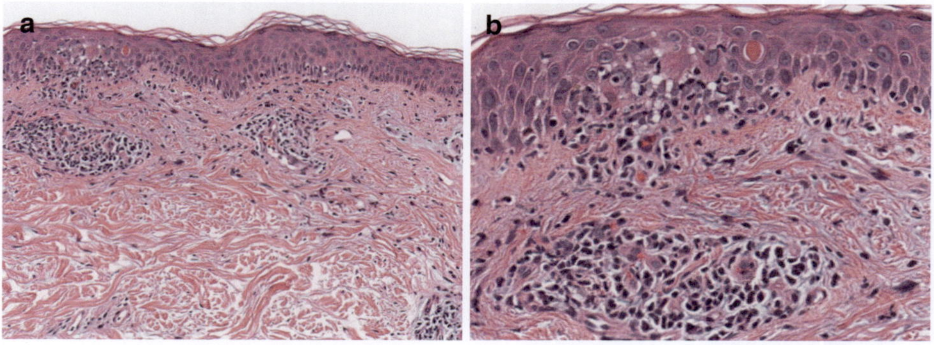

Fig. 18.2 Graft versus host disease (GVHD) (*5×, 20×; H&E*): (**a**) Characterized by a typically mild inteface dermatitis and associated dyskeratosis. (**b**) There is a vacuolar interface dermatitis with satellite-cell necrosis (an epidermal lymphocyte adjacent to a necrotic keratinocyte).

Chronic Graft Versus Host Disease

19

Natalie Spaccarelli

Overview

- Graft versus host disease (GVHD) is caused by the introduction of immunologically competent donor cells into a recipient whose tissues display antigens that the donor cells view as foreign; causing the donor cells to attack the host
- GVHD most commonly occurs following allogeneic hematopoietic stem cell transplant (SCT)
  - Can also occur following the transfusion of non-irradiated blood products into an immunocompromised host or after solid organ transplant (particularly liver)
- Pathogenesis of cGVHD is less well defined that that of aGVHD but donor T-cells are viewed as a key mediator in both, though regulatory cells and a mismatch between antigen presenting cells and effector cells may be involved
  - The potential role of B cells and humoral (antibody mediated) immunity in cGVHD is an area of active investigation
- Although classically acute graft versus host disease (aGVHD) was defined as reactions occurring less than 100 days following SCT, and chronic graft versus host disease (cGVHD) occurring after 100 days, these entities are better distinguished by their clinical presentations than by their timing
  - Lichen planus–like and scleroderma-like skin manifestations are considered diagnostic of cGVHD in the appropriate clinical context
- Onset of chronic GVHD can be progressive (acute GVHD merging into chronic GVHD), quiescent (resolution of acute GVHD followed by appearance of chronic GVHD), or de novo (chronic GVHD starting in the absence of any history of acute GVHD)
- cGVHD is seen in ~60% of SCT recipients with skin being the most commonly affected organ

Clinical Presentation

- Cutaneous presentations of cGVHD are more varied than in aGVHD (Fig. 19.1)
  - Early cutaneous cGVHD can manifest as a subtle morbilliform rash similar to aGVHD, though this is rarely seen

N. Spaccarelli, MD
University of Pennsylvania, Philadelphia, PA, USA
e-mail: natalie.spaccarelli2@uphs.upenn.edu

M. Rosenbach et al. (eds.), *Inpatient Dermatology*,
https://doi.org/10.1007/978-3-319-18449-4_19

- More established cGVHD is most often characterized by a lichen-planus like eruption of erythematous-to-violaceous papules, or tight bound-down sclerotic/sclerodermoid cutaneous changes similar to systemic sclerosis or eosinophilic fasciitis
  - Sclerotic/sclerodermoid changes include: subtle dimpling of the skin with deep tissue firmness and thickening, or the "dry riverbed" sign of collapsed veins in extremities when elevated, due to persistent subcutaneous fibrosis,
- Dyspigmentation (depigmentation, hypopigmentation, and/or hyperpigmentation), nail dystrophy or loss, alopecia, poikiloderma, mucosal inflammation, and genital ulcers can also occur
- Skin changes can be accompanied by other manifestations of cGVHD
  - Oral: xerostomia, lichen-planus-like changes, ulcers
  - Ocular: dry eyes, cicatricial conjunctivitis, and sicca syndrome
  - Muscle/fascia/joint: contractures of joints, myositis, and fasciitis
  - Gastrointestinal: characterized by diarrhea, difficulty swallowing, and/or appetite loss
  - Hepatic: characterized by abnormal LFTs, hepatomegaly, and/or jaundice
  - Lung: characterized by restrictive or obstructive pulmonary function defects

Histopathology

- Lichen-planus like eruptions are most often characterized by hypergranulosis, hyperkeratosis, and dense band-like infiltrate of lymphocytes at the dermal-epidermal junction with necrotic keratinocytes and pigment dropout (Fig. 19.2)
- Sclerotic changes are most often characterized by superficial vessel dilation, atrophy of epidermis, dermal collagen homogenization, hair follicle loss, and peri-eccrine fat loss

Differential Diagnosis

- Lichenoid drug eruption: can be hard to distinguish and timing/history is important; this will more often be transient
- Lichen planus: can closely resemble cGVHD, though in the post-transplant setting cGVHD is more common
- Morphea: these flat, dull-brown, bound-down patches can resemble areas of sclerodermoid GVHD, though morphea is often more localized
- Systemic sclerosis: there is extensive clinical and histological overlap, though if observed in the post-transplant setting cGVHD is the more likely diagnosis
- Eosinophilic fasciitis: if observed in the post-transplant setting cGVHD is the more likely diagnosis

Work-Up

- Diagnosis is usually based on clinical criteria, but histological confirmation with biopsy should be sought when possible and is ideally obtained prior to starting treatment
- In patients with non-sclerotic lesions, punch biopsy is sufficient
- In patients with sclerotic lesions, particularly deep forms of fasciitis, incisional biopsy is sometimes necessary in order to include enough tissue from the subcutis and possibly the fascia
  - Avoid biopsying the lower legs as wound healing can be poor; imaging, particularly contrast MRI, may demonstrate fascial enhancement and obviate the need for biopsy
- CBC with differential, CMP should be performed and pulmonary functions tests may be considered
- All patients should be referred back to their oncologist and managed jointly

Treatment

- Treatment, particularly when scleroderma-like, is often challenging as there is no consistently effective therapy

- Mild cGVHD may respond to topical treatments alone
  - Topical steroids must usually be high potency at first (attempt to gradually reduce their intensity) and may be applied under occlusion or in combination with wet wraps in the short term
  - Topical tacrolimus and pimecrolimus (calicineurin inhibitors) can be used alone or together and, if using tacrolimus, start with 0.1% and taper to 0.03% depending on the response
  - If topicals are not effective after 2 weeks of daily use, other treatments should be considered
- Systemic therapies such as oral corticosteroids, tacrolimus, mycophenolate mofetil, imatinib, sirolimus, hydroxychloroquine, rituximab, janus kinase-inhibitors, and low-dose IL-2 can be effective in more severe or non-responsive cases
- Phototherapy (primarily PUVA and UVA1), extracorporeal photopheresis can be also beneficial and are usually used in combination with systemic therapies
- All patients with scleroderma-like disease should have their joint mobility closely monitored, and physical therapy is an essential part of treatment regimens

Suggested Readings

1. Ferrara J, Levine JE, Reddy P, et al. Graft-versus-host disease. Lancet. 2009;373:1550–61.
2. Peñas PF, Zaman S. Many faces of graft-versus-host disease. Australas J Dermatol. 2010;51:1–10.
3. Sundram U. A review of important skin disorders occurring in the posttransplantation patient. Adv Anat Pathol. 2014;21:321–9.
4. Ziemer M. Graft-versus-host disease of the skin and adjacent mucous membranes. J German Soc Dermatol. 2013;11:477–95.

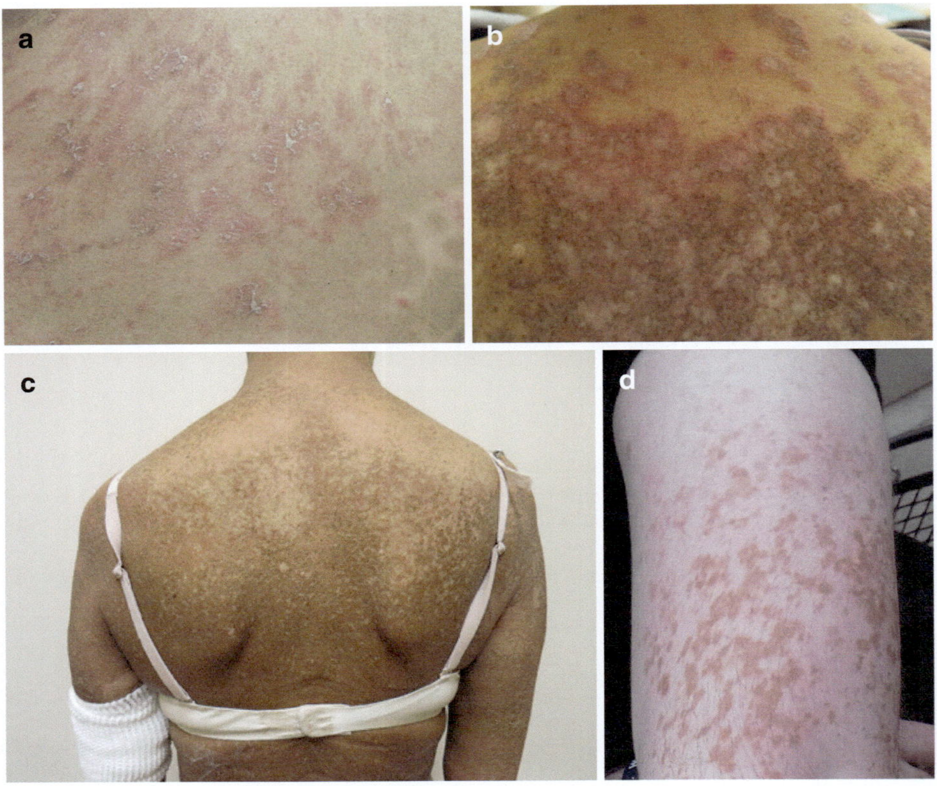

Fig. 19.1 Chronic graft versus host disease (cGVHD): (**a**) The pink-to-violaceous flat papules of lichen planus-like cGVHD have extensive scaling, a clinical clue to the presence of an interface reaction. (**b**) Purple papules and plaques with superficial scale and dyspigmentation in a patient with lichen planus-like cGVHD. (**c**) Hypo and hyperpigmentation creating a "salt and pepper" appearance in a patient with chronic cutaneous graft-versus-host disease. (**d**) Extensive dyspigmentation in a patient with widespread lichenoid cGVHD. (**e**) Deep sclerosis of the fascia resulting in a "pseudocellulite" appearance of the upper arm in a patient with chronic cutaneous GVHD. (**f**) Shiny sclerotic plaques of chronic cutaneous GVHD resembling morphea. (**g**) This sclerodermatous change is often pronounced at sites of pressure, such as the waist-band area. (**h**) Sclerosis resulting in reduce range of motion in the "prayer sign" in a patient with chronic scleroderma-like GVHD. (**i**) Extensive sclerosis and fibrosis resembling linea morphea on the feet of a patient with severe cGVHD.

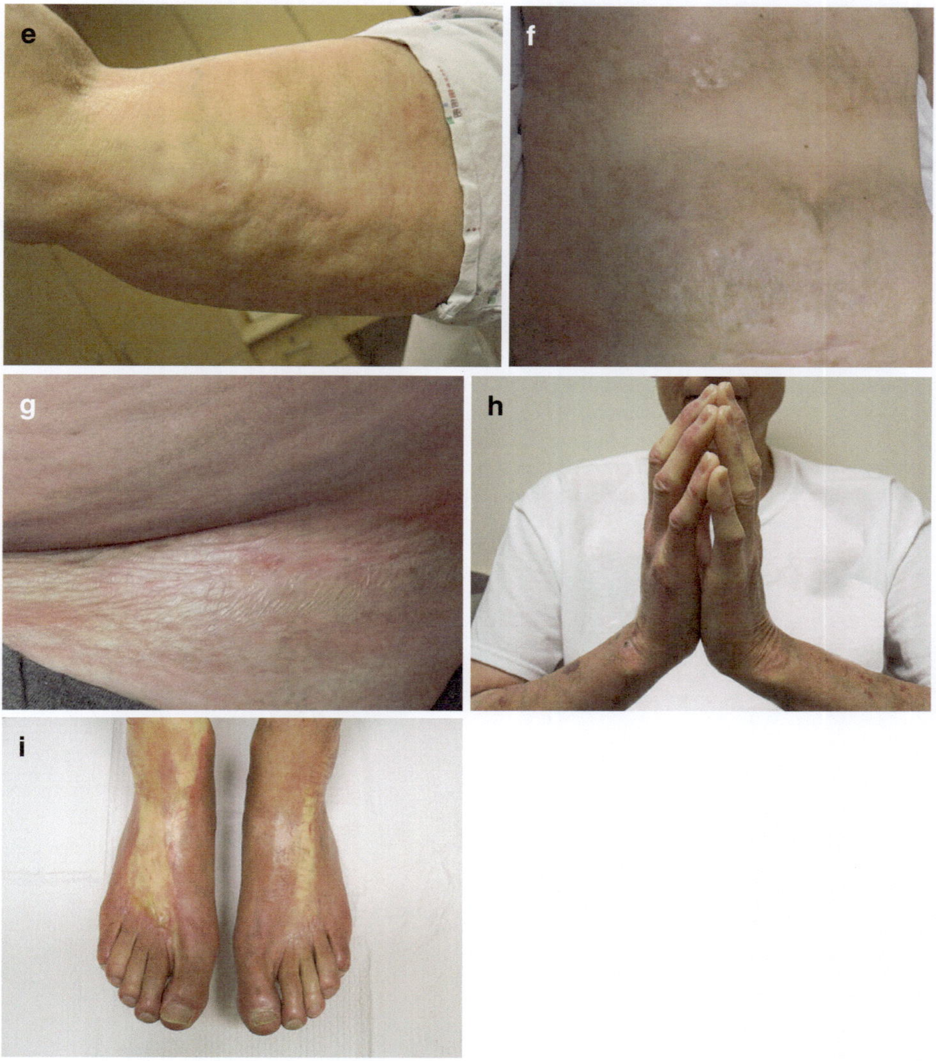

Fig. 19.1 (Continued)

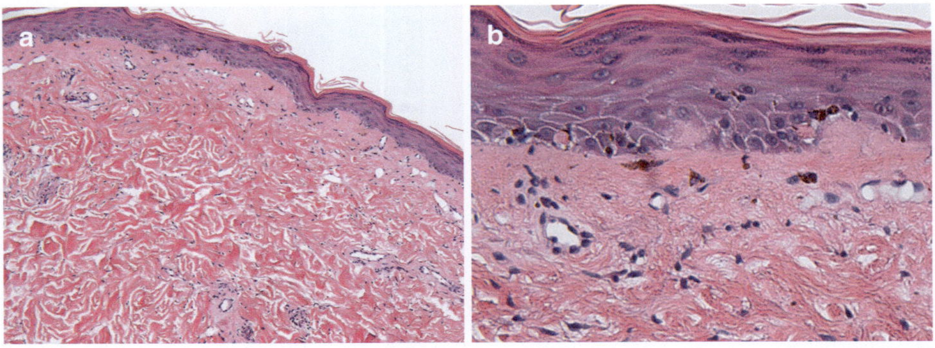

Fig. 19.2 Chronic graft versus host disease (cGVHD) (*5×, 20×; H&E*): Chronic GVHD can be subdivided into lichenoid and sclerodermoid types. Both often show evidence of a mild interface dermatitis and pigment incontinence. (**a**) In sclerodermoid GVHD, the biopsy is often squared off due increased, homogenized dermal collagen, and there may be loss of follicular structures and peri-eccrine fat. (**b**) With lichenoid GVHD, parakeratosis and a slight increase in the inflammatory infiltrate at the dermal-epidermal junction can be observed.

Part IV

Bacterial Infections

Infections can be a significant cause of morbidity and mortality if not rapidly and accurately diagnosed and treated. In the inpatient setting, patients can be extremely ill, immunocompromised, or have multiple comorbidities complicating their ability to fight infections resulting in atypical or overlapping presentations. Dermatologists play an instrumental role in the initial diagnosis and management of infections with cutaneous manifestations. In the upcoming chapters we will cover the cutaneous findings in bacterial, viral, fungal, and ectoparasitic infections.

Infections can manifest in the skin as a primary cutaneous infection from direct inoculation, with secondary cutaneous involvement as part of a systemic infection with hematogenous spread, or with reactive phenomena in the skin as a result of systemic infection or inflammation. The skin findings may vary not just due to the underlying pathogen, but also due to the host's immune status. A small bland lesion in an immunosuppressed patient may actually represent a serious deeper infection with a poor host inflammatory response.

Most infectious processes are acute, with rapid onset of symptoms and skin findings; some, however, can be slower to develop (such as mycobacterial infections, endemic deep fungal infections, or Kaposi sarcoma), and the history and timing of the eruption is often just as important as the pattern of skin findings. If an infection is suspected, it is often important to empirically broadly cover the patient for all possible etiologic agents, and to rapidly initiate a diagnostic workup.

Skin-specific diagnostic tests can include superficial skin swabs (while nonspecific, this can confirm a suspected superficial infection, as in impetigo, and also provide sensitivity data to allow targeted antibiosis), KOH preps to look for dermatophytes, Tzank smears for clues to herpes infections, skin scrapings to evaluate for scabies, sterile incision and drainage of deeper abscesses (which can be both diagnostic and therapeutic), or skin biopsy and tissue cultures. Sometimes specific cutaneous eruptions will prompt consideration for additional testing, such as serologic evaluation for antibodies or targeted systemic workup to look for internal infectious sources. Patients with systemic infections often require rapid diagnosis and coordinated, multidisciplinary management with multiple experienced physicians.

Superficial Staphylococcal and Streptococcal Infections

20

Grant Ghahramani

Overview

- Skin infections are commonly secondary to infection of *Streptococcus pyogenes* (Group A β-hemolytic streptococci), *Stapylococcus aureus*, or a combination of the two gram positive organisms
- Polymorphous presentation depending on organism, virulence factors, host, depth of infection, and skin structure(s) involved
  - Folliculitis: suppurative inflammation of the hair follicle
  - Furuncle: folliculitis with extension into adjacent dermis/subcutis resulting in an abscess
  - Carbuncle: multiple adjacent furuncles
  - Abscess: localized and contained "walled off" collection of pus
  - Impetigo: Superficial bacterial infection which can be primary (arising in normal skin) or secondary (arising at sites of skin damage from local trauma or underlying dermatosis); bullous or nonbullous
    Impetiginization may be used to refer to secondary impetigo over a preexisting dermatitis or other skin process
  - Ecthyma: superficial bacterial infection with a thick crust; ulcerative non-bullous form of impetigo
  - Cellulitis: suppurative inflammation of the deep dermis and subcutis causing expanding erythema
  - Erysipelas: suppurative inflammation of the upper dermis ("superficial cellulitis") and often lymphatics resulting in a well demarcated erythematous plaque
  - Staphylococcal scalded skin syndrome (SSSS): extensive exfoliative dermatitis caused by bacterial toxins typically from a distant *S. aureus* (phage group 2) infection

Clinical Presentation

- Folliculitis: hair-follicle based pustules which can involve any hair-bearing skin location but chest, back, buttocks, and intertriginous areas are favored (Fig. 20.1)
- Furuncle: perifolicullar fluctuant tender dermal to subcutaneous nodule (abscess) that may develop into multifocal communicating lesions with draining sinus tracts (carbuncle)
  - Carbuncles are more common in areas like the back and thigh which have thicker skin and tend to scar with resolution

G. Ghahramani, MD
Cotton O'Neil Dermatology, Topeka, KS, USA

M. Rosenbach et al. (eds.), *Inpatient Dermatology*,
https://doi.org/10.1007/978-3-319-18449-4_20

- Abscess: Fluctuant dermal to subcutaneous red plaque or nodule with a possible "head" or focal pustule
- Impetigo: characterized by distinct honey-colored dried adherent crusting over damaged skin
  - Nonbullous form (impetigo simplex, impetigo contagiosa, nonbullous impetigo):
    Highly contagious common skin infection typically seen in children that often presents as golden-yellow crusted skin lesions with thin honey to straw-colored exudate on the face, especially around the nose and mouth, or extremities Affected immunocompetent adults often had contact with an infected child
  - Bullous impetigo: Classically seen in neonates/infants secondary to exposure to toxins associated with *S. aureus* infections (exfoliative toxin A), patients develop fragile vesicles which quickly evolve into bullous lesions which may become generalized; honey-yellow crusts form over ruptured bullae
    Due to bacterial exfoliative toxin which targets desmoglein 1 (shared target with SSSS and pemphigus)
- Ecthyma: punched out ulcerations filled with yellow to dark brown to black crusted eschar resembling a crust-filled "volcano"
- Cellulitis: deep pyogenic infection involving the dermis and subcutis resulting in ill-defined streaking erythema (lymphangitis) with associated edema tenderness and warmth; patients may have a fever, leukocytosis, and/or lymphadenopathy
  - As lesions tend to expand marking the borders can aid in visual assessment of progression/improvement
- Erysipelas: sharply demarcated bright red to violaceous patches and thin plaques with localized pain, heat, swelling, and raised indurated border on the face or legs; prominent lymphatic involvement can occur
- SSSS: acute, febrile, rapid desquamation syndrome due to exfoliative toxin seen in young children or in adults often with renal insufficiency on dialysis
  - Associated with immunosuppression, diabetes, trauma, lymphedema, poor hygiene; children frequently affected
  - Exfoliative toxin A targets desmoglein 1 (shared target with bullous impetigo and pemphigus)

Histopathology

- Furunculosis/Carbuncle: acute inflammatory infiltrate involving and surrounding the follicle along with associated necrosis
- Impetigo: superficial acute inflammatory infiltrate at or above the granular layer consisting of neutrophils and gram positive bacteria; later lesions may evolve into a vesicle or pustule with separation at the granular layer (Fig. 20.2)
- Abscess: a dermal collection of mixed neutrophilic and necrotic debris (Fig. 20.3)
- Ecthyma: superficial ulceration or vesicopustule with a thick serous crusting extending into the dermis with numerous bacteria. The deeper processes generally show similar features of an acute inflammatory reaction within the dermis with vascular dilation, edema, and infiltration of neutrophils
- Gram stain can be performed and will highlight gram positive cocci

Differential Diagnosis

The differential diagnosis varies somewhat by the clinical morphology.

- Folliculitis:
  - Eosinophilic folliculitis: pruritic lesions on the chest/face of patients with HIV
  - Steroid acne: monomorphic fine pustules and pinpoint papules on the chest, shoulders, back, in setting of chronic steroid use

- Impetigo:
  - Allergic contact dermatitis: can also be weepy with serous fluid that dries as a crust; less distinctly yellow/honey colored, and always pruritic
  - Tinea infection: should have more of a flaky fine white scale, and annular character
  - If bullous may resemble varicella, herpes simplex virus infection, scabies, autoimmune bullous dermatoses, insect bites: culture and ancillary testing can differentiate
- Ecthyma:
  - Deep fungal infection: usually there is some purulence around the crust in ecthyma which will culture gram positive organisms; histology may also distinguish
  - Medium vessel vasculitis (MVV): patients should lack the systemic symptoms and serologic evidence of MVV
- Erysipelas and cellulitis:
  - Contact dermatitis: contact is pruritic whereas infections are often painful, and contact dermatitis often has epidermal change, whereas these infections are deeper—but patients may have more than one process (e.g., applying neomycin to a wound and getting both infection and contact dermatitis)
  - Stasis dermatitis: stasis is bilateral, whereas cellulitis is unilateral, and far more acute
  - Rosacea: can closely mimic erysipelas but the rosacea is chronic, and often has more telangiectasias and papulopustular lesions
- Staphylococcal scalded skin syndrome:
  - SJS/TEN: SJS/TEN almost invariably involves mucosa, whereas SSSS does not affect it

Work-Up

- For superficial infections (with crusts or pustules), bacterial culture can be performed by cleansing with alcohol, nicking a lesion with a needle or blade, and sending bacterial cultures
- Abscesses should be incised and drained as this is in some cases curative, and material can be sent for culture to tailor antimicrobial therapy appropriately
- Skin biopsy with tissue culture can be performed if atypical presentation or non-response to therapy; tissue culture has a low yield, but has higher sensitivity than blood cultures
- In cellulitis it is challenging to identify the organism; if there are breaks in the skin cultures can be sent but those often identify superficial colonizers
  - Tissue culture or aspiration of the leading edge of the infection may be higher yield than blood culture, but still are only positive in the minority of cases.
  - Often performed if infection fails to improve, recurs, or the host is immunosuppressed
- Titers such as ASO and DNAse B may be used as ancillary evidence for a recent streptococcal infection
- Monitoring of neonates with bullous lesions for dissemination of exfoliative toxin and development of SSSS

Treatment

- Warm compresses and topical antimicrobial (such as mupirocin, bleach baths) for early cases of impetigo
- Regular wound care with removal of crust and acetic acid soaks or bleach baths
- Incision and drainage followed by warm compresses for abscesses, furuncles, and carbuncles may be sufficient in immunocompetent hosts without surrounding cellulitis
- First generation oral cephalosporins such as dicloxacillin or cephalexin are first line therapy in areas with low rates of MRSA, but one should check local epidemiologic data and tailor thearpy
- Penicillin therapy is indicated if Streptococcal infection suspected
- Consider either trimethoprim–sulfamethoxazole, doxycycline, or clindamycin if MRSA suspected or cultured or in high incidence areas or high risk populations (athletes, patients with recent hospitalization, nursing home)

- Patients with cellulitis should be evaluated for risk factors—such as tinea pedis or abnormal veno-lymphatic return, which if addressed appropriately may reduce repeat infections.
- Monthly decolonization if methicillin resistant S. aureus occurs with recurrent episodes
- Intravenous antibiotics are indicated if systemically ill

Suggested Readings

1. Stevens DL, et al. Practice guidelines for the diagnosis and management of skin and soft tissue infections: 2014 update by the infectious diseases society of America. Clin Infect Dis. 2014;59(2):147.
2. Weng QY, Raff AB, Cohen JM, et al. Costs and consequences associated with misdiagnosed lower extremity cellulitis. JAMA Dermatol. 2017;153(2):141–6.
3. Swartz MN. Cellulitis. N Engl J Med. 2004;350:904–12.
4. Raff AB, Kroshinsky D. Cellulitis: a review. JAMA. 2016;316:325–37.

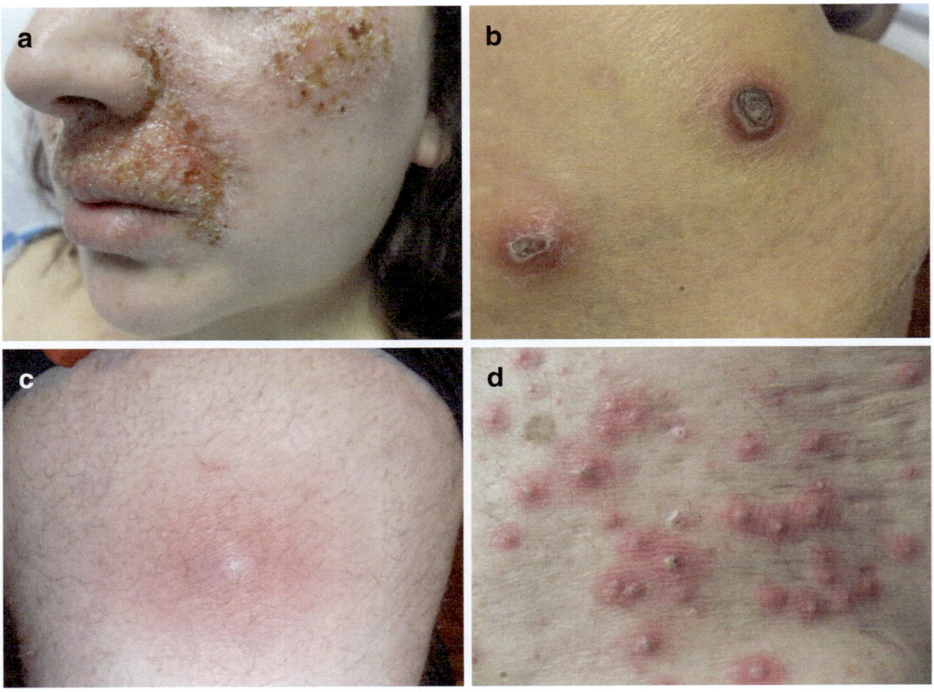

Fig. 20.1 Staph and strep bacterial infections of the skin: (**a**) Impetigo: Honey colored crust and superficial weepy erosions typical of impetigo. (**b**) MRSA ecthyma: Round red nodules with central core crusts resembling "volcanos" typical of chronic ecthyma due to *Staph* or *Strep*. (**c**) Abscess: A small abscess with surrounding erythema consistent with cellulitis on the thigh due to *Staph aureus*. (**d**) Folliculitis: folliculocentric pustules with visible hairs coming through the pustules.

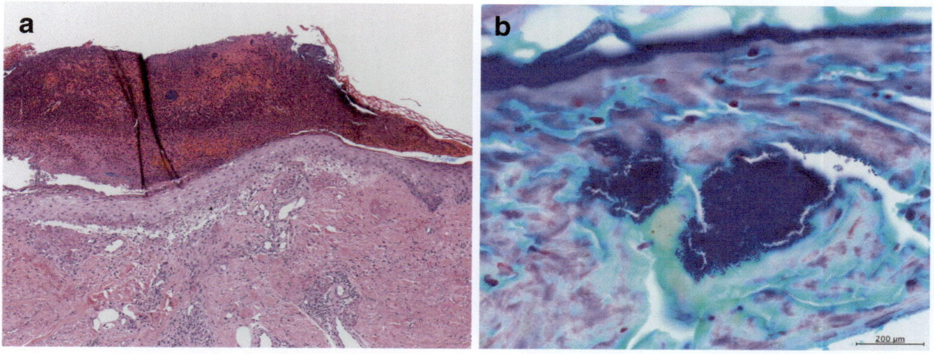

Fig. 20.2 Impetigo: (**a**) On lower power, there is crusted serous exudate with neutrophils, and epidermal spongiosis and a dermal inflammatory infiltrate. (**b**) On higher power, numerous Gram positive cocci in collections are noted within the serum crust (Courtesy of Brian Swick, MD).

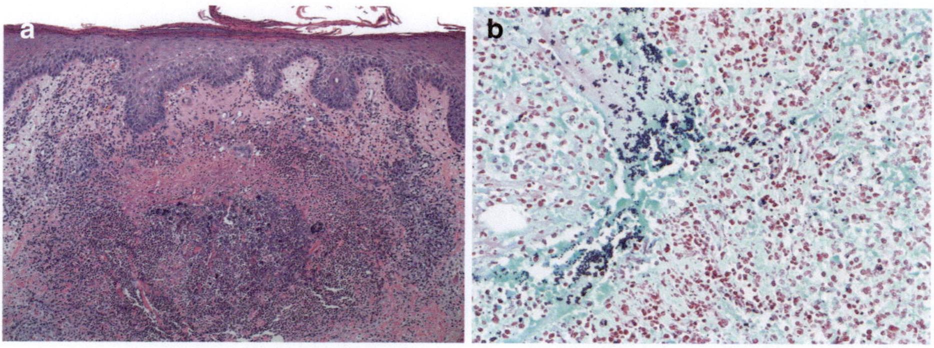

Fig. 20.3 Abscess: (**a**) On low power, there is a collection of neutrophils and neutrophilic debris (Courtesy of Brian Swick, MD). (**b**) On Gram stain, numerous Gram positive cocci among the neutrophilic inflammatory infiltrate is observed scattered.

Cellulitis

21

Campbell L. Stewart

Overview

- Suppurative inflammation involving the dermis and subcutis resulting in an expanding area of erythema with nonpalpable borders and associated edema, tenderness, and warmth
  - Ill-defined ascending linear red streaks represent underlying acute lymphangitis
- Cellulitis is a clinical diagnosis as cultures of both the blood and skin are often negative
- Commonly secondary to inoculation with skin flora following trauma
- Streptococci species (~90%), methicillin sensitive Staphylococcus aureus (MSSA) (~10%), rarely methicillin resistant Staphylococcus aureus (MRSA), and gram negative bacteria
  - Trauma may be mild and includes: penetrating injuries, intravenous drug use (IVDU), insect bites, iatrogenic secondary to lines, ports, or catheters
  - Nontraditional organisms are more commonly seen in immunocompromised hosts
  - Risk factors include pre-existing conditions that result in skin barrier disruption (e.g.intertrigo and tinea pedis), venous/lymphatic stasis (post-surgery, venous insufficiency), obesity, chronic liver disease and diabetes
- Associated septis/septic emboli and gangrene/necrosis more commonly occur in immunocompromised patients and children

Clinical Presentation

- Initial lesions and predisposing sites of trauma may appear innocuous but will quickly expand forming ill-defined erythematous lesions with non-palpable borders which can be exquisitely tender and warm to the touch; progressive pitting edema is typically evident especially on the lower extremities (Fig. 21.1)
  - Severe cases may develop necrosis or associated vesiculobullous lesions
- In adults the lower extremities are most commonly involved except in cases of IVDU where lesions tend to develop on the arms at prior injection sites; presentations vary based on site and source of infection
  - Children more commonly develop cellulitis of the head and neck
  - Recurrent cellulitis may occur in the setting of lymphatic insufficiency, immunodeficiency, or repeat inoculation injuries (IVDU)

C. L. Stewart, MD
Division of Dermatology, Department of Medicine, University of Washington,
Seattle, WA, USA

M. Rosenbach et al. (eds.), *Inpatient Dermatology*,
https://doi.org/10.1007/978-3-319-18449-4_21

- In severe neutropenia/immunosuppression consider gram negative rods, atypical mycobacteria, opportunistic fungi including *Cryptococcus, Mucor, Aspergillus*, in addition to nosocomial organisms (*Pseudomonas,* MRSA)
  - Patients with pseudomonas or *Stenotrophomonas maltophilia* septiciemia may present with subcutaneous cellulitic nodules
- Pseudomonas infections following puncture wounds, classically of the foot, may result in cellulitis ± osteomyelitis
- Patients with soil contaminated open wounds/open fractures may develop anaerobic crepitis cellulitis following contamination with *Clostridium perfringens* (thick gram positive rods); deeper infection can lead to necrotizing fasciitis and myonecrosis (gas gangrene)
  - Lesions have a thin malodorous dark exudate; in the setting of myonecrosis patients experience intense pain associated with necrosis extending from the skin to the muscle
  - Spontaneous (nontraumatic) gas gangrene/cellulitis can occur secondary to *C. septicum*
- Gram negative cellulitis from *Pasteurella* species (*P. multocida*) and/or *Capnocytophaga canimorsus* may follow animal bites; *Eikenella corrodens* may follow human bites
- Puncture wounds associated with aquatic enviroments or exposure to prior open wounds may be secondary to *Aeromonas ssp, Edwardsiella tarda, Erysipelothrix rhusiopathiae* (also common in farmers), *Vibrio vulnificus*, and *Mycobacterium marinum*
- Preseptal cellulitis (anterior eyelid infection) or orbital cellulitis (inflammation of ocular muscles and associated fat but not the globe) are typically caused by staph and strep
  - fungal cellulitis can occur and may be life threatening; may follow trauma, surgery, or infections typically of the face, oral cavity or ear
    - *Mucorales*: diabetic ketoacidotic patients
    - *Aspergillus*: typically patients are severely immunocompromised

Histopathology

- Dilated lymphatics and capillaries
- Marked dermal edema, occasionally inducing subepidermal blisters
- Primarily neutrophilic inflammation which may be diffuse or angiocentric (Fig. 21.2)
- Low burden of bacteria may be seen
- Tissue cultures and bug stains are often negative
- In immunocompromised and/or septic patients necrosis is more common with underlying ectatic vessels, fibrin thrombi; in this setting numerous organisms are often evident

Differential Diagnosis

- Deep vein thrombosis: a palpable cord and history of risk factors (immobility, malignancy, birth control pills), though ultrasound may be needed to distinguish
- Venous stasis dermatitis: bilateral involvement, slowly developing, evidence of chronicity (dilated veins, red-brown discoloration from hemosiderin deposition)
- Panniculitis: multiple discrete areas of inflammation with uninvolved skin between, sometimes with deep palpable nodules
- Erythema migrans: history of tick exposure, possibly a central punctum/bite site, less acutely ill
- Contact dermatitis: sharply demarcated, more epidermal change with oozy, crusted appearance, very pruritic

Work-Up

- A thorough history and physical to evaluate for mimics of cellulitis, and to determine if the patient requires a hospital stay for treatment
- Evaluate for portal of entry for the infectious agent, examine interdigital toe webspaces for evidence of maceration and scale
- Complete blood count with differential, erythrocyte sedimentation rate, C-reactive protein
- Blood cultures (positive in ≤5% of cases) in immunocompromised, if obvious portal of entry, or admitting to hospital
- Needle aspiration and/or punch biopsy in immunocompromised patients, patients unresponsive to therapy

Treatment

- If immunocompentent, not systemically ill, and have no co-morbidiites: outpatient treatment directed at streptococcal species and MSSA (dicloxacillin, cephalexin)
- If purulent collection is present, incision and drainage must be performed; broaden coverage for MRSA
- Hospitalize if 'purulent cellulitis' develops, if they are seriously ill, immunocompromised, or if unresponsive to MSSA coverage
- Leg elevation reduces pain and inflammation, prevents scarring of the lymphatics, lessens chance of recurrence
- Oral steroids (prednisone 40 mg daily for seven days) may reduce the pain and inflammation, shorten the course of the disease, reduce hospital stay, and may decrease chance of recurrence
- Recurrent cellulitis:
  - Treat/control predisposing conditions if possible (e.g. diabetes, HIV, lymphedema, venous insufficiency)
  - Consider decolonization, such as in the setting of MRSA
  - Consider prophylactic antibiotics

Suggested Readings

1. Hirschmann JV, Raugi GJ. J Am Acad Dermatol. 2012 Aug;67(2):163.e1–12.
2. Hirschmann JV, Raugi GJ. J Am Acad Dermatol. 2012 Aug;67(2):177.e1–9.
3. Thomas KS et al. N Engl J Med. 2013 May 2;368(18):1695–703.
4. Stevens DL, et al. Practice guidelines for the diagnosis and management of skin and soft tissue infections: 2014 update by the infectious diseases society of America. Clin Infect Dis. 2014;59(2):147.

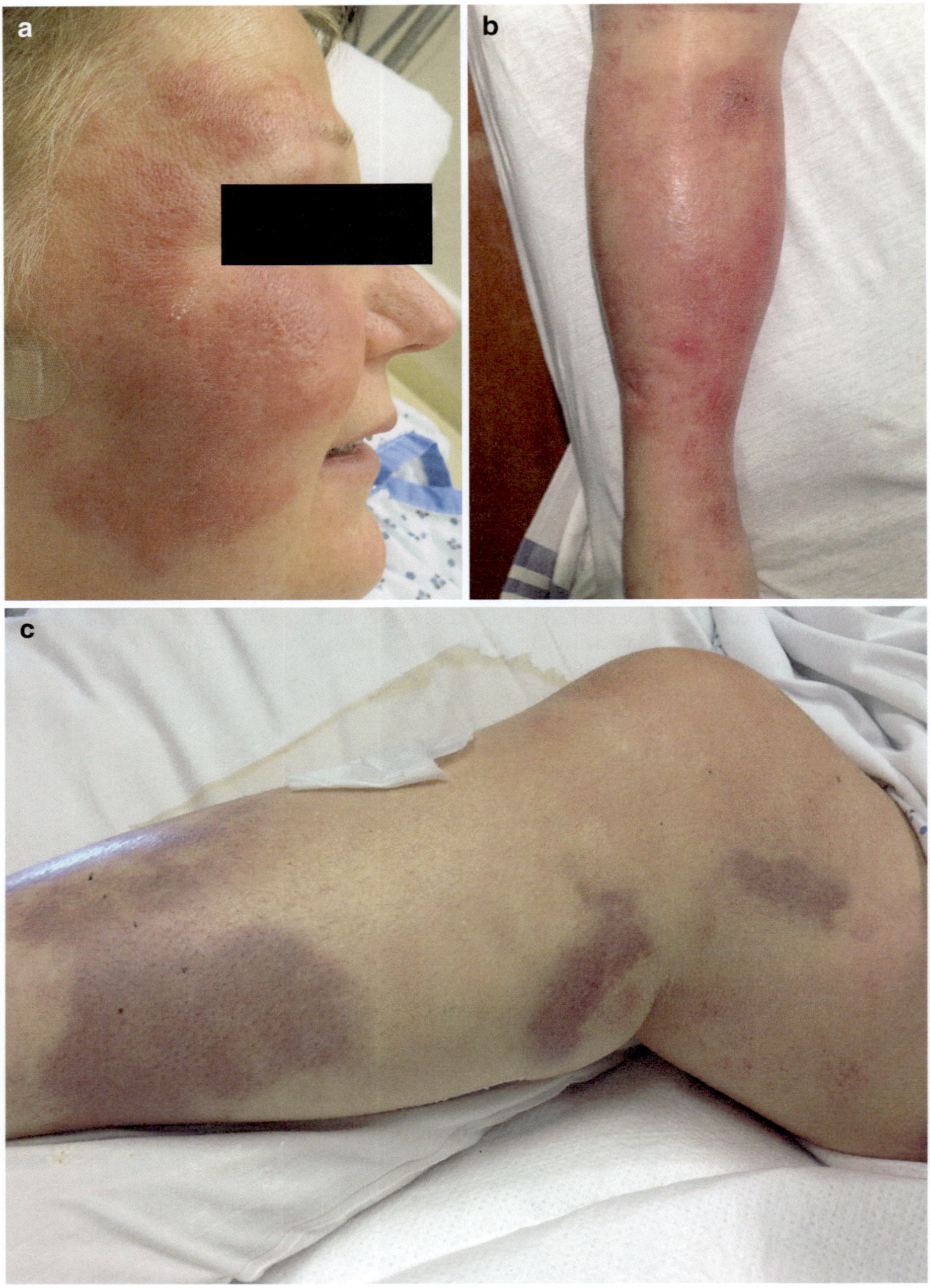

Fig. 21.1 (**a**) Erysipelas: Bright red, warm, indurated, and tender plaque of facial cellulitis and superficial lymphatic inflammation. (**b**) Cellulitis: Bright red, tender erythema with defined borders involving a single leg. Unilaterality is key to a diagnosis of cellulitis. (**c**) Immunosuppressed patients may get cellulitis from unusual organisms, including gram negative cellulitis, which can manifest with violaceous, ecchymotic-like patches. This patient with leukemia has severe pseudomonas cellulitis.

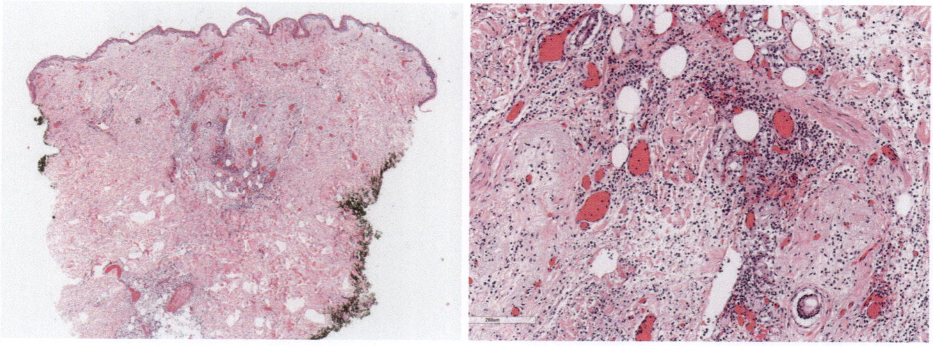

Fig. 21.2 Cellulitis (*2.5*×, *10*×): There is diffuse neutrophilic inflammation in the dermis with edema and vascular congestion.

Necrotizing Fasciitis

22

Laura A. Taylor

Overview

- Necrotizing fasciitis (NF) is a potentially life threatening deep microbial infection of the subcutaneous fat and fascia which rapidly spreads along facial planes
- NF is an emergency necessitating immediate antibiotic use and surgical intervention
  - Mortality rates are up to 40%, and increased in the setting of delayed debridement/treatment, group A streptococci (GAS) infection, older patients, pre-existing comorbidities with associated organ dysfunction/failure
  - Fascia is particularly susceptible to necrosis due to its poor blood supply; this allows rapid extension of subcutaneous infection to surrounding tissues; the muscle is often spared due to its ample blood supply
- NF is categorized based on the presence of mono- or polymicrobial infections; of note the list of potential causative organisms is extensive but GAS is most common
  - Type 1: polymicrobial infections (aerobic and anaerobic bacteria)
  - Type 2: monomicrobial infection (can be used to refer to combined GP infections, commonly *S. aureus and S. pyogenes*)
    - Predominant type seen in children and immunocompetent adults
    - In patients with GAS/*S. aureus* infections there is an associated risk of toxic shock syndrome (TSS)
  - Type 3: gas gangrene: typically caused by clostridium spp. which produce subcutaneous gas and clinical crepitus
- Predisposing factors include: immunosuppression, intravenous drug abuse, diabetes, kidney failure, recent penetrating injury/surgery, ulcers (decubitus or ischemic)

Clinical Presentation

- Classically presents as "pain out of proportion to exam," with a mild clinical lesion (potentially resembling a bruise) with severe pain and signs of sepsis (Fig. 22.1)
- Early lesions may be difficult to differentiate from cellulitis; intense pain and necrosis with dusky lesions, evolving anesthesia, crepitis, blistering, and lack of response to antibiotics are clues to deeper involvement

L. A. Taylor, MD
Department of Pathology and Laboratory Medicine, University of Pennsylvania, Philadelphia, PA, USA
e-mail: Laura.Taylor@uphs.upenn.edu

M. Rosenbach et al. (eds.), *Inpatient Dermatology*,
https://doi.org/10.1007/978-3-319-18449-4_22

- Rapidly evolving exquisitely painful warm edematous erythematous ill-defined lesions which abruptly progress (24–48 h) to gray-blue necrotic lesions extruding malodorous exudates which evolve into fulminant gangrene within 4–5 days
  - Subcutaneous fat necrosis can feel firm, "woody", or nodular on palpation
  - Subcutaneous gas may be appreciated on imaging or exam (crepitus)
  - Hemorrhagic bullae may form
  - Although initially associated with intense pain patients classically lose sensation as nerves are destroyed
  - Associated extensive "tense" edema can lead to compartment syndrome
- Patients will develop sepsis/septic shock if infection is inadequately controlled
- NF is most common on the lower extremities; less common locations include the perineum, upper extremities, and trunk but can occur anywhere
  - Fournier's gangrene: perineum/perianal/genital involvement
  - Omphalitis (umbilical stump infection) can lead to abdominal wall NF in neonates
  - Cervical (neck) NF has been reported following oropharyngeal surgery in patients with odontogenic infections
  - Abdominal surgery is a risk factor for type 1 abdominal wall NF

Histopathology

- The diagnosis is clinical and because of the acuity, there is generally not sufficient time to obtain a biopsy
  - Although a biopsy is typically not warranted in this setting debridement tissue sent for histology will show extensive necrosis with variable degrees of inflammation; septic vasculitis with abundant organisms are often seen (Fig. 22.2)
  - Gram stains, and Grocott/PAS/Fite in atypical cases, can be used to help highlight organisms

Differential Diagnosis

- Erysipelas: acute superficial skin infection is more red, sharply demarcated, and patients, while sick, are not as hemodynamically unstable as patients with NF
- Cellulitis: generally acute onset, red, hot, tender extremity with fever and a white count; can have overlap with early NF but patients are more hemodynamically stable, with less pain, and less ecchymoses/duskiness/signs of tissue breakdown
- Necrotizing neutrophilic dermatoses: both PG and Sweets can be mistaken for NF, and vice-versa; generally NF as an overwhelming infection will be culture positive, whereas neutrophilic dermatoses are culture negative; pathergy, or worsening after surgery, may suggest neutrophilic dermatoses

Work-Up

- NF is a true medical emergency which requires recognition of the clinical signs
- Suspected cases of NF warrant emergency surgery consultation for bedside cut-down, where a 2 cm incision is made to the fascia and blunt dissection is performed by the surgeon with their finger; lack of bleeding and evidence of necrosis are concerning and indicative of NF
- CBC, CMP, CK, Lactate
  - Often nonspecific, depending on immune status patients may exhibit leukocytosis with a left shift
  - CK: indicative of muscle necrosis may be elevated; more commonly elevated in the setting of type 2 infection (GAS); may elevate if compartment syndrome develops
  - Lactate may be elevated due to necrosis, breakdown, hypoperfusion, and sepsis
- If the diagnosis is in doubt, tissue may be sent for histology to exclude mimics (PG/Sweets)
- Blood and wound cultures with susceptibilities (make sure to order aerobic and anaerobic cultures)
- Radiography can help determine extent and depth of disease but diagnosis should not be delayed while waiting imaging studies—a bedside emergency surgery consultation is the diagnostic test of choice

Treatment

- Emergency consultation with surgery and infectious disease is recommended, and patients should be moved to an intensive care unit
  - Prompt fasciotomy (surgical debridement) can be life-saving; in more advanced cases further surgical intervention such as amputation may be necessary
  - Surgery should not be delayed for ancillary testing
- Establish IV access and provide fluids and IV antibiotics (broad spectrum pending susceptibility results from blood/wound cultures)
  - Pseudomonas coverage should be included for neutropenic patients
  - Some forms of NF may be worsened by bacterial toxin production; occasionally antibiotics or alternate agents are employed in an attempt to limit bacterial toxin production

Suggested Readings

1. Stevens DL, et al. Practice guidelines for the diagnosis and management of skin and soft tissue infections: 2014 update by the Infectious Diseases Society of America. Clin Infect Dis. 2014;59(2):147.

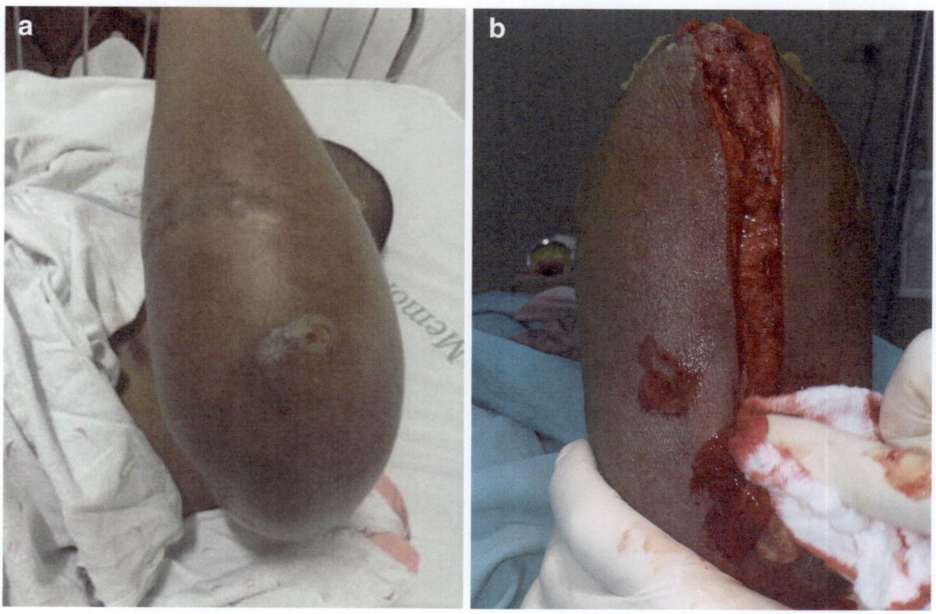

Fig. 22.1 Necrotizing fasciitis: Necrotizing fasciitis often presents after incidental trauma, leading to a mild-appearing eruption, such as a bruise or ecchymosis, with pain out of proportion to exam and physiologic signs of sepsis; shown here (**a**) before and (**b**) after fasciotomy and surgical debridement.

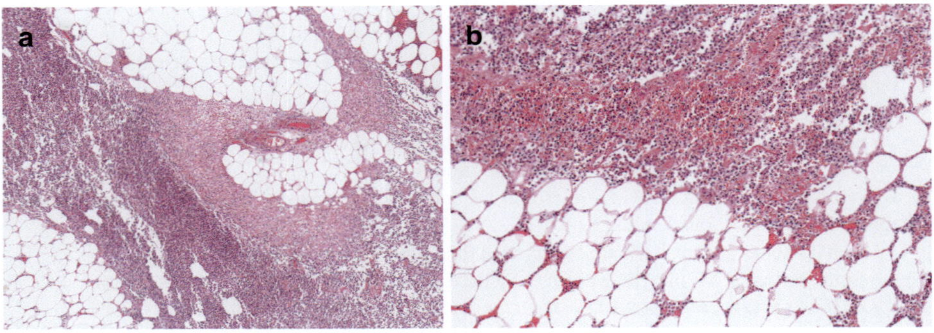

Fig. 22.2 Necrotizing fasciitis (*10×, 40×; H&E*): A deep biopsy is necessary to obtain fascia and make the diagnosis. (**a**, **b**) There is extensive acute inflammation and tissue necrosis spreading along fascial planes. Gram stain can be used to highlight the associated organisms but a tissue culture should be performed for speciation and susceptibilities.

Staphylococcal Scalded Skin Syndrome 23

Laura A. Taylor

Overview

- Staphylococcal scalded skin syndrome (SSSS) is caused by systemic effects of circulating exfoliative toxins released by phage II strains of *S. aureus* (MRSA or MSSA). The exfoliative toxins target desomoglein 1 (Dsg1) resulting in generalized superficial blister formation and desquamation
- Dsg1 is involved in keratinocyte cell adhesion and concentrated in the superficial epidermis. In mucosal sites, Dsg3 is expressed extensively and can compensate for loss of Dsg1. Toxin-mediated cleavage of Dsg1 results in superficial flaccid fragile bullae of non-mucosal skin
  - Both bullous impetigo and SSSS are caused by bacterial released toxins targeting Dsg1; pemphigus foliaceus and some forms of pemphigus vulgaris are caused by autoantibodies targeting Dsg1
    - In bullous impetigo the infection is local and cultures of the lesion are commonly positive
    - In SSSS the infection is distant with only toxins present at the lesional site, so tissue cultures are negative
- More common in young children, especially infants, as they have poor renal clearance (allowing toxin buildup) and immature immune systems. Adults can develop SSSS in the setting of renal insufficiency and/or immunodeficiency
  - In children the infectious source may be conjunctivitis or nasapharygeal in origin; blood cultures are rarely positive
  - In adults pneumonia is a typical source and bacteremia is common
- SSSS has a good prognosis overall in children with spontaneous recovery occurring within days likely coinciding with the formation of neutralizing antibodies; adults have significant associated morbidity and mortality as a function of their underlying disease and high rate of septicemia

Clinical Presentation

- Patients may exhibit symptoms associated with primary infection
- Fever, malaise, and intense diffuse skin tenderness may proceed cutaneous manifestations

L. A. Taylor, MD
Department of Pathology and Laboratory Medicine,University of Pennsylvania, Philadelphia, PA, USA
e-mail: Laura.Taylor@uphs.upenn.edu

M. Rosenbach et al. (eds.), *Inpatient Dermatology*,
https://doi.org/10.1007/978-3-319-18449-4_23

- Erythema appears on the head/neck and intertriginous area with abrupt development of large areas of flaccid sterile bullae which rupture almost as quickly as they form, causing a generalized erosive and exfoliative dermatitis (Fig. 23.1)
  - The epidermis is shed as large sheets; mucosa is spared, and palms and soles are often less affected
  - The skin may appear crinkled from diffuse superficial keratinocyte separation prior to actual blister-roof sloughing
- Patients may have perioral and periocular erosions/fissuring with crusting but all exhibit mucosal sparing
- As the epidermal cleavage is superficial, once treated patients may heal quickly and without scarring

Histopathology

- Bullae will be evident with separation at or below the granular layer (superficial epidermis); as there is no infection (only toxins) at the site there will be little to no associated inflammation (Fig. 23.2)

Differential Diagnosis

- Bullous impetigo: More localized and often with thick honey crusting, but as this is caused by the same processed there is extensive overlap
- SJS/TEN: will almost always involve mucosa, whereas SSSS always spares the mucosa; biopsy (often performed as STAT frozen section) can help differentiate the two when in doubt
- Pemphigus foliaceus: clinically and histologically can be nearly identical; the concomitant symptoms, rapidity, and proof of an infection can distinguish the two

Work-Up

- The first step is often confirming the diagnosis and excluding some of the potential emergencies on the differential (particularly SJS/TEN), which can sometimes be distinguished clinically
  - Biopsy may help confirm the diagnosis
- In some centers, there is confirmatory testing which can demonstrate the presence of the toxin; this is uncommon, and more often the work-up is geared at finding the potential infection
- All patients should undergo a thorough physical exam and often multiple cultures—not simply skin swabs and blood cultures, but urine and lung examination as well
  - Children should be cultured in the throat/nasopharynx, umbilicus, areas of abnormal/raw/inflamed skin, perianal/gluteal region

Treatment

- Patients should undergo supportive care with repletion of fluid and electrolyte losses
- Careful skin care with moisture and non-stick dressings where appropriate
- Systemic antibiotics should be initiated to treat identified (or suspected) infections and should cover potential resistant organisms
  - Dual antibiotic therapy may be used including clindamycin as its mechanism of action includes ribosomal targeting which may limit bacterial protein/toxin production
- Intravenous immunoglobulin (IVIG) therapy may be utilized in severe cases

Suggested Reading

1. Stevens DL, et al. Practice guidelines for the diagnosis and management of skin and soft tissue infections: 2014 update by the Infectious Diseases Society of America. Clin Infect Dis. 2014;59(2):147.

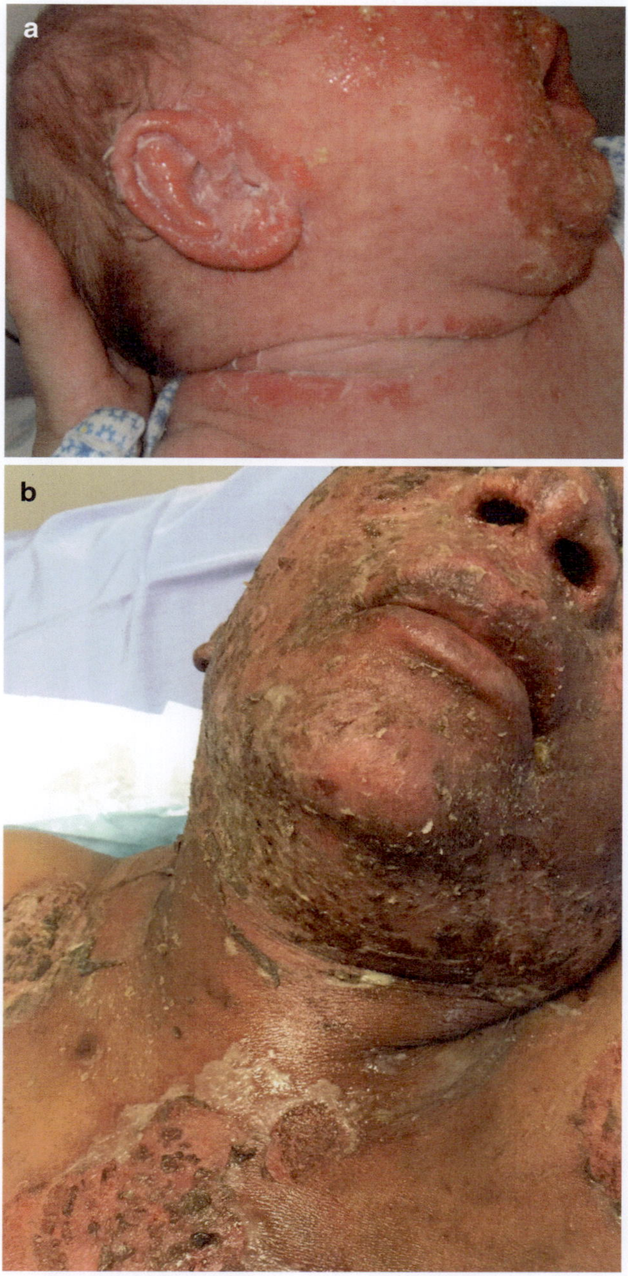

Fig. 23.1 Staphylococcal scalded skin syndrome: (**a**) Seen in an infant due to severe localized impetigo with honey-colored crusts on the face, and superficial peeling of the top layer of the skin distant from the infection on the neck. (**b**) Severe staphylococcal staph scalded skin in an immunosuppressed adult with widespread superficial blistering.

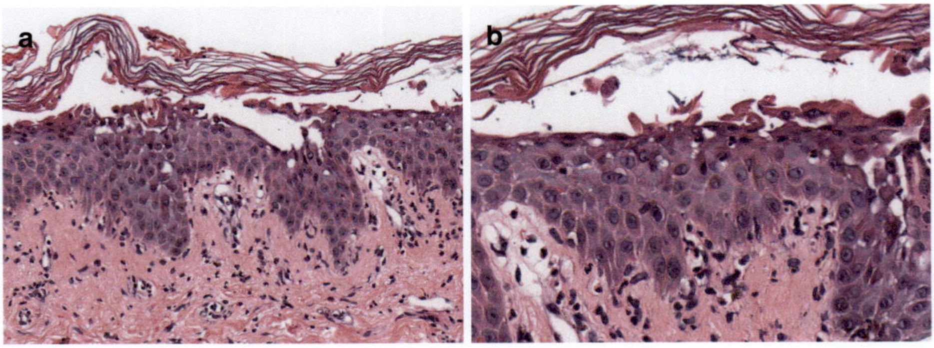

Fig. 23.2 Staphylococcal scalded skin syndrome (*10×*, *20×*; *H&E*): (**a**) The biopsy shows superficial acantholysis with subcorneal separation leading to blister formation. The intracorneal acanthoslysis can have scattered neutrophils but often is pauci-inflammatory.

Ecthyma Gangrenosum

24

Campbell L. Stewart

Overview

- Clinical term used to describe a cutaneous infection, classically secondary to *Pseudomonas aeruginosa* sepsis, in an immunocompromised patient
  - *Pseudomonas aeruginosa* is responsible in the majority of cases with the remainder caused mostly by other gram negative bacteria
  - May occasionally be secondary to fungal infections (*Aspergillus fumigatus* and *Candida albicans),* or gram positive bacteria (*Staphyloccus aureus)* and very rarely without associated bacteremia
- Almost all cases represent hematogenous seeding with an embolus of bacteria which fills a small dermal vessel and seeds the skin; this causes the cutaneous phenotype (angulated necrosis) and the histology (intense bacterial infiltration of the skin with a limited host response)
  - Rarely, direct primary cutaneous infection with virulent pathogens (such as *pseudomonas*) can cause a localized ecthyma gangrenosum lesion
- Worse outcomes are associated with a delay in treatment, multiple lesions, and continued neutropenia

Clinical Presentation

- Lesions classically start as an angulated dusky purple-gray hypoperfused patch which may blister or expand to a necrotic ulcer with or without eschar (Fig. 24.1)
- Many patients will have one lesion or a cluster of only a handful of lesions; widespread involvement is rare
- Primary skin direct infection without antecedent bacteremia can present with an erythematous nodule or hemorrhagic vesicle
- Slight predilection for the lower extremities and buttocks, but may be seen anywhere on the body

C. L. Stewart, MD
Division of Dermatology, Department of Medicine, University of Washington, Seattle, WA, USA

M. Rosenbach et al. (eds.), *Inpatient Dermatology*,
https://doi.org/10.1007/978-3-319-18449-4_24

Histopathology

- Epidermal necrosis with papillary dermal edema, hemorrhage, bacterial colonies, and a mixed inflammatory infiltrate of variable density (Fig. 24.2)
  - The inflammatory infiltrate is often less robust than expected due to patients' underlying immunosuppression
- Bacterial colonies can typically be seen on standard sections as intravascular infectious emboli or as dermal infiltrates and can be highlighted by a Gram stain; classically will stain the gram negative bacilli of *Pseudomonas*

Differential Diagnosis

- Herpes simplex/Varicella zoster viral infection: usually will have clustered monomorphic vesicles or punched-out erosions
- Pyoderma gangrenosum: will usually have a rim of edema and an overhanging border of intact-epidermis over the expanding ulcer
- Angioinvasive fungal infections: may show more violaceous discoloration studded with black areas of necrosis, and/or a "bull's eye" appearance, but can be clinically indistinguishable; histopathology and culture is important
- Vasculitis (small-medium vessel): may show other signs such as livedo reticularis or nodules, and may be more widespread and affect other organ systems
- Vasculopathy (antiphospholipid antibodies (APLA), cryoglobulinemia): may show a predilection for more distal sites, and may have more of a fine retiform purpura appearance with angulated areas, but there is significant overlap; histopathology will distinguish these

Work-Up

- A complete history and physical exam, particularly evaluating for immunosuppression
- Complete blood count with differential
- Blood and urine cultures should also be performed
- Skin biopsy from the ulcer (typically the edge) should be performed for H&E, gram stain, and tissue culture (from a more central portion of the lesion may be higher yield)
- Ultrasonography or MRI imaging may be considered if deeper soft tissue involvement is suspected

Treatment

- Antimicrobial treatment must be initiated immediately (ideally following procurement of tissue and blood cultures)
- Anti-pseudomonal penicillin, such as piperacillin, should be combined with an aminoglycoside (gentamycin) barring comorbid contraindications
- Broad spectrum treatment is indicated and may need to include anti-fungal agents (voriconazole or amphoteracin B) initially in the immunosuppressed
- G-CSF should be considered in neutropenic patients where appropriate
- If lesions fail to respond to medical treatment, surgical excision may be indicated for limited disease

Suggested Readings

1. Vaiman M, et al. Ecthyma gangrenosum and ecthyma-like lesions: review article. Eur J Clin Microbiol Infect Dis. 2014;34(4):633–9.
2. Reich HL, et al. Nonpseudomonal ecthyma gangrenosum. J Am Acad Dermatol. 2004;50(5 Suppl):S114–7.
3. Chang AY, et al. Nonpseudomonal ecthyma gangrenosum associated with methicillin-resistant staphylococcus aureus infection: a case report and review of the literature. Cutis. 2012;90(2):67–9.

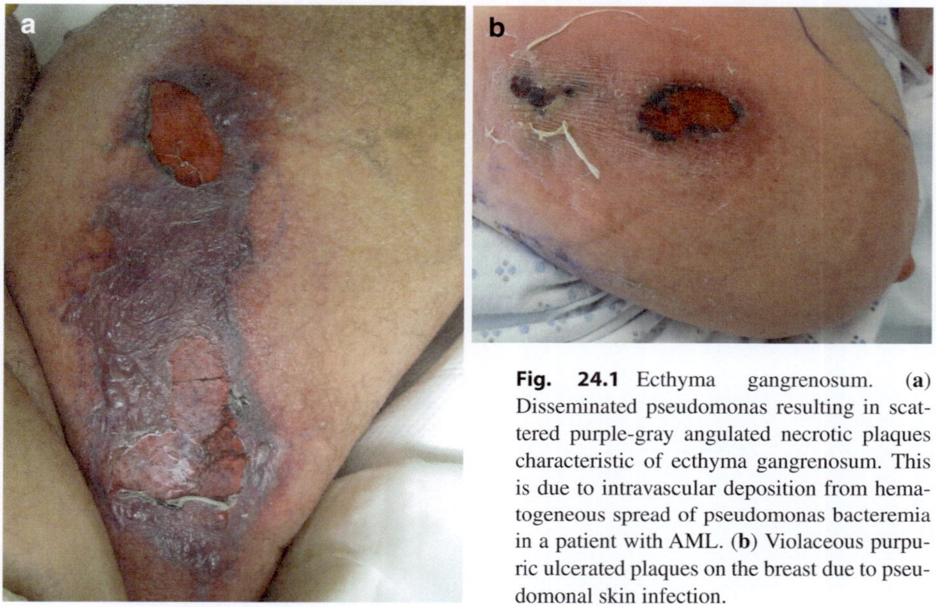

Fig. 24.1 Ecthyma gangrenosum. (**a**) Disseminated pseudomonas resulting in scattered purple-gray angulated necrotic plaques characteristic of ecthyma gangrenosum. This is due to intravascular deposition from hematogeneous spread of pseudomonas bacteremia in a patient with AML. (**b**) Violaceous purpuric ulcerated plaques on the breast due to pseudomonal skin infection.

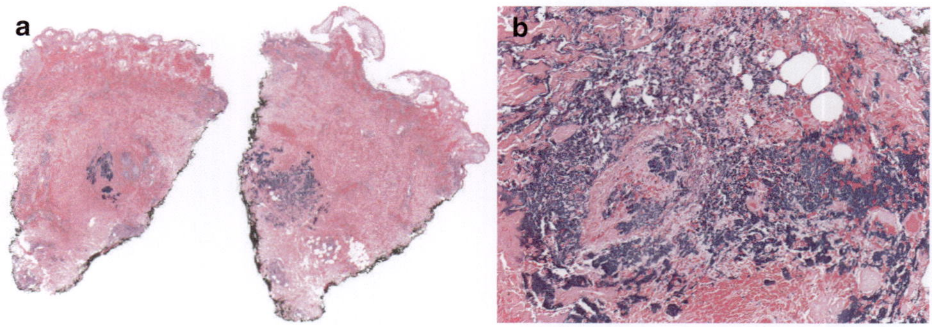

Fig. 24.2 Ecthyma gangranosum (*2× to 10×; H&E*): (**a**) Low power demonstrates epidermal necrosis with inflammation and hemorrhage within the dermis. Thrombi are typically present. (**b**) Numerous bacteria are present in the deep dermis with associated necrosis and hemorrhage with minimal inflammatory infiltrate.

Purpura Fulminans

25

Karolyn A. Wanat

Overview

- Purpura fulminans is a dermatologic emergency of widespread vasculopathy secondary to intravascular thrombosis resulting in sudden, progressive cutaneous hemorrhage and necrosis, with high morbidity and mortality
- Syndrome presents in three different settings:
  - Neonatal purpura fulminans: Rare hereditary deficiency of protein C or S which leads to intravascular collapse within the first days of life
  - Acquired purpura fulminans: Most often occurs 1–2 weeks after Group A Strep or varicella infection and is caused secondary to production of antibodies that interfere with the function of natural anticoagulants
    - Also can be secondary to trauma, malignancy, obstetric complications, hepatic failure, toxins
  - Acute infectious purpura fulminans: The most common form, is typically associated with bacteremia (meningococcemia, streptococcal/staphylococcal sepsis)
    - Pathogenesis depends on the infectious agent; for example, in the setting of meningococcemia sepsis, bacterial endotoxins consume anti-coagulant proteins leading to a prothrombotic state
    - Cases secondary to other infections including rickettsia, malaria, leptospirosis, and viruses have been reported

Clinical Presentation

- Rapidly progressive large, often distal, symmetric purpuric patches and plaques with features of angulated, stellate, and/or retiform (net-like) purpura that progress to develop overlying bullae and/or skin necrosis with eschars (Fig. 25.1)
- Predilection for buttocks and lower extremities
- Patients are ill with fever, shock, and/or disseminated intravascular coagulation (DIC)

K. A. Wanat, MD
Department of Dermatology, Medical College of Wisconsin, Milwaukee, WI, USA
e-mail: karolyn-wanat@uiowa.edu

M. Rosenbach et al. (eds.), *Inpatient Dermatology*,
https://doi.org/10.1007/978-3-319-18449-4_25

Histopathology

- Within the small vessels of the skin, fibrin thrombi are seen with a mild perivascular infiltrate and extensive hemorrhage (Fig. 25.2)
- Later lesions often have epidermal necrosis or subepidermal bullae
- No vasculitis is observed

Differential Diagnosis

Other causes of retiform purpura: these can share many clinical phenotypic elements (angulated, retiform purpura) and can be hard to distinguish clinically; history, lab testing, and pathology are all essential

- Antiphospholipid antibody syndrome (APLA): can display angulated/stellate purpura and cause internal clots; lab testing may be necessary to distinguish
- Cryoglobulinemia: tends to be more distal and not as sudden or severe, with patients less frequently as critically ill, but lab testing may be necessary to distinguish
- Cholesterol emboli: tends to follow intravascular procedures and typically affects the kidneys predominantly, with more mild skin findings of livedo reticularis in most cases
- Calciphylaxis: usually in the setting of end-stage renal disease and more chronic than purpura fulminans, the lesions often have time to develop a thick black eschar
- Warfarin necrosis: tends to occur shortly after warfarin initiation and preferentially in high-fat proximal areas, often with less diffuse retiform changes and less critically ill patients
- Septic vasculitis (bacteria, fungus): more often distal with palpable purpura and signs of embolic phenomena

Work-Up

- A complete history and physical exam
- Blood cultures
- Tissue biopsy and tissue culture to confirm diagnosis
- CBC, PT, PTT, d-dimer, fibrinogen, haptoglobin to evaluate for coagulation defects:
  - Prolonged prothrombin time and partial thromboplastin time is consistent with disruption of the clotting cascade via consumption/decreased factor synthesis
  - Low level fibrinogen level is consistent with a consumptive process; however, it may be normal/elevated in the setting of infection because it is an acute phase reactant
  - Increased fibrin split products such as D-dimer
  - Thrombocytopenia secondary to platelet consumption
  - Leukocytosis evident in the setting of infection
  - Anemia in the setting of red cell lysis and hemorrhage: peripheral blood smear review may demonstrate schistocytes and fragmented red blood cells.
- Other causes of hypercoagulability, such as Factor V Leiden mutations, have been reported in the setting of purpura fulminans; therefore in the appropriate clinical context a hypercoagulability workup with associated molecular testing may be indicated
- Extended testing to exclude entities on the differential is often required, such as comprehensive hypercoaguability workup, APLA testing, cryoglobulin testing (including RF/complements) and more

Treatment

- Patients are critically ill an require high level supportive care in an experienced ICU setting with goal directed therapy and close internal organ monitoring
- Targeting underlying cause (infection vs. inherited or acquired abnormality in clotting) and supportive treatment are the mainstay

- In cases of infection, broad spectrum antibiotics and aggressive management of sepsis are recommend
- In cases where DIC is present, treatment with fresh frozen plasma may be used
- When soft tissue necrosis has occurred, surgical removal of tissue, fasciotomy, or amputation may be necessary
- Blood or platelet transfusions also may be necessary
- Adjuvant therapies (heparin, antithrombin III, recombinant tissue plasminogen activator, and hyperbaric oxygen) have inconsistent results

Suggested Readings

1. Talwar A, Kumar S, Gopal MG, Nandini AS. Spectrum of purpura fulminans: report of three classical prototypes and review of management strategies. Indian J Dermatol Venereol Leprol. 2012;78(2):228.
2. Thornsberry LA, LoSicco KI, English JC 3rd. The skin and hypercoagulable states. J Am Acad Dermatol. 2013;69(3):450–62.
3. Gunawardane ND, Menon K, Guitart J, Cotliar JA. Purpura fulminans from meningococcemia mimicking Stevens-Johnson syndrome in an adult patient taking etanercept. Arch Dermatol. 2012;148(12):1429–31.

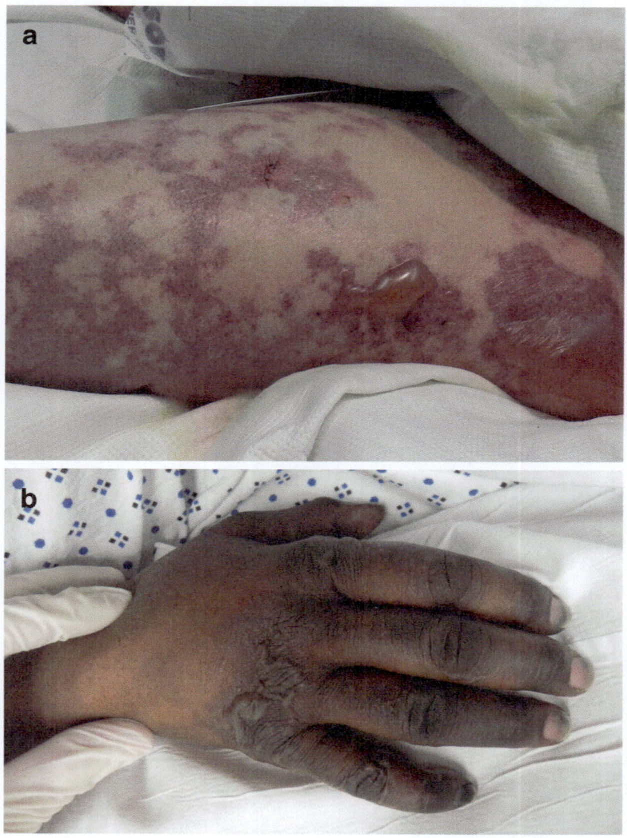

Fig. 25.1 Livedo racemosa: (**a**) Extensive angulated purpura with "incomplete jagged links" consistent with livedo racemosa, indicative of intravascular clot formation. The extensive vasculopathy leads to tissue ischemia, and overlying bullae, as shown here in a liver transplant patient with pseudomonas sepsis and DIC resulting in purpura fulminans. (**b**) Intravascular clotting leads to distal purpura and can lead to dusky digits and peripheral ischemia, as shown here with extensive angulated purpura and early blister formation on the hands.

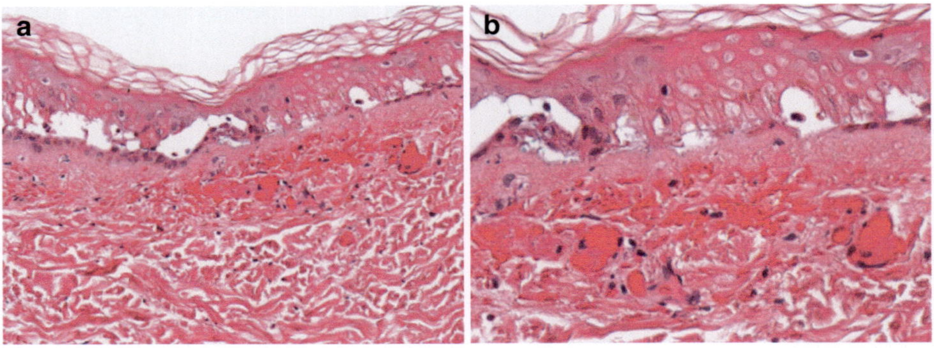

Fig. 25.2 Purpura fulminans (*10×, 20×; H&E*): (**a**) There is extensive epidermal necrosis secondary to ischemic damage. (**b**) There are congested vessels with fibrin thrombi and red blood cell extravasation in the superficial dermis.

Meningococcal Infections

26

Campbell L. Stewart

Overview

- *Neisseria meningitides* is a gram negative bacterium which causes meningitis and rapidly progressive sepsis resulting in fatal shock in 70–90% of untreated patients, with treatment mortality rates still as high as 10–20%
- Epidemics are associated with crowded settings such as college dormitories, and are most common in winter and spring
  - Patients with immunodeficiency, asplenia, or C5–C9 complement deficiencies are at increased risk
- Virulence depends on the serogroup, which determines capsule expression as well as the outer membrane lipo-oligosaccharide endotoxin
  - Serogroups B, C, Y are most common in the United States
  - Serogroup B is most common in infants
  - Serogroup C is associated with major epidemic outbreaks in adolescents and young adults

Clinical Presentation

- Meningitis is the most common presentation of meningococcal disease; patients often present with concomitant sepsis
  - Headache, nausea, vomiting, photophobia, nuchal tenderness and mental status changes are indicative of meningitis
- Occasionally patients may present with hemorrhagic skin lesions and fever, without obvious signs of sepsis or meningitis
  - These cases can rapidly progress (<24 h) without appropriate treatment making it imperative for the clinician to consider meningococcal disease in this setting
- Cutaneous lesions are typically an early manifestation of meningococcal sepsis and are characterized by scattered petechiae on the trunk and extremities which rapidly evolve into confluent patches of often-angulated purpura with deep gray centers; mucous membranes may also be affected (Fig. 26.1)
- Thrombi cause ischemia in the skin and soft tissues which can result in loss of digits and limbs in addition to multi-organ failure

C. L. Stewart, MD
Division of Dermatology, Department of Medicine, University of Washington, Seattle, WA, USA

M. Rosenbach et al. (eds.), *Inpatient Dermatology*,
https://doi.org/10.1007/978-3-319-18449-4_26

Histopathology

- Biopsies demonstrate a thrombo-occlusive septic vasculopathy with fibrin thrombi and various degrees of endothelial damage (although this is not a true vasculitis) (Fig. 26.2)
- Gram stain will highlight gram negative diplococci in and around the microvasculature and surrounding tissue necrosis
- Ischemic type changes will be evident in more established lesions

Differential Diagnosis

- Rocky Mountain Spotted Fever (RMSF): while patients are often systemically ill in both diseases, RMSF patients are less critically ill. RMSF tends to develop on the ankles and wrists and spread both proximally and distally with pink papules and petechiae
- Endocarditis: patients may have small distal purpuric lesions due to emboli, and usually display less confluent lesions and a less rapidly catastrophic course
- Henoch-Schonlein purpura, vasculitis, and other systemic vasculitidies: will often start with characteristic palpable purpura and not the broad angulated gray-centered purpuric patches
- Antiphospholipid syndrome (APLA): may have a tendency to be more distal initially, involving fingers and toes, but catastrophic APLA may require lab and biopsy findings to distinguish
- Gram-negative or Gram-positive sepsis with purpura fulminans: can have overlapping features and may require culture data to distinguish

Work-Up

- A complete history and physical examination are necessary
  - A full skin exam including mucous membranes must be performed
  - The patient's mental status should also be assessed and serial monitoring for meningeal signs
- CBC with differential typically reveals a leukocytosis with a left shift
- Coagulation studies to investigate for disseminated intravascular coagulopathy (DIC)
- Lumbar puncture with gram stain and culture are essential; PCR testing of the plasma or cerebrospinal fluid may be used where available
- Blood cultures

Treatment

- Early antibiotic treatment is the mainstay and helps reduce morbidity and mortality
  - Benzylpenicillin, cefotaxime, ceftriaxone, or chloramphenicol may be used
- Patients in septic shock require treatment in an intensive care unit with aggressive fluid resuscitation and mechanical respiratory support
- Patients should be isolated if meningococcemia is suspected
- Patients may require systemic steroids, especially if adrenal hemorrhage occurs

Prevention

- Chemoprophylaxis with rifampin or fluoroquinolones can be used in close contacts of infected patients and helps control small outbreaks
- A tetravalent vaccine (serogroups A, C, W-135 and Y) is available

Suggested Readings

1. Stephens DS, et al. Epidemic meningitis, meningococcaemia, and Neisseria meningitidis. Lancet. 2007;369(9580):2196–210.
2. Drage LA, et al. Clinical pearls in dermatology. Mayo Clin Proc. 2012;87(7):695–9.

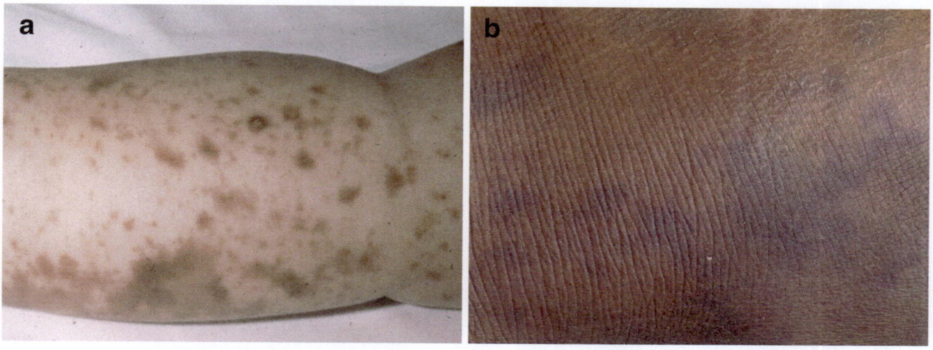

Fig. 26.1 Meningococcal rash: (**a**) Retiform purpuric macules and patches in a patient with meningococcemia (Courtesy of W. Van Stoecker). (**b**) Dusky angulated retiform purpura in a child with fulminant meningococcemia.

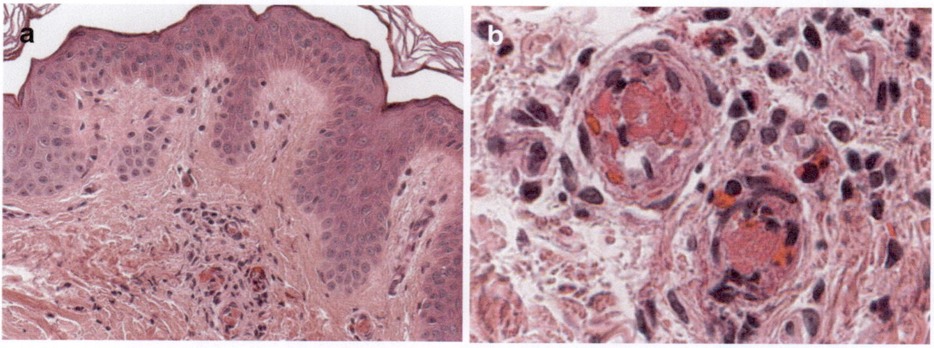

Fig. 26.2 Meningococcemia (*20×, 40×; H&E*): (**a**) The epidermis is relatively spared with the key pathology in the dermis. (**b**) There is a mixed inflammatory infiltrate, including eosinophils, in the superficial dermis, and fibrin thrombi are evident (Courtesy of Children's Hospital of Philadelphia, Department of Pathology).

Atypical Mycobacterial Infection

27

Megan H. Noe

Overview

- Atypical mycobacteria refers to mycobacterial infection by species other than *M. tuberculosis* or *M. leprae*
- Mycobacterial species are ubiquitous in nature, especially in soil, vegetation, and water. Skin disease can follow direct inoculation while disseminated disease tends to occur in immunocompromised hosts following inhalation, ingestion or inoculation injury
  - Historically classified based on growth rate (slow growers/rapid growers) and light-induced pigmentation (photochromogens/nonchromogens); a subset of species which more commonly cause cutaneous disease are listed below
    - Rapid growers: require 3–5 days to grow
      - *M. abscessus, M. fortuitum,* and *M. chelonae*
    - Slow growers: require 2–3 weeks to grow
      - Photochromogens: *M. kansasii*, *M. marinum*
      - Nonchromogens: *M. avium, M. intracellulare*, *M. ulcerans*
- *M. avium* and *M. intracellulare* are highly similar and jointly referred to as *M. avium* complex (MAC)
  - The incidence of MAC has risen dramatically since the AIDS epidemic and represents a leading cause of opportunistic infections in immunocompromised hosts

Clinical Presentation

- Atypical mycobacterial infections can present with a variety of cutaneous findings, depending on the acuity of infection, the species, the mechanism of exposure, and the immune status of the host.
  - Most patients will present with a skin nodule on the extremity, which may be red and crusted and can ulcerate and drain purulent discharge. Step-wise proximal extension through superficial venolymphatics can lead to a sporotrichoid pattern of multiple nodules of varying ages tracking upwards from an infected limb (Fig. 27.1).
  - Multiple interconnected draining sinuses, purulent abscesses and carbuncle-like collections of multiple pustules, and fluctuant subcutaneous nodules may be seen
  - Immunocompromised patients may have an atypical presentation or a more aggressive infection

M. H. Noe, MD, MPH
Department of Dermatology, University of Pennsylvania,
Philadelphia, PA, USA
e-mail: Megan.Noe@uphs.upenn.edu

M. Rosenbach et al. (eds.), *Inpatient Dermatology*,
https://doi.org/10.1007/978-3-319-18449-4_27

- One of the most common atypical mycobacterial infections is with *M. marinum*
  - Patients develop red-to-purple inflammatory or verrucous nodules at the site of prior skin trauma/abrasion following contact with contaminated water (swimming pools, fish tanks) or fish (fishermen, cooks)
  - Lesions tend to occur on the upper extremities, commonly the fingers, and can demonstrate sporotrichotic spread, with nodules developing in a distal-to-proximal pattern along regional lymphatics
- *M. ulcerans* tends to cause a somewhat distinct presentation
  - Typically an isolated subcutaneous nodule forms, after a couple of months the lesion ulcerates forming a deep painless ulcer ("Buruli ulcer") with the propensity for extensive lateral expansion may lead to associated osteomyelitis
  - When severe they can cause marked morbidity/deformity
- The rapidly growing mycobacteria (*M. abscessus*, *M. fortuitum*, and *M. chelonae*) can present with more acute lesions
  - Pustular lesions, multiple draining interconnected abscesses, numerous small ulcerations, and distal purulent plaques may be seen due to the more rapid spread

Histopathology

- Histopathology can vary from non-specific neutrophilic and/or lymphohistiocytic inflammation to well-formed tuberculoid granulomas (Fig. 27.2)
  - Mixed inflammation with poorly-formed granulomas, histiocytes, and neutrophils, with debris and tissue necrosis is often noted
- Organisms are usually difficult to identify, especially in immunocompetent hosts, even with appropriate special stains
  - AFB and modified acid-fast stains (FITE) should be performed and repeated if suspicious

Differential Diagnosis

- Sporotrichosis: Clinically may overlap; if histology demonstrates AFB+ organisms it can help distinguish the two, but often exposure history is the key
- Staphylococcus abscess: While there may be clinical overlap, staph should be easy to culture and thus differentiate
- Leishmaniasis: Can rarely cause sporotrichoid nodules, but more often crusted ulcerated lesions especially on the ears, with a different exposure history
- Nocardia: Again, there may be clinical overlap, but histopathology and special stains should differentiate this

Work-Up

- Biopsy for histopathology and tissue culture
- Tissue culture requirements vary by species; if there is a strong index of suspicion for mycobacterial infection, it is best to contact the microbiology lab and alert them
  - Most mycobacterial infections are slow growing and cultures should be maintained for 4–6 weeks
  - Some species (including *M. marinum*) grow best at 30–32 °C instead of the typical 37 °C, whereas others (such as *M. haemophilum*) have special growth medium requirements
- PCR analysis can be performed if there is high clinical suspicion, or if AFB+ organisms are seen in the biopsy specimen, but is not widely available
- Tuberculin skin test (can cross react with multiple mycobacterial species) or interferon gamma release assay (can cross react with a select set of mycobacterial species) may be positive in an active infection, but negative testing does not exclude the diagnosis

- Blood cultures may be performed if there is concern for hematogenous spread (particularly in compromised hosts), and requires special culturettes
- Organ specific imaging may be performed if concerned for systemic infection (such as a pulmonary or endovascular source); skin and soft tissue imaging may be indicated to evaluate for deep tissue involvement, abscesses, or underlying osteomyelitis

Treatment

- Management of atypical mycobacterial infections can be challenging and it is reasonable to consult with an experienced clinician or infectious disease colleague
- Immunosuppressed patients should have their suppression tapered if clinically appropriate
- Decisions to treat depend on the pattern of infection, and history of exposure; as mycobacteria are generally slow growing, treatment requires long duration of antibiotics, and inappropriate management can lead to microbial resistance
- Most infections require treatment with more than 1 active agent, and duration for 1–2 months past resolution of symptoms, typically at least 3–4 months total. Immunocompromised patients may require longer treatment.
- Selection of antimycobacterial antibiotics usually requires speciation of the infection; once available, empiric antibiotics may be selected based on historical resistance patterns of that species
  - Susceptibility testing may help demonstrate antimicrobial resistance and allow for optimization of the antibiotic regimen
- Typical agents used include: tetracycline class antibiotics (particularly minocycline), trimethoprim/sulfamethoxazole, clarithromycin, ethambutol, rifampin, clofazamine, and more, depending on the particular species, extent of infection, and medical comorbidities of the patient
- Surgical debridement may be indicated depending on the organism and pattern of infection

Suggested Readings

1. Bhambri S, Bhambri A, Del Rosso JQ. Atypical mycobacterial cutaneous infections. Dermatol Clin. 2009;27:63–73.
2. Griffith DE, Aksamit T, Brown-elliot BA, et al. An official ATS/IDSA statement: diagnosis, treatment and prevention of nontuberculous mycobacterial disease. Am J Respir Crit Care Med. 2007;175:367–416.
3. Lewis FMT, Marsh BJ, von Reyn CF. Fish tank exposure and cutaneous infections due to Mycobacterium marinum: Tuberculin skin testing, treatment and prevention. Clin Infect Dis. 2003;37(3):390–7.

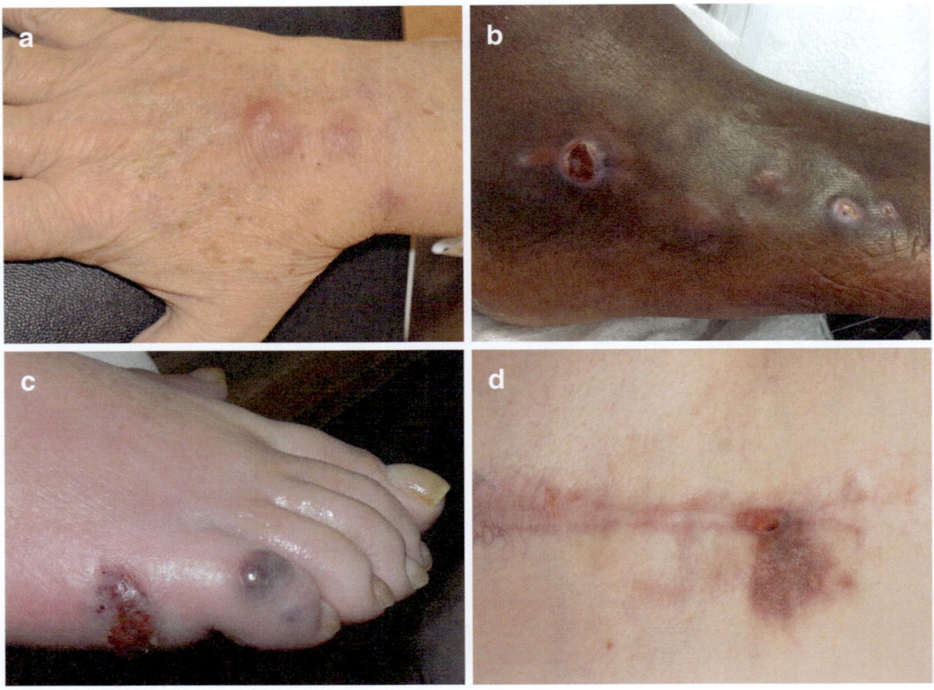

Fig. 27.1 Atypical mycobacterial infections: (**a**) Erythematous nodules of *Mycobacterium marinum* exhibiting sporotrichoid, lymphocutaneous spread. (**b**) Tumefaction and draining sinus tracks due to infection with *Mycobacterium chelonae* resembling Madura foot. (**c**) Hematogenous infection can result in distal red to violaceous papulonodules at sites of embolized globules of mycobacteria. (**d**) Mycobacterial infection of a median sternotomy site following lung transplantation.

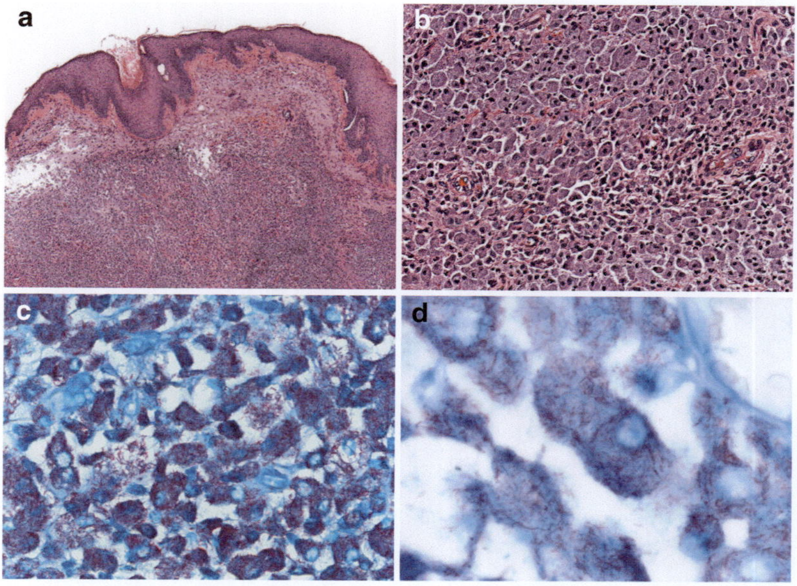

Fig. 27.2 Mycobacteria (*5×, 10×; H&E–40×, 100×; AFB*): This biopsy was obtained from an AIDS patient with a severe disseminated *mycobacterium avium intracellular* infection. (**a**) Low power demonstrates a dermal abscess with neutrophilic and granulomatous inflammation, and necrosis. (**b**) On higher power, the inflammatory infiltrate is composed of both neutrophils and histiocytes. (**c**, **d**) The Acid Fast Bacilli (AFB) stain highlights numerous organisms engulfed by histocytes.

Lyme Disease

28

Karolyn A. Wanat

Overview

- Tick borne illness secondary to infection by spirochete *Borrelia burgdorferi*
- Transmitted by Ixodes scapularis tick
- 96% of confirmed cases reported from 14 states: Northeast United States and Midwest States (specifically Minnesota and Wisconsin) with highest rates
- Reports of infection increasing in other states every year, including notable northward progression due to climate change
- Early diagnosis and treatment is important to help prevent long-term sequalae

Clinical Presentation

- Presentation can be divided into early localized, early disseminated, and late Lyme disease. Early localized presents with cutaneous manifestations whereas early disseminated and late Lyme disease less commonly has skin findings but have neurologic, cardiac, and musculoskeletal complaints (Fig. 28.1)
- An embedded tick may be seen, and careful inspection of the entire surface, including creases and the scalp, should be conducted
- Early localized Lyme:
  - Characteristic eruption: erythema migrans, which occurs in 80% of patients
  - Erythema migrans: Expansion of erythematous patch with central clearing and "bull's eye appearance" 7–14 days after a tick bite; vesicular, hemorrhagic, and pustular components have been described
  - Predilection for intertriginous areas but can be anywhere that tick bites
  - May have other associated viral symptoms (fever, arthalgias, myalgias, fatigue, lymphadenopathy, headache)
- Early disseminated disease: multiple erythema migrans lesions may be present due to spirochetemia
- Borrelial lymphocytoma: more commonly reported in Europe and presents as a single bluish-erythematous swelling that can be up to several centimeters

K. A. Wanat, MD
Department of Dermatology, Medical College of Wisconsin, Milwaukee, WI, USA

M. Rosenbach et al. (eds.), *Inpatient Dermatology*,
https://doi.org/10.1007/978-3-319-18449-4_28

Histopathology

- Histopathology is not necessary if characteristic lesion or embedded *Ixodes* tick is observed in an endemic area (Fig. 28.2)
- Erythema migrans: superficial and deep lymphoplasmacytic infiltrate with variable number of eosinophils and mast cells; can have associated epidermal or dermal necrosis
- Borrelia lymphocytoma: dense lymphocytic infiltration of the dermis and subcutaneous tissue that may have recapitulation of lymph nodes and can be difficult to distinguish from primary cutaneous B cell lymphoma

Differential Diagnosis

- Southern tick-associated rash illness (STARI), which is found in the southeast and south central regions of the United States can present with erythema migrans that can be challenging to distinguish and if suspected often empiric treatment is initiated
- Cellulitis: usually has rapid onset of painful, bright red, hot leg with fever and leukocytosis, without the characteristic "ringed" appearance of erythema migrans
- Urticaria: wheals are smaller in size, higher in number, and more rapidly develop and resolve than typical erythema migrans lesions
- Contact dermatitis: should be pruritic, geometric, and with serous drainage and crust due to the epidermal edema
- Fixed drug eruption: dusky violaceous center and occurs repeatedly at the same site(s), but individual lesions can closely mimic erythema migrans

Work-Up

- A thorough history and physical exam should be obtained, including travel to endemic areas and potential tick exposure with exam forpotential ticks on individuals
- If characteristic lesion of erythema migrans is present in a patient in an endemic area, serologic testing is not required or recommended and treatment should be initiated
- Serologic testing should be reserved for patients with a recent history of having resided in or traveled to an area endemic for Lyme disease, risk factor for tick exposure, and have symptoms of early disseminated or late Lyme disease (neurologic, cardiac symptoms, or arthritis). In these patietns, CDC recommends two-step process with first step being enzyme immunoassay; if positive or indeterminate, the second test, a Western blot is performed

Treatment

- Treatment of choice is doxycycline 100 mg twice daily for 14–21 days; for children under 8 years, pregnant women, or allergic patients, then amoxillin should be substituted.

Suggested Readings

1. Sehgal VN, Khurana A. Lyme disease/borreliosis as a systemic disease. Clin Dermatol. 2015;33(5):542–50.
2. Müllegger RR, Glatz M. Skin manifestations of lyme borreliosis: diagnosis and management. Am J Clin Dermatol. 2008;9(6):355–68.
3. https://www.cdc.gov/lyme/.

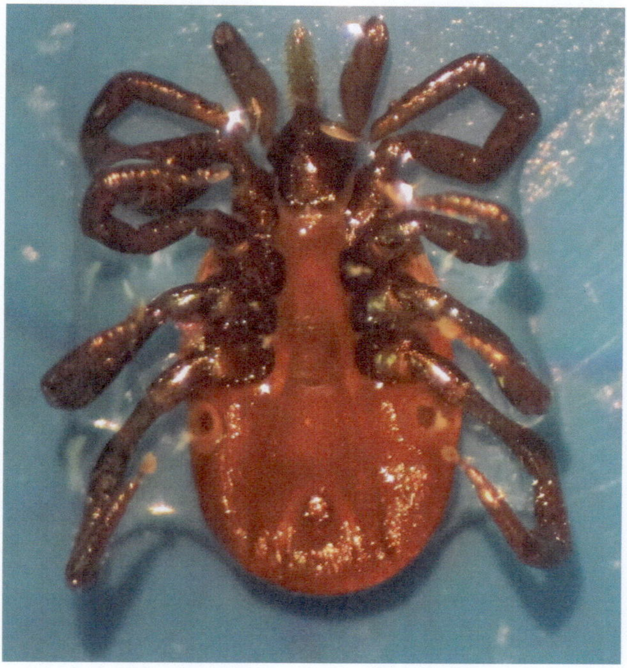

Fig. 28.1 *Ixodes scapularis* tick with characteristic dark legs (ventral aspect pictured).

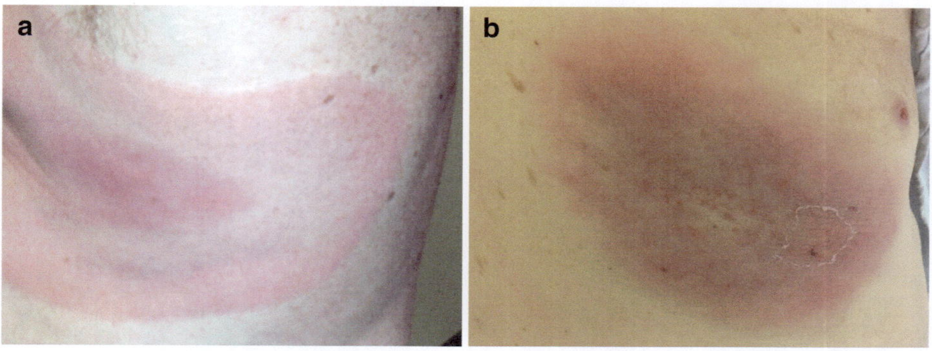

Fig. 28.2 (**a**) Erythema chronicum migrans is a pink-erythematous plaque which expands outward from the bite site; the center may be clear or show a redder central plaque. (**b**) This patch of ECM is less distinct, but the bite site is visible with some superficial desquamation around the tick insertion site.

Spotted Fever

29

Reid W. Masters

Overview

- Spotted fever refers to a group of diseases, includes Rocky Mountain spotted fever (RMSF) and Mediterranean spotted fever, which are caused by *Rickettsiae*, a gram-negative bacterium that is transmitted during feeding by the arthropod vector (tick, flea, or mite)
  - *Rickettsiae* is also the causative organism for Typhus (epidemic, endemic, and scrub) and Rickettsialpox, which will not be discussed in this section
- Diagnosis is a clinical and epidemiologic one based on signs, symptoms, and vector exposure
- Misdiagnosis and delayed treatment are responsible for most fatalities, so high index of suspicion and low threshold for empiric coverage is required
  - Cutaneous findings cannot be relied on exclusively for diagnosis since treatment maybe sought prior to the development of a rash and some patients will develop only mild skin findings or none at all, known as "spotless spotted fever"
- RMSF is the most lethal tick-vectored illness in the United States with a mortality rate of 25% in untreated patients
  - RMSF is most common in the Southeast and Central/Midwest USA but has been reported in 46 states and should be considered endemic in the contiguous United States
  - Inappropriate exclusion based on geography is a common pitfall
  - Most commonly seen in the summer-spring months (corresponding to a surge in numbers of its primary vector, the *Dermacentor* tick), may linger due to climate change
  - Many patients will not recall a prior tick bite (40%) and inoculation sites can be difficult to find, therefore a diagnosis should not be discounted if there is no evidence of an exposure

Clinical Presentation

- Headache, myalgia, and gastrointestinal distress are common early symptoms
- Rash usually appears on day 3–5 of the illness
  - RMSF: 1–2 week incubation period followed by a macular eruption which presents on wrists, ankles and forehead with centrifugal and centripetal spread (<24 h) (Fig. 29.1)
  - Once the rash is generalized it becomes petechial and hemorrhagic with common involvement of the palms and soles (~72 h)

R. W. Masters, MD
Department of Dermatology, Virginia Mason Medical Center, Seattle, WA, USA

M. Rosenbach et al. (eds.), *Inpatient Dermatology*,
https://doi.org/10.1007/978-3-319-18449-4_29

- Although eschar (tache noir) is not typically associated with RMSF, it is commonly present at the site of inoculation in other riskettsial infections, including Mediterranean spotted fever, and serves as a helpful diagnostic clue
- Without proper treatment, spotted fever can progress to cutaneous necrosis/gangrene, pulmonary hemorrhage and edema, acute respiratory distress syndrome, myocarditis, acute renal failure, meningoencephalitis, and cerebral edema

Work-Up

- A thorough history that elicits exposure to ticks or tick-infested habitats, rat exposure, or concurrent illness in household pets (especially dogs) or in similarly exposed family members can be extremely helpful to establish a presumptive diagnosis
- Skin exam to assess rash and look for potential inoculation site
- CBC, CMP
  - Leukopenia, thrombocytopenia, and elevated liver enzyme levels may occur; hyponatremia can be seen in RMSF
- Biopsy specimen of the eschar is preferred if eschar is present, otherwise the center of a petechial macule or papule is the biopsy site of choice, though pathology is not required to make the diagnosis or to initiate therapy if diagnosis is suspected
  - Immunofluorescence of immunohistochemistry may identify *Rickettsiae,* though it is not be widely available
  - Biopsy may assist in narrowing the differential diagnosis
- Serologic diagnosis is retrospective
  - Antibodies typically remain undetectable until around day 7
  - PCR is not a sensitive marker of early disease due to initial low levels of circulating organisms (blood or tissue)

    If tissue is used: biopsy of the eschar site, where there is the highest concentration of organisms, is ideal, but this is rarely done in practice
- Appropriate consultation and workup based on symptomatology including potentially neurologist, pulmonologist, and/or nephrologist along with an infectious disease specialist

Histopathology

- The histology is nonspecific but classically a lymphohistiocytic vasculitis is present, but other common findings include perivascular edema and extravasated erythrocytes (Fig. 29.2)
- Advanced lesions may show necrosis with an associated necrotizing vasculitis ± thrombosis
- Organisms measure 0.3–0.5 μm and are too small to be seen by traditional light microscopy and H&E methods
  - Fluorescent antibodies or immunohistochemistry can aid in visualization, although these will typically require a send-out test since they are available only at limited locations, including through the CDC

Differential Diagnosis

- Small vessel vasculitis (including Henoch-Schonlein purpura): discrete, distinctive palpable purpura
- Ehrlichiosis: shared distribution (common in central and SE USA), often presents with fever and headache and more commonly presents without an associated rash (patients diagnosed with RMSF In the absence of rash may actually have ehrlichiosis); when skin finding are present they are variable in appearance but may mimic RMSF
- Kawasaki disease: fever preceeding a rash characterized by strawberry tongue, conjunctivitis, and often peeling of the creases/folds

- Early secondary syphilis: scale-rimmed ham-colored macules usually involving the palms and soles
- Measles: cephalo-caudad spread of a morbilliform eruption, versus the ankles/wrists and then centripetal and centrifugal spread as in RMSF
- Meningococcemia: broad areas of rapidly developing gray-centered purpura may distinguish this, but early in the disease there is significant overlap and if in doubt, patients should be empirically treated for both entities
- Disseminated gonococcal infection: hemorrhagic pustules over joints with arthralgias
- Immune or thrombotic thrombocytopenic purpura: petechial lesions may predominate, along with some distal livedoid discoloration and potentially renal dysfunction

Treatment

- Empiric treatment is essential and must be started if the diagnosis is considered; treatment should not be held for results/confirmation
- Doxycycline is the first line therapy for all non-pregnant patients regardless of age
  - Of note, although Doxyclicline is typically avoided in the pediatric patient it should be used in the case of RMSF as the potential lethality of the illness outweighs the risk of associated side effects in this population
- Chloramphenicol is less effective and should only be prescribed to patients when Doxycyline is contraindicated
- Management of children and pregnant women should include multidisciplinary care
- Patients should be educated about tick-preventive measures and self-exam after hiking through tick-prone areas

Suggested Readings

1. Chapman A, Bakken JS, Folk SM, et al. Tickborne Rickettsial Diseases Working Group. Diagnosis and management of tickborne rickettsial diseases: Rocky Mountain spotted fever, ehrlichiosis, and anaplasmosis—United States. MMWR Recomm Rep. 2006;55:1–27.
2. Masters EJ, Olson GS, Weiner SJ, Paddock CD. Rocky Mountain spotted fever: a clinician's dilemma. Arch Intern Med. 2003;163(7):769–74.
3. Walker DH. Rickettsiae and rickettsial infections: the current state of knowledge. Clin Infect Dis. 2007;45S:39–44.

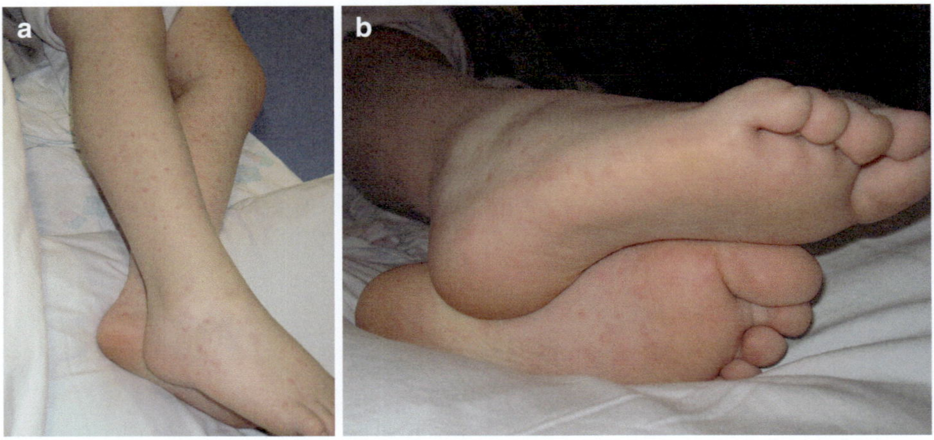

Fig. 29.1 RMSF: (**a**, **b**) Petechial macules on the ankles and soles in a patient with rocky mountain spotted fever. Lesions start on the ankles and wrists and spread both centrifugally and centripetally. By the time cutaneous manifestations develop, most patients are febrile and systemically ill.

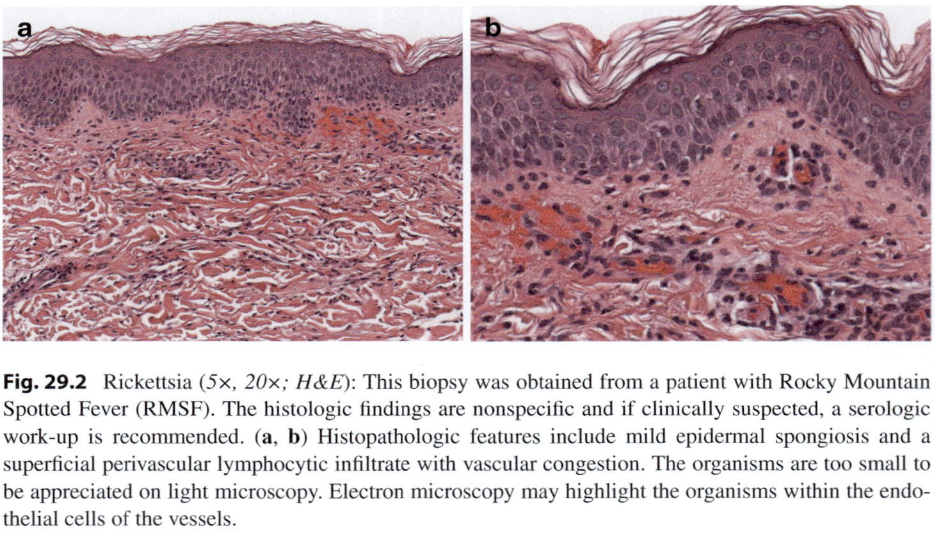

Fig. 29.2 Rickettsia (*5×, 20×; H&E*): This biopsy was obtained from a patient with Rocky Mountain Spotted Fever (RMSF). The histologic findings are nonspecific and if clinically suspected, a serologic work-up is recommended. (**a**, **b**) Histopathologic features include mild epidermal spongiosis and a superficial perivascular lymphocytic infiltrate with vascular congestion. The organisms are too small to be appreciated on light microscopy. Electron microscopy may highlight the organisms within the endothelial cells of the vessels.

Syphilis

30

Karolyn A. Wanat

Overview

- An infectious disease caused by the spirochete *Treponema pallidum*, transmitted primarily by sexual contact and *in utero*
- If left untreated, it progresses through four stages: primary, secondary, latent, and tertiary
- The incidence of infection has been on the rise since 2000, particularly in the men who have sex with men population

Clinical Presentation

- Primary syphilis occurs 10–90 days after contact with an infected person. A firm, red papule (or papules) rapidly erodes to form a painless ulcer with raised borders, usually on the genitalia
  - The primary lesion can be missed as it is usually asymptomatic, depending on the anatomic site (vaginal mucosa, perianal, certain parts of the male genitalia)
- Secondary syphilis usually presents with a pityriasiform eruption 2–10 weeks after the chancre
  - Patchy alopecia can develop
  - Condyloma lata can present with moist verrucous papules or plaques
  - Mild constitutional symtpoms are common
  - Diffuse ham-colored macules with fine scale erupt variably across the trunk and extremities, and notably frequently involve the palms and soles (Fig. 30.1)
  - Palm and sole lesions can vary from a few millimeter diameter macules to large centimeter-sized smooth plaques
  - Syphilitic eruptions can be seen as part of immune reconstitution inflammatory syndrome (IRIS) in HIV+ patients when starting anti-retroviral therapy
- Early latent syphilis describes the first year following self-resolution of untreated primary or secondary syphilis; late latent syphilis may last a few to many years
- Tertiary syphilis may affect any organ, leading to focal and global neurological problems, aortic aneurysms, and granulomatous lesions (gummas) of the bone or skin
- Early congenital syphilis (diffuse exfoliative rash, radial perioral scarring, epiphysitis) occurs within the first two years of life, while late congenital syphilis (interstitial keratitis, Clutton joints, ulcerating gummas, seizures) manifests in those older than 2 years

K. A. Wanat, MD
Department of Dermatology, Medical College of Wisconsin, Milwaukee, WI, USA
e-mail: karolyn-wanat@uiowa.edu

M. Rosenbach et al. (eds.), *Inpatient Dermatology*,
https://doi.org/10.1007/978-3-319-18449-4_30

Differential Diagnosis

- Syphilis is one of the "great mimickers," and because its manifestations are variable, the differential diagnosis of syphilis is extensive
- Primary syphilitic chancre: herpes, simplex virus, chancroid, granuloma inguinale, Lipschutz ulcer; specific diagnostic testing and often empiric treatment for multiple entities is performed
- Secondary syphilis: pityriasis rosea (which may have a herald patch preceeding the widespread eruption, and characteristically spares the palms and soles), drug eruption, or viral exanthem

Histopathology

- Perivascular and lichenoid infiltrate of lymphocytes, plasma cells, and histiocytes in primary and secondary syphilis; organisms can be highlighted using *T pallidum* immunoperoxidase staining (Fig. 30.2)
- Granulomatous inflammation, palisaded macrophages, central necrosis, and plasma cells in tertiary syphilis; treponemes are rarely present

Work-Up

- Biopsy is not always necessary but may be helpful in some cases
- Initial screening: nontreponemal tests (RPR or VDRL) become positive 1–2 weeks after chancre appears and become nonreactive over time after treatment
  - RPR may be falsely negative in the setting of extensive infection (such as in immunosuppressed patients including HIV/AIDS), termed the "prozone phenomenon," serial dilutions should be performed if infection is suspected and RPR is negative
- Confirmatory testing: treponemal tests (FTA-ABS, MHA-TP, TPPA, etc.)
- Darkfield microscopy and immunofluorescence (DFA-TP) are options where available
- Test all patients with syphilis for other STDs, including HIV

Treatment

- Penicillin remains the drug of choice Benzathine PCN G 2.4 million units IM × 1 for primary, secondary, or early latent disease; late latent syphilis requires 3 doses at 1-week intervals
- Doxycycline can be considered in PCN-allergic patients; desensitization is usually necessary in pregnancy, congenital, tertiary, and neurosyphilis
- Patient partners should receive benzathine PCN G 2.4 million units IM × 1
- Patients should be monitored and followed with repeat RPR or VDRL testing over 12–24 months
- All patients should be counseled about safe sex practices and screened for other STDs

Suggested Reading

1. Workowski KA, Bolan GA. Centers for disease control and prevention sexually transmitted diseases treatment guidelines. MMWR. 2015;64(RR3):1–137.

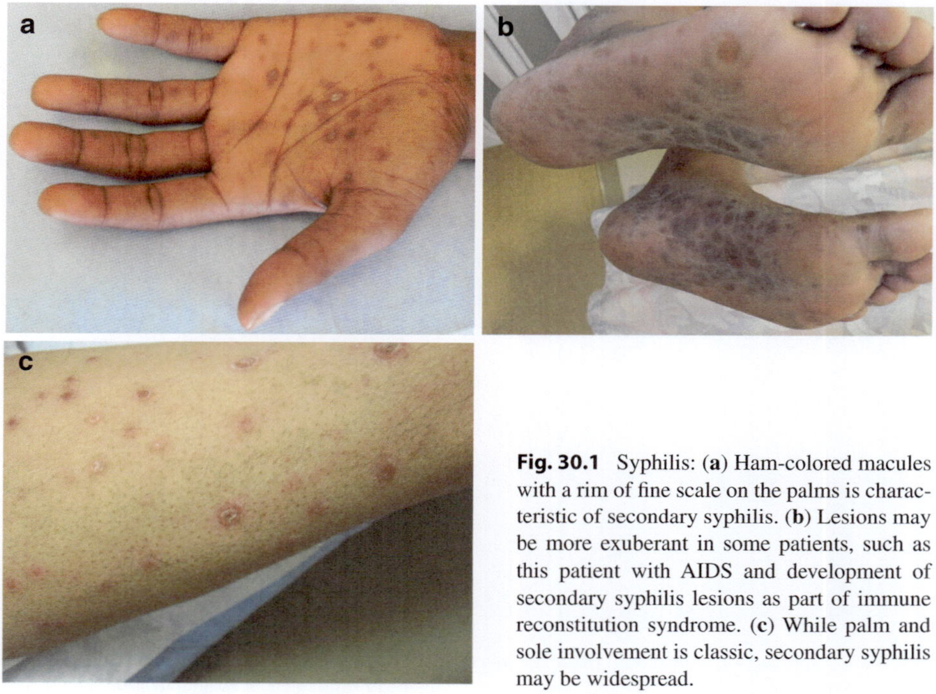

Fig. 30.1 Syphilis: (**a**) Ham-colored macules with a rim of fine scale on the palms is characteristic of secondary syphilis. (**b**) Lesions may be more exuberant in some patients, such as this patient with AIDS and development of secondary syphilis lesions as part of immune reconstitution syndrome. (**c**) While palm and sole involvement is classic, secondary syphilis may be widespread.

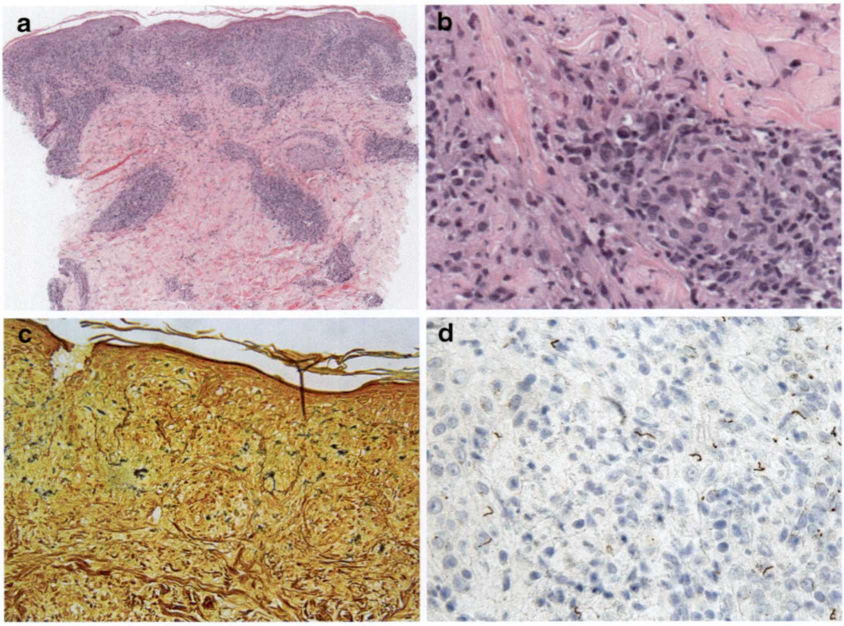

Fig. 30.2 Syphilis (*4×, 40× H&E, Warthin Starry 20×, Treponemal Ab Immunostain, 10×*): (**a**) Low power demonstrates a superficial and deep intense mixed infiltrate with a lichenoid component. (**b**) Higher power highlights the characteristic plasma cell-rich infiltrate. (**c**) Silver-based stains can highlight the treponemal organisms, shown here as globules of spirochetes. (**d**) Newer techniques including Treponemal-specific immunohistochemistry can help identify organisms in less exuberant cases.

Part V

Infections: Viral

Herpes Simplex Virus

31

Molly Moye

Overview

- Herpes simplex virus (HSV) causes painful vesicular eruptions with distribution classically differing based on the infectious serotype (1 vs. 2); However, both types of HSV can cause serious manifestations including keratoconjunctivitis (leading cause of corneal blindness in the US), oropharyngitis, encephalitis/meningitis, pneumonia, and potentially fatal neonatal infections
- Herpes simplex virus 1 (HSV-1) typically causes recurrent oral, lip, and facial eruptions and often is acquired via non-sexual contact, but is an increasing cause of genital herpes
- HSV-2 typically causes recurrent genital and perianal eruptions and is one of the most common sexually transmitted diseases
- Pathogenesis:
  - Following primary infection, HSV resides in sensory dorsal root ganglia, most often in the trigeminal, cervical or lumbrosacral nerves, and periodically causes painful eruptions that tend to recur on the same body site with each episode
  - HSV reactivation can occur spontaneously or secondary to an illness, immunosuppression, tissue damage or stress and is a common cause of recurrent erythema multiforme

Clinical Presentation

- HSV lesions typically present as painful clear vesicles on an erythematous base, which may occur as isolated lesions or in clusters, which may become pustular and/or develop crusts; vesicles may not be evident on mucosal surfaces as they erode quickly (Fig. 31.1)
  - Recurrent lesions can also present as very painful, non-healing erosions or as verrucous or vegetative lesions
  - As lesions evolve the vesicles can rupture leading to shallow, punched-out erosions; these can form larger clusters but usually have a scalloped border and satellite circular erosions around the main cluster
  - Lesions are prone to secondary bacterial infections

M. Moye, MD
Forefront Dermatology, Louisville, KY, USA
e-mail: mollymoye@me.com

M. Rosenbach et al. (eds.), *Inpatient Dermatology*,
https://doi.org/10.1007/978-3-319-18449-4_31

- Primary HSV-1 infection can be asymptomatic or can present with a prodrome of fever, malaise and headache followed by either a painful cutaneous/oral eruption of vesicles, or as pharyngitis
  - Acute gingivostomatis may occur with primary infection (10%), typically in childhood
- Primary HSV-2 infection typically presents as painful genital or backside vesicles or erosions
  - Often associated with inguinal lymphadenopathy and in females dysuria/urinary retention is common
- Disseminated HSV can infect established dermatoses, commonly poorly controlled atopic dermatitis, resulting in a vesicular and ulcerative eruption known as eczema herpeticum
- Immunosuppressed patients may develop atypical presentations of HSV
  - HSV should be suspected in any immunosuppressed patient with punched out or scalloped ulcers, vesicles, or erosions, but in immunosuppressed hosts, single lesions, crusted/chronic hyperkeratotic lesions, and infection of broad, irregular ulcerations may be seen
  - Generally HSV should be considered for any vesicle, erosion, ulcer, or vegetative lesion in an immunosuppressed host
- HSV can manifest slightly differently on atypical sites, such as folliculitis on the face from beard involvement, or tightly clustered small deep-seated vesicles (perhaps due to the thick acral skin) on the finger, which is referred to as herpetic whitlow

Histopathology

- Keratinocytes infected with HSV become enlarged and pale ("ballooning degeneration") with nuclear viral cytopathic changes including multinucleation, chromatin peripheral margination with a central blue-grey glassy appearance, and nuclear molding; eosinophilic round nuclear inclusion bodies surrounded by a clear halo maybe identified (Fig. 31.2)
- Prominent acantholysis with an subepidermal/intraepidermal vesicle formation and adjacent spongiosis can be a histopathologic clue; cytopathic multinucleated cells and neutrophils are typically found floating within the vesicle
- HSV immunohistochemistry can be utilized to confirm etiology (histologically indistinguishable from VZV)

Differential Diagnosis

Note that HSV is so common, with so much clinical overlap, testing is often indicated and necessary to distinguish these entities

- For oral lesions:
  - Aphthous stomatitis: generally broader and deeper, and less clustered, but can be challenging to distinguish
  - Drug-induced mucositis: usually more diffuse epithelial inflammation, sloughing, and crusting, but the two may coexist
  - Herpangina: may be more localized on the posterior oropharynx, but can be challenging to distinguish
- For genital lesions:
  - Genital aphthae: generally broader and deeper, and less clustered, but can be challenging to distinguish
  - Syphilis: often a painless larger ulcer than the grouped smaller lesions of HSV, but verrucous HSV can resemble syphilitic chancres
  - Chancroid: characteristic HSV grouped vesicles can be distinguished, but chronic verrucous HSV can closely resemble chancroid
- For cutaneous lesions:
  - Varicella Zoster Virus: a linear eruption of slightly umbilicated vesicles on an erythematous base sparing the midline favors VZV, but there can be significant overlap
  - Bullous impetigo: often a honey-colored crust will be present, but it is not uncommon for eroded HSV to develop secondary staph superinfection and for both to be present

Work-Up

- Tzanck smear obtained by scraping from base of a new vesicle or erosion is often performed as a bedside test, allowing for rapid results if multinucleated giant cells are present
  - Tzanck smear cannot differentiate HSV from VZV
- PCR testing for HSV from a swab of a lesion is rapid and is highly sensitive and specific
  - PCR testing is becoming the most common means of testing for HSV, especially in the hospital setting
- Direct fluorescent-antibody (DFA) testing and viral culture are older, less sensitive methods used to diagnose active herpes infections
- Viral culture may be performed, particularly if patients are suspected to have anti-viral resistant strains of HSV, which require sensitivity testing to demonstrate
- Serum testing for antibodies is not helpful at distinguishing between active and latent infection
- Skin biopsy can be performed if the diagnosis is unclear and is often recommended for more atypical presentations of herpes, such as verrucous lesions

Treatment

- Acyclovir and valacyclovir can be used interchangeably
  - The benefits of valacyclovir are slightly increased bioavailability and the need for fewer daily doses compared with acyclovir
  - Oral bioavailability is excellent, so intravenous drug delivery is only necessary in cases of critically ill individuals such as neonates, immunosuppressed patients or patients with systemic disease
- For each medication, multiple treatment regimens exist; refer to the CDC's latest guidelines for up-to-date information
- For acyclovir-resistant HSV, foscarnet and cidofovir are treatment options

Suggested Readings

1. Xu F, Sternberg MR, Kottiri BJ, et al. Trends in herpes simplex virus type 1 and type 2 seroprevalence in the United States. JAMA. 2006;296:964–73.
2. Simmons A. Clinical manifestations and treatment considerations of herpes simplex virus infection. J Infect Dis. 2002;186(suppl 1):S71–7.
3. Bolognia JL, Jorizzo JJ, Rapini RP, editors. Chapter 79: Human herpes viruses. In: Dermatology. 2nd ed: Elsevier; 2008. p. 1199–217.

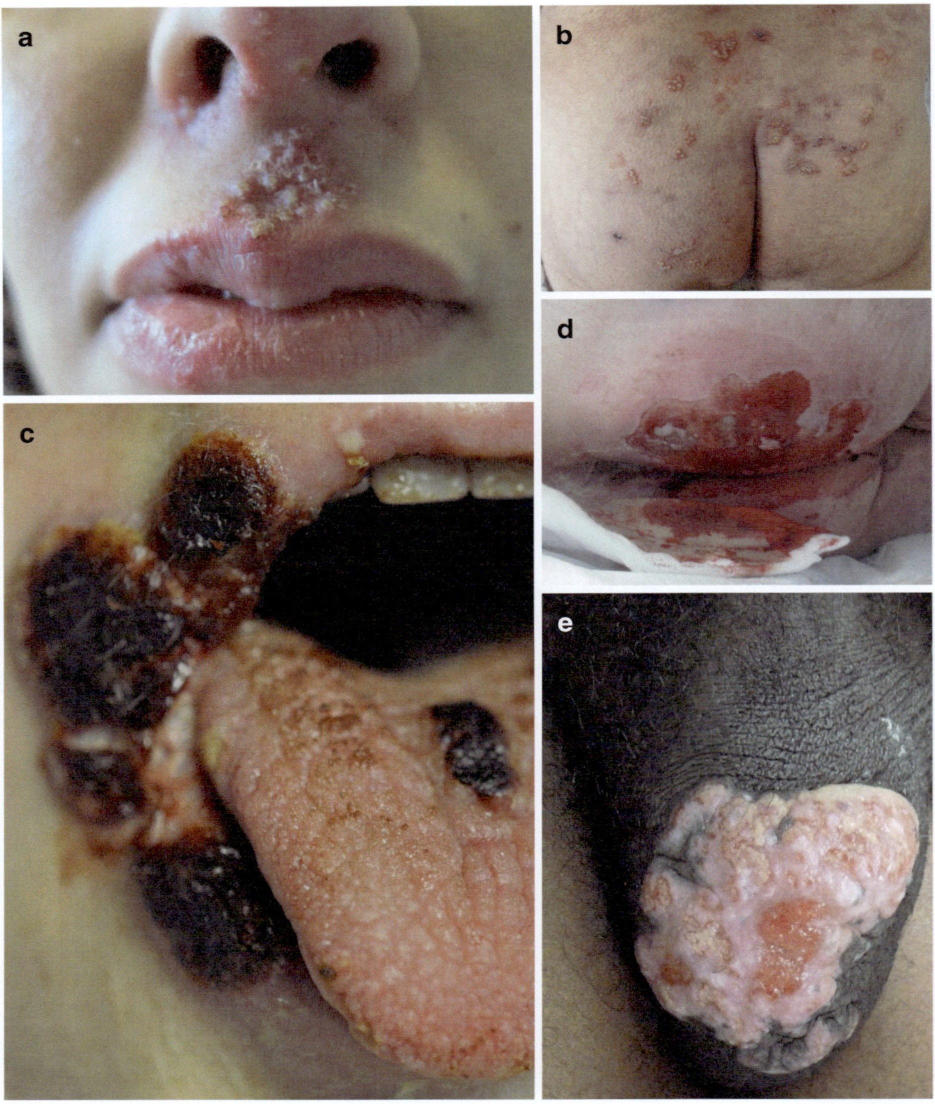

Fig. 31.1 Herpes simplex virus. Herpes can present with multiple morphologies, particularly in the immunosuppressed host. (**a**) Clustered vesicles on an erythematous base is classic; involvement of the perioral area. (**b**) Grouped vesicles on the buttocks/groin. (**c**) Crusted, verrucous lesions can develop in chronic disease when patients are suppressed. (**d**) Ulcers can develop; examination of the edge can reveal punched out erosions or scalloped borders. (**e**) Longstanding lesions can develop a vegetative, heaped up appearance.

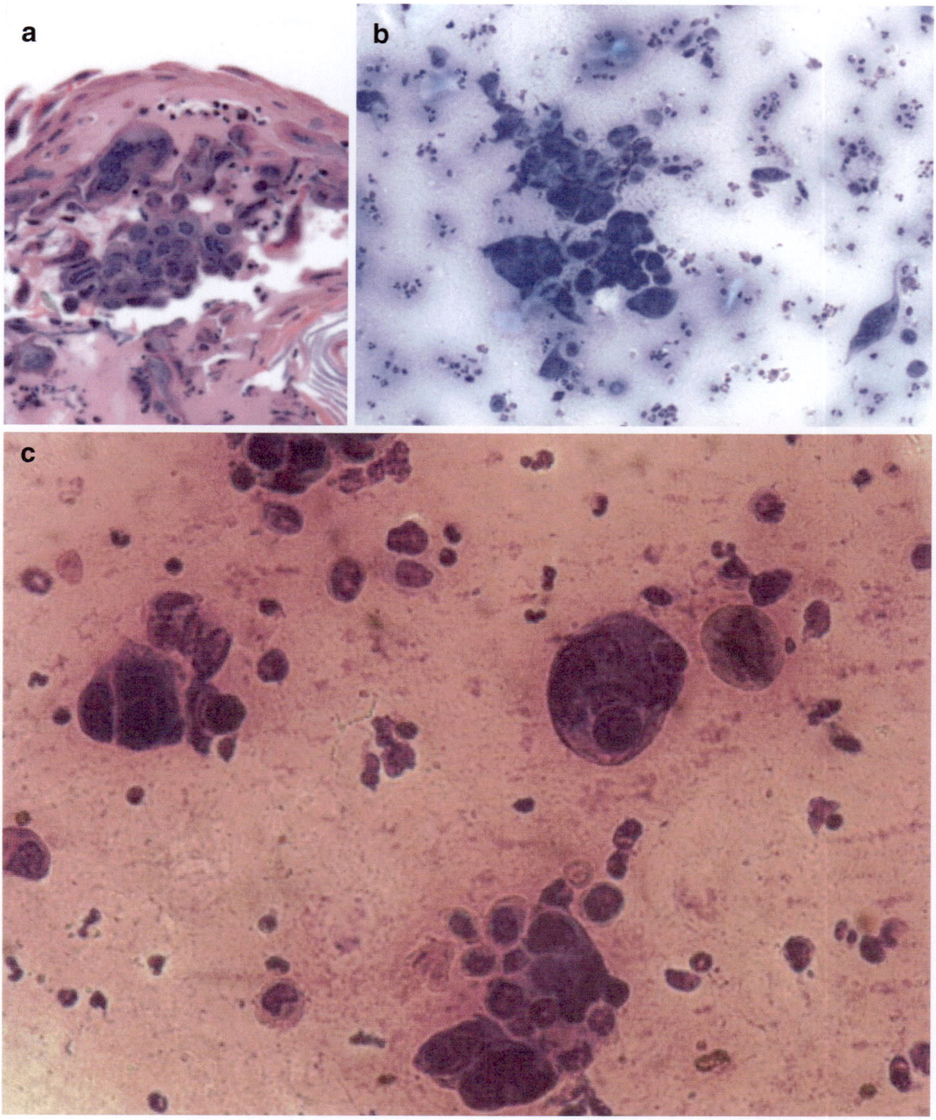

Fig. 31.2 Herpes simplex virus (*10× H&E, 4× Tzanck smear, 20× Tzanck smear*): (**a**) Histopathology will demonstrate acantholysis and intraepidermal vesicles, often with single acantholytic keratinocytes within the blister cavity. Overlying epidermal necrosis also can occur. The associated inflammatory infiltrate is mixed, with predominantly lymphocytes and neutrophils. Differentiating between HSV and VZV can be done with immunohistochemical stains. (**b**, **c**) Tzanck smear will demonstrate enlarged, ballooned keratinocytes; multiple cells will mold together and show multinucleation, molding of adjacent nuclei to one another, and nuclear margination with a rim of chromatin.

Eczema Herpeticum

32

Joy Wan

Overview

- Painful vesicles and erosions in the setting of a disseminated herpes simplex virus (HSV) infection superimposed on an a pre-existing dermatosis, classily seen in the setting of atopic dermatitis (AD)
  - Can be associated with any condition that leads to epidermal barrier dysfunction and thus increased susceptibility to viral invasion
    - Less common underlying dermatoses include: Darier's disease, cutaneous T-cell lymphoma (CTCL), pemphigus foliaceus or vulgaris, burns, etc.
  - More generally referred to as Kaposi varicelliform eruption which also encompasses similar cutaneous manifestations secondary to vaccinia, coxsackie A16, and other viruses
- Affects 3–6% of patients with AD, with the highest risk among children
  - Associated risk factors include: increased severity of AD, earlier onset of AD, higher rate of asthma and allergic rhinitis, higher immunoglobulin E levels, deficiency in skin antimicrobial peptides
- Systemic viremia can occur, leading to multi-organ involvement, including meningitis and encephalitis, which is associated with a mortality rate of up to 10%
- May result from either primary or recurrent infection and can recur with subsequent viral re-exposures or reactivations; typically secondary to HSV-1
  - Primary type more commonly presents in infants/children and accounts for most associated fatalities; there will not be circulating antibodies present
- Can be complicated by bacterial superinfection, usually *Staphylococcus aureus*, *Streptococcus pyogenes,* or *Pseudomonas aeruginosa*

Clinical Presentation

- Can range from a mild, localized infection to a widespread, severe illness depending on the extent, timing, and host immune status
- Monomorphic dome-shaped vesicles which progress to painful, crusted, punched-out erosions that usually heal over 2–6 weeks; depending on the time of presentation, vesicles may be absent, and 1–2 mm punched-out or even linear erosions may be the sole sign of HSV (Fig. 32.1)

J. Wan, MD
Children's Hospital of Philadelphia, University of Pennsylvania, Philadelphia, PA, USA
e-mail: joy.wan@uphs.upenn.edu

M. Rosenbach et al. (eds.), *Inpatient Dermatology*,
https://doi.org/10.1007/978-3-319-18449-4_32

- Primarily involves areas affected by the underlying inflamed skin and can subsequently spread to non-involved regions
- Most commonly affects the head, neck, and trunk
- Usually accompanied by fevers, chills, malaise, and regional lymphadenopathy
- Involvement of the skin around the eye can lead to ocular involvement and is an ophthalmologic emergency

Histopathology

- Early nuclear swelling of keratinocytes with margination of nuclear chromatin, multinucleated keratinocytes with nuclear molding, and late ballooning degeneration of keratinocytes resulting in acantholysis and vesicle formation
- Immunohistochemical stains for HSV-1 or HSV-2 can be used to highlight infected cells and confirm the type of viral infection

Differential Diagnosis

- Primary or disseminated varicella infection: can be clinically similar though VZV may be less confluent and tightly packed, however PCR may be required to distinguish
- Widespread impetigo or other bacterial superinfection: frequently follows eczema herpeticum as bacteria gets in the eroded skin, and cases of dual infection are common; bacterial infection may be more weepy or show an orange/honey colored serous crust
- Contact dermatitis: usually more localized and not as monomorphic, without true vesicles and lacking punched out erosions

Work-Up

- Often can be diagnosed by its clinical features and supported by confirmatory viral studies
  - A biopsy may be indicated in an atypical case, a nonresponsive patient, or to assess for herpetic infection when viral cultures are negative but clinical suspicion is high
- Tzanck smear may demonstrate large multinucleated cells but does not differentiate HSV from VZV
- Diagnosis can be confirmed by polymerase chain reaction for HSV DNA, viral culture, or direct fluorescent antibody staining
  - Cultures should be taken from the edge of the ulcer
- Serologic testing and biopsy are of little diagnostic value and not routinely recommended
- If bacterial superinfection is suspected, cultures should be performed
- Monitor patients closely for systemic symptoms, and seek ophthalmologic consultation if eye involvement is suspected

Treatment

- Promptly initiate systemic antiviral therapy (do not delay while awaiting lab results)
- Intravenous antiviral therapy, usually high-dose acyclovir
- Oral antiviral therapy can be used for those with milder disease not requiring hospitalization (valacyclovir, acyclovir, or famciclovir)
- All treatment is given for a minimum of 7–10 days
- Acyclovir resistance is uncommon, but intravenous foscarnet (or cidofovir) should be used in such cases
- Consider suppressive therapy with oral antivirals (acyclovir, valacyclovir, or famciclovir) in patients with recurrent HSV infection
- If bacterial superinfection is suspected, anti-staphylococcal antibiotics should be administered
- Topical calcineurin inhibitors are contraindicated in the acute phase
- Many also avoid topical corticosteroids in the acute phase to actively infected skin, although there is no convincing evidence of harm to date

Suggested Readings

1. Cathcart SD, Theos A. Inpatient management of atopic dermatitis. Dermatol Ther. 2011;24(2):249–55.
2. Gordon R, Tyring S. Vesicular eruption. JAMA. 2012;307(14):1528–9.
3. Luca NJ, Lara-Corrales I, Pope E. Eczema herpeticum in children: clinical features and factors predictive of hospitalization. J Pediatr. 2012;161(4):671–5.

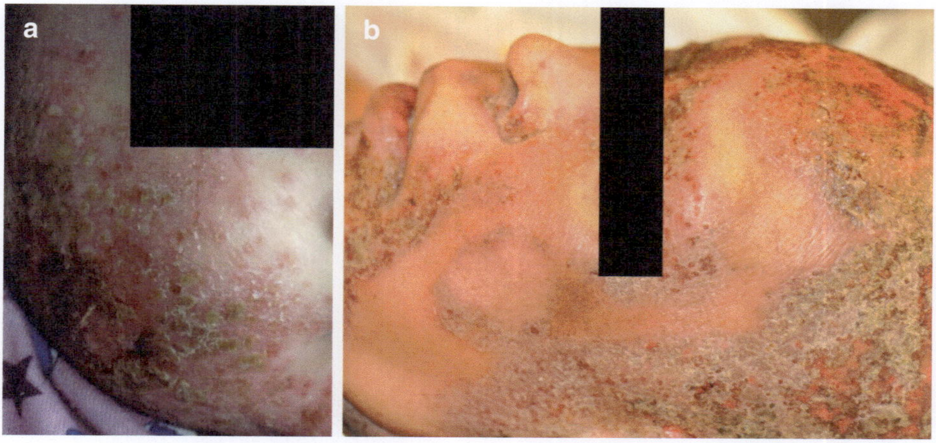

Fig. 32.1 Eczema herpeticum: (**a**) Disseminated 1–2 mm vesicles and punched-out erosions; this case also shows secondary impetiginization due to staph superinfection, resulting in honey colored crusting. (**b**) Herpes can widely infect any preexisting dermatosis or damaged skin, as shown in this patient with erythroderma from CTCL and widespread punched out erosions due to HSV infection.

Varicella Zoster Virus

33

Aileen Y. Chang

Overview

- Varicella zoster virus (VZV) is a DNA virus in the herpesvirus family which manifests with a generalized vesicular eruption (primary varicella, chickenpox) or painful unilateral vesicles confined to a dermatome (dermatomal zoster, herpes zoster, shingles)
- Primary varicella typically occurs in children under the age of 10; when it occurs in adults the course is often worse with a higher rash burden and increased risk of systemic complications
- Following primary infection the virus remains dormant in the dorsal root ganglia; viral reactivation can occur years later; risk of reactivation increases with age, trauma or immunosuppression
  - Reactivation leads to new viral synthesis which infects skin innervated by the sensory nerve it travels along causing dermatomal distribution of the rash; V1 (facial) and T3-L2 (thoracolumbar) are the most common dermatomes involved
- Primary varicella can lead to intrauterine infection and fetal complications early in pregnancy; infections occurring late in pregnancy may be passed onto the child causing neonatal varicella
- Of note, reactivated VZV infection is not associated with fetal/neonatal complications likely secondary to maternal protective antibodies

Clinical Presentation

- Primary varicella:
  - A prodrome of fever, malaise, or pharyngitis precedes the generalized vesicular rash, which appears in successive crops such that lesions are in different stages of development
  - New vesicle formation generally stops within 4 days, and most lesions crust over within 6 days
  - The rash is highly pruritic and typically starts on the head with diffuse spread, although the proximal involvement remains more pronounced
  - Complications include pneumonia, hepatitis, and encephalitis

    Reye syndrome: potentially fatal encephalopathy and hepatitis, often associated with aspirin use in children with chickenpox

A. Y. Chang, MD
Department of Dermatology, University of California, San Francisco, CA, USA
e-mail: aileen.chang@ucsf.edu

M. Rosenbach et al. (eds.), *Inpatient Dermatology*,
https://doi.org/10.1007/978-3-319-18449-4_33

- Herpes zoster:
  - Burning or throbbing pain often precedes the rash, which begins as erythematous papules, evolves into vesicles/bullae, and crusts in 7–10 days, at which point it is no longer infectious (Fig. 33.1)
  - Complications include bacterial superinfection; uveitis/keratitis; aseptic meningitis; motor neuropathy (such as facial palsy/Bell palsy); vertigo, tinnitus, or hearing loss (Ramsey-Hunt syndrome); and post-herpetic neuralgia
- Disseminated Zoster:
  - Begins similar to dermatomal zoster, with a localized prodrome of pain and eruption of grouped vesicles
  - There is secondary generalization beyond the initial dermatome, with >20 discrete vesicles outside the primary dermatome. VZV may spread to involve the CNS (encephalitis), liver (hepatitis), and lungs (pneumonia/pneumonitis)

Histopathology

- Ballooning degeneration, acantholysis, and multinucleation of keratinocytes with molding and margination of nuclear chromatin are visible on Tzanck smear and biopsy (Fig. 33.2)
- Surrounding inflammatory infiltrate and underlying leukocytoclastic vasculitis may also be seen
- Immunohistochemical staining for VZV can aid in diagnosis as the histology is indistinguishable from a HSV infection

Differential Diagnosis

- Herpes simplex: HSV is more often recurrent and usually localized to the orolabial, genital, or buttock region, but clinically the lesions are quite similar to VZV and PCR testing may be necessary
- Measles: Measles involves the buccal mucosa with characteristic Koplik spots (white papules opposite the first and second molars that are classically present early in the course of measles), and the exanthem generally lacks vesicles
- Contact dermatitis: Should be more localized with a geometric, sharply demarcated, generally nondermatomal shape, and lack true vesicles (epidermal spongiosis can lead to pseudovesicles)
- Hand foot mouth disease (HFMD): should involve the mouth/mucosa and have more oval shaped vesicles following dermatoglyphs, with prominent hand/foot involvement
- Secondary syphilis: Vesiculopustular lesions are an atypical presentation of secondary syphilis that can present similarly to disseminated zoster or primary varicella. Nontreponemal tests (e.g. VDRL, RPR) and specific treponemal antibody tests (e.g., FTA-ABS, TP-PA) should be used to confirm the diagnosis

Important Work-Up

- This is a clinical diagnosis and advanced studies are often not required; further work-up may be warranted if the presentation is atypical or in an immunocompromised or pregnant host
- Tzanck smear is operator-dependent but rapid and inexpensive
- PCR is an extremely sensitive and increasingly available means of confirming VZV from skin lesions and body fluids
- Direct fluorescent antibody (DFA) staining of scrapings from active vesicular lesions is less sensitive than PCR but on-par with Tzanck
- Viral culture is slow and insensitive but is necessary in the rare case that antiviral resistance is suspected

Treatment

- Antiviral therapy (acyclovir, valacyclovir) is recommended within 72 h of symptom onset for herpes zoster in order to decrease duration/severity of lesions and decrease post-herpetic neuralgia
  - IV acyclovir may be necessary in immunosuppressed patients and for those with disseminated disease

- Supportive care:
  - NSAIDs, acetaminophen, and opioids may be useful for acute pain
  - Ophthalmologic care is important in the case of suspected ocular involvement or V1 dermatomal zoster
  - Steroids may be used for Bell palsy or Ramsey-Hunt syndrome
  - Gabapentin and tricyclic antidepressants may be beneficial for post-herpetic neuralgia, and early initiation may be preventative
- Varicella vaccine and herpes zoster vaccine are available
  - Non-immune pregnant women exposed to VZV should be treated with varicella-zoster immune globin (VZIG) or prophylactic acyclovir
- VZV is highly contagious and patients with active vesicles should be on appropriate isolation, which may vary by hospital.
  - Generally the virus is spread by direct contact, but immunosuppressed patients or those with disseminated disease, negative pressure airborne isolation may be required

Suggested Readings

1. Dworkin RH, Johnson RW, Breuer J, et al. Recommendations for the management of herpes zoster. Clin Infect Dis. 2007;44(Suppl1):S1.
2. Gnann JW Jr, Whitley RJ. Clinical practice. Herpes zoster. N Engl J Med. 2002;347(5):340.

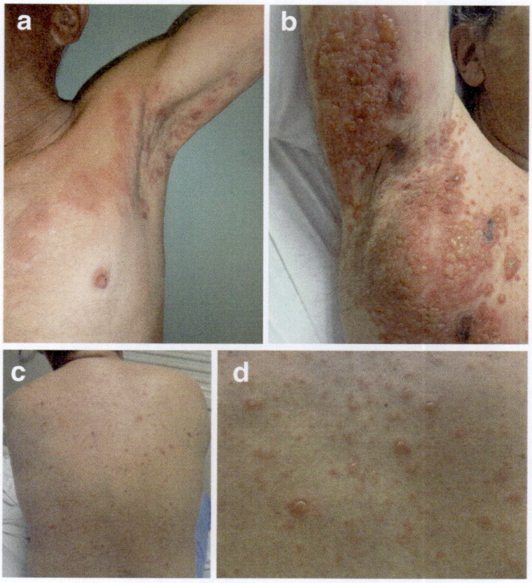

Fig. 33.1 Varicella zoster virus. (**a**, **b**) Grouped vesicles in a dermatomal distribution consistent with herpes zoster (shingles) due to reactivation VZV infection. (**c**, **d**) Generalized vesicles and erythematous crusts consistent with disseminated zoster or primary VZV infection.

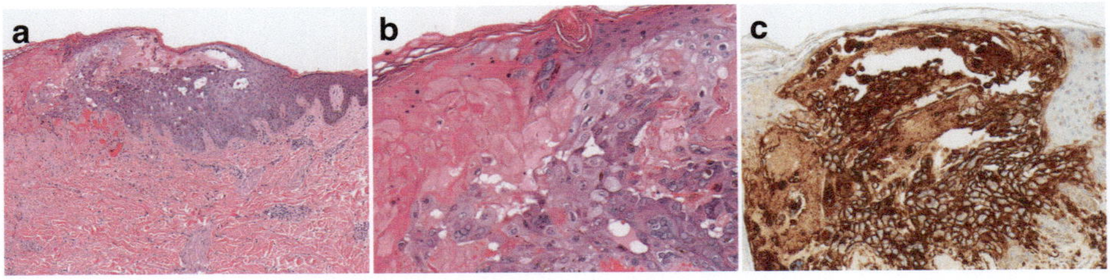

Fig. 33.2 Varicella infection (*5×, 20×: H&E; 10×: VZV IHC*). (**a**) At low power vesicle formation can be appreciated along with epidermal necrosis with acantholysis. (**b**) On higher power, there is epidermal necrosis with underlying cells demonstrating the cytopathic features of the cells with multinucleated cells and nuclear molding. (**c**) The cytopathic features of HSV and VZV infections are indistinguishable and so immunohistochemical staining can help determine the type of infection. Immunohistochemical stains on this case were strongly positive for VZV.

Coxsackie Virus: Hand-Foot-Mouth Disease

34

Nkanyezi N. Ferguson

Overview

- Hand-foot-and-mouth disease (HFMD) is a highly contagious viral illness characterized by fever and mucocutaneous vesiculopapules on the palms, soles, mouth, and buttocks, commonly caused by coxsackievirus-A16, enterovirus 71, and less commonly other members of the Picornavirus group
- Seasonal outbreaks typically occur in the spring to fall months
  - The virus is contagious for weeks after initial outbreak and remote exposures may be common, particularly in adults
- Commonly affects younger children ages 5 and below; atypical disease and adult infection is becoming more common
  - Atypical disease presentation has been observed with coxsackievirus-A6 which occurs in the late fall to winter, affects older individuals and has more widespread cutaneous involvement (often involving the scalp and groin)
  - Large blisters or vesiculobullous lesions with palm and sole desquamation and eczema herpeticum-like reactions ("eczema coxsackium") may be seen
  - More severe disease courses may be associated with enterovirus-71 infection with reports of encephalitis, myocarditis, pulmonary edema and death

Clinical Presentation

- Mucocutaneous symptoms are preceded by fever, malaise, sore throat and diarrhea
- Erythematous papules evolve into oval shaped gray vesicles ("football shaped") with an erythematous halo, typically present on the palms and soles with less common involvement of the buttocks, dorsal hands, and feet; the vesicles often follow the dermatoglyphs of the fingers (Fig. 34.1)
  - Buttock involvement is common in younger diaper-wearing patients and are composed of macules and papules more often than vesicles
  - The rash is relatively asymptomatic and is not usually associated with pruritis or pain
- Vesicles and erosions are present in the mouth, affecting the hard and soft palate, buccal mucosa, gingiva and tongue

N. N. Ferguson, MD
University of Iowa Hospital and Clinics, Iowa City, IA, USA
e-mail: nkanyezi-ferguson@uiowa.edu

M. Rosenbach et al. (eds.), *Inpatient Dermatology*,
https://doi.org/10.1007/978-3-319-18449-4_34

- Spontaneous resolution often occurs within 7–10 days
- Onychomadesis (temporary nail matrix arrest resulting in shedding of the nail plate) can occur during convalescence and may present weeks to months later

Histopathology

- Epidermal necrosis with reticular degeneration and the formation of intraepidermal often multilocular vesicles (Fig. 34.2)
  - While intraepidermal vesicles are seen with early lesions biopsies of older lesions may demonstrate subepidermal seperation
  - Absence of inclusion bodies or multinucleated giant cells
- Superficial perivascular lymphocytic inflammation with occasional areas of interface dermatitis

Differential Diagnosis

- Eczema herpeticum: can be challenging to distinguish clinically; bedside Tzank smear or PCR testing may be necessary
- Varicella: primary VZV or disseminated VZV can share overlapping clinical features; PCR testing should be confirmatory
- Erythema multiforme: the target lesions of EM should have three true zones of distinctly different color, and are often larger than the small oval vesicles of HFMD
- Differential for oral mucosal involvement:
  - Herpangina: similar to the oral lesions of HFMD, but widespread mucocutaneous involvement is less common
  - Aphthous stomatitis: the oral lesions will be larger, deeper ulcers, and there is not hand or foot involvement

Work-Up

- Diagnosis can be made through history and physical examination alone
- RT-PCR can detect virus from vesicular fluid; material from throat swabs and stool samples can be used if vesicular fluid is not available
- Testing blood samples is not routinely performed given the transient nature of viremia; results are often negative by the time patients present with skin findings

Treatment

- Treatment is supportive as disease is usually self-limited
- Education regarding hygiene precautions to prevent respiratory or fecal-oral spread is important
- High risk groups including young children, immunocompromised adults, elderly and pregnant woman are at risk for rare severe complications including pulmonary edema, myocarditis, meningitis and encephalitis

Suggested Readings

1. Lott JP, Liu K, Landry ML, Nix WA, Oberste MS, Bolognia J, King B. Atypical hand-foot-and-mouth disease associated with coxsackievirus A6 infection. J Am Acad Dermatol. 2013;69(5):736–41.
2. Feder HM Jr, Bennett N, Modlin JF. Atypical hand, foot, and mouth disease: a vesiculobullous eruption caused by Coxsackie virus A6. Lancet Infect Dis. 2014;14(1):83–6.
3. Kaminska K, Matinetti G, Lucchini R, Kaya G, Mainettia C. Coxsackievirus A6 and hand, foot and mouth disease: three case reports of familial child-to-immunocompetent adult transmission and a literature review. Case Rep Dermatol. 2013;5(2):203–9.

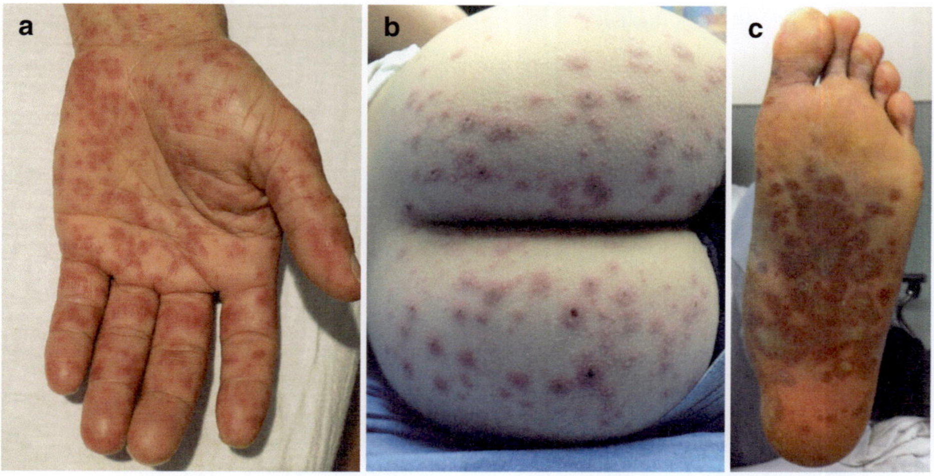

Fig. 34.1 Hand-foot-mouth disease: (**a**) Painful erythematous papules and oval gray vesicles on the palm of an adult with hand-foot-mouth disease; the vesicles often lay in parallel to the dermatoglyphs of the fingerprints. (**b**) Gray vesicles and excoriated erythematous papules and crusts on the buttocks of a child with hand-foot-mouth disease. (**c**) Dusky violaceous patches and vesicles on the feet of an African-American adult with widespread coxsackie-A6 infection affecting the hands, feet, mouth, and buttocks.

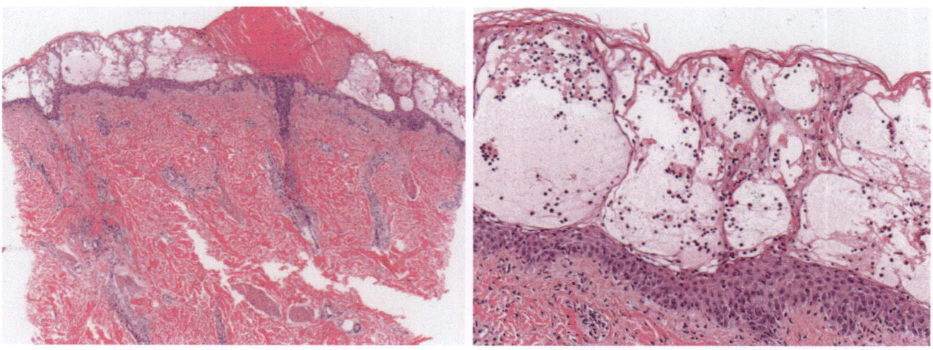

Fig. 34.2 HFMD: Histopathology is not necessary for classic infections. For atypical presentations, histopathology will demonstrate basketweave stratum corneum with underlying epidermal necrosis, dyskeratosis, and intraepidermal vesiculation with papillary dermal edema. The superficial dermis demonstrates a lymphocytic infiltrate.

Human Immunodeficiency Virus

35

Jack Abbott

Overview

- Human immunodeficiency virus (HIV) retrovirus causes progressive immunosuppression secondary to impaired cell-meditated immunity and decreased CD4 count resulting in an extensive spectrum of infectious, inflammatory, and neoplastic manifestations
- Cutaneous findings can be seen in a variety of forms throughout a patient's disease course and ranging from a morbilliform rash associated with acute viral infection and seroconversion to hyperpigmented skin with lichenification from photosensitivity seen in advanced disease
  - Cutaneous eruptions are typically associated with the immunosuppressed state caused by the virus rather than damage done by the virus itself
- Due to the patient's immunosuppression they are more susceptible to infection and a more aggressive course
- Patients with HIV/AIDS are at increased risk for drug reactions due to the variety of medications they are exposed to; for example, many patients are treated with TMP-SMX for PCP prophylaxis and sulfonamides are a common cause of DRESS, EM, SJS/TEN

Clinical

- 80–90% of patients with HIV have cutaneous manifestations; often seen as the first presentation of systemic disease
- Suspect HIV infection in in patients with unexplained immunosuppression which may manifest as skin disease with severe or widespread involvement, atypical skin eruptions, and refractory disease, especially in the setting of risk factors or known exposures

J. Abbott, MD
Department of Dermatopathology, University of Pennsylvania, Philadelphia, PA, USA
e-mail: james.abbott@uphs.upenn.edu

M. Rosenbach et al. (eds.), *Inpatient Dermatology*,
https://doi.org/10.1007/978-3-319-18449-4_35

Histopathology

- The pathology varies based on what type of lesion is biopsied; a biopsy of an opportunistic infection may reveal disease-specific pathology related to that infectious agent, while a biopsy of a pruritic papule from immune dysregulation can show nonspecific features of eczematous dermatitis with eosinophils. Severely suppressed patients with AIDS may have evidence of multiple processes within a single lesion (such as crypotococcus and Kaposi's). When evaluating HIV-related lesions, it is important to be cognizant of what lesion is biopsied and to utilize clinical/pathologic correlation to arrive at a diagnosis

Differential diagnosis

- Often a differential diagnosis is based around $CD4^+$ count and viral load (see Table 35.1):
  - $CD4^+ > 500$ (cells/mm^3): Acute retroviral syndrome, Oral hairy leukoplakia
  - $CD4^+ < 500$ (cells/mm^3): Oropharyngeal candidiasis, Herpes Zoster, Kaposi sarcoma
  - $CD4^+ < 250$ (cells/mm^3): Eosinophilic folliculitis, Molluscum contagiosum (severe), Herpes simplex (disseminated), Cryptococcosis (disseminated)
  - $CD4^+ < 50$ (cells/mm^3): Severe mucocutaneous herpes simplex, Mycobacterium avium complex (MAC)
  - At any $CD4^+$ count (severity dependent on immune status): scabies, varicella, staph, lymphoma

Table 35.1 Dermatologic manifestations of HIV based on CD4 count

	Manifestations	$CD4^+$ count (cells/mm^3)	Work-up	Treatment
Acute retroviral syndrome	2–4 weeks after infection: fever, lymphadenopathy, pharyngitis, morbiliform rash (trunk > palms, soles), may be oral erosions; similar to acute mononucleosis	>500	False negative HIV antibodies (ELISA), Positive: HIV RNA/DNA, p24 antigen	Symptomatic therapy, consider ART
Oropharyngeal Candidiasis (thrush)	MC fungal infection, white creamy plaques on buccal mucosa or tongue that bleed or display atrophic red macules when scraped off Four types: Pseudomembranous candidiasis, erythematous candidiasis (red patches), hyperplastic candidiasis (smooth white dorsum of tongue), and angular cheilitis (corner of mouth with erythema, cracking, and erosions)	<500	Oral exam, scrape plaques (hyperplastic forms does not scrape off) Confirm with culture or microscopy—pseudohyphae and yeast forms	ART, Oral: local nystatin or clotrimazole
Varicella zoster virus (VZV)	Primary infection: variable course from pruritic vesicles on erythematous macules to severe pulmonary involvement Zoster: HIV patients with unusual multi-dermatomes, dissemination, and verrucous lesions	<500, severity dependent	Tzanck smear, DFA, PCR, serology, biopsy	ART (may worsen disease due to immune recovery syndrome), Acyclovir, varicella zoster immune globulin (VZIG) Vaccination with live attenuated VZV is contraindicated

Table 35.1 (continued)

	Manifestations	CD4⁺ count (cells/mm³)	Work-up	Treatment
Kaposi Sarcoma	Vascular spindle cell neoplasm associated with human herpesvirus 8 (HHV 8) infection, most commonly involving the skin as red to brown papules, patches, plaques, or nodules that can ulcerate	<500	Biopsy with HHV8 IHC	ART Local destructive therapies (cryotherapy, intralesional chemotherapy, superficial radiation, topical retinoid)
Eosinophilic folliculitis (Figs. 35.1 and 35.2)	Common folliculocentric erythematous pruritic papules and pustules that primarily involve the upper trunk, face, and scalp	<250	Biopsy and culture; CBC may show peripheral eosinophilia	Symptomatic therapy—topical corticosteroids, oral antihistamines, UVB ART—effect varies
Disseminated Cryptococcosis	Encapsulated yeast found in high concentration in bird feces and decaying plant matter Potential sites of involvement: lungs, skin, CNS (meningitis), GU Papulonodular lesions with rolled borders; can mimic molluscum contagiosum (dome papules with central umbilication)	<250	Cutaneous—biopsy and culture CSF—culture, latex agglutination for capsular polysaccharide antigens	IV amphotericin B and oral flucytosine ART
Molluscum Contagiosum (Fig. 35.1)	Poxvirus; flesh colored papules with central umbilication that coalesce into large lesions	<250 (extensive) <50 (giant)	Culture and biopsy or microscopy of cyst contents (Fig. 35.3)	ART Local destructive therapies (curettage, imiquimod, topical cidofovir)
Scabies	Ectoparasite that burrows on the hands, wrists, ankles, and interdigital webbing resulting in pruritic papules and plaques Crusted scabies—hyperkeratotic pruritic lesions due to extensive mite load	Any level	Skin biopsy or microscopy—mites, eggs, and feces (scybala)	Ivermectin and topical permethrin 5%; Patients are contagious, must isolate Monitor for secondary infection (increased risk for sepsis)
HIV photodermatitis) (Fig. 35.1)	Photosensitivity that can develop in patients, generally with chronic disease, leading to lichenified, hyperpigmented skin in sun exposed areas May be a component of medication-induced photosensitivity in some patients	(<200)	History and physical exam with sharp demarcation at clothing lines; biopsy may be nonspecific but supportive	ART Photoprotective measures Topical steroids

Work-Up

- In patients without a known diagnosis of HIV/AIDS when it is suspected a thorough history related to potential exposures is very important; this should cover high risk behaviors such as unprotected sex and intravenous drug use (IVDU)
- In patients without an established diagnosis of HIV/AIDS appropriate testing; ELISA tests are used for antibody screening with confirmation testing
  - With fourth generation HIV ELISA testing patients are tested for IgG, IgM, and p24
    - p24 antigen is produced approximately 2–3 weeks after exposure and its inclusion allows for detection earlier than previous testing which was only antibody dependent
    - The testing does not differentiate between HIV1/2 so additional immunoassays are need for confirmation and specific diagnosis
  - HIV viral load testing, done with RNA, can be used to detect disease even earlier, as early as 5–15 days post infection and can be used to track disease after a diagnosis is made
  - CD4 counts should also be ordered and trended

Management

- Antiretroviral therapy (ART) regimens control HIV infection, thereby decreasing opportunistic infections and severe skin manifestations; however, the medications can lead to cutaneous drug reactions
  - ART management is an area of rapid change and patients' treatment regimen should be managed by an experienced infectious disease specialist
- Most lesions will resolve with improved CD4 counts in the setting of proper ART management; more specific management will depend on the specific manifestation (see Table 35.1)

Suggested Readings

1. Khambaty MM, Hsu SS. Dermatology of the patient with HIV. Emerg Med Clin North Am. 2010;28(2):355–68. https://doi.org/10.1016/j.emc.2010.01.001.
2. Tappero JW, Perkins BA, Wenger JD, Berger TG. Cutaneous manifestations of opportunistic infections in patients infected with human immunodeficiency virus. Clin Microbiol Rev. 1995;8(3):440–50.
3. Uihlein LC, Saavedra AP, Johnson RA. Cutaneous manifestations of human immunodeficiency virus disease. In: Goldsmith LA, Katz SI, Gilchrest BA, Paller AS, Leffell DJ, Wolff K, editors. Fitzpatrick's dermatology in general medicine, 8e. New York: The McGraw-Hill; 2012. http://mhmedical.com/content.aspx?aid=56089773.
4. Rieger A, Chen TM, Cockerell CJ. Cutaneous manifestations of HIV infection. In: Bolognia J, Jorizzo JL, Schaffer JV, editors. Dermatology. 3rd ed. Philadelphia: Elsevier Saunders; 2012. p. 1285–302.

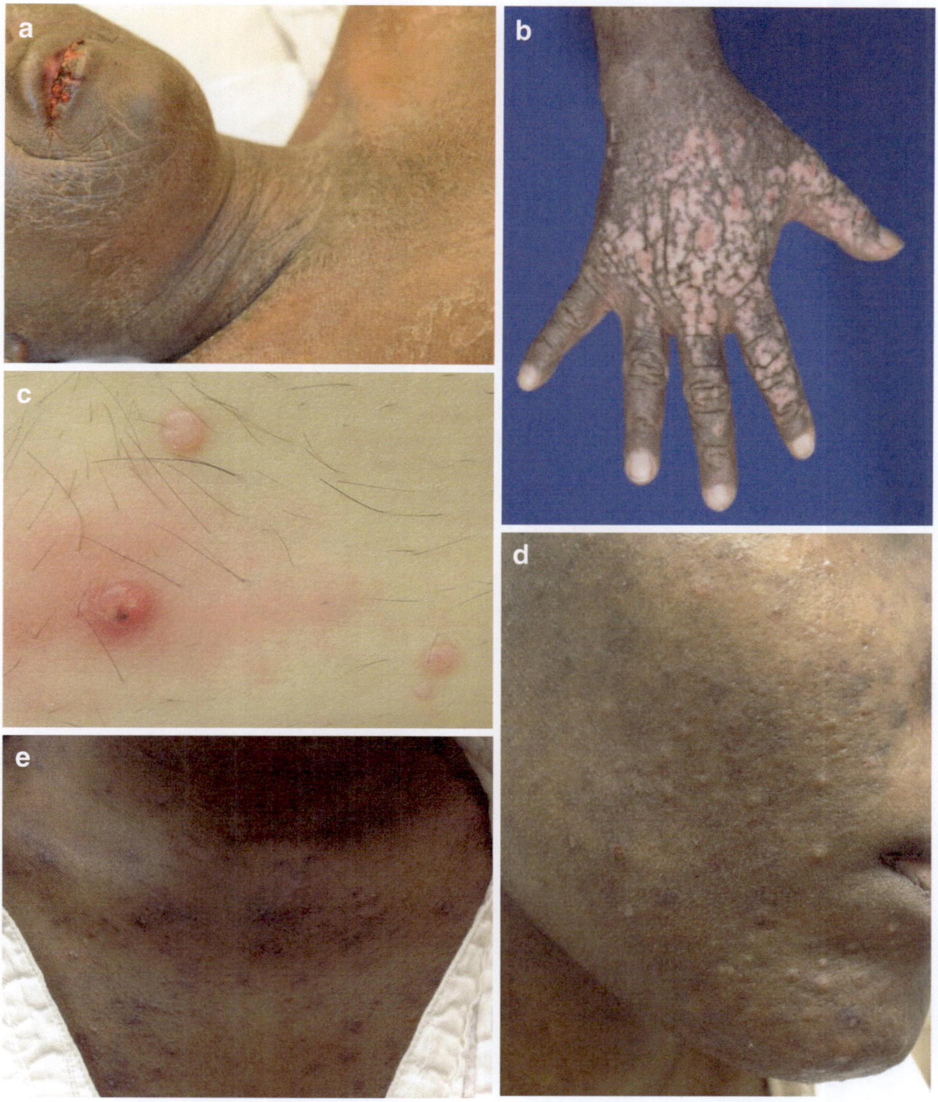

Fig. 35.1 HIV photodermatitis: (**a, b**) Patients with HIV can develop a lichenoid eruption in photoexposed areas leading to hyperpigmented, pruritic patches and plaques. Note slight sparing under the chin, and the involvement of the V-neck of the chest. This patient also has generalized xerosis (**b**). (**c**) Molluscum contagiosum. These flesh colored to pink papules often have a white core and umbilication; when inflamed they can turn red and resemble infection. (**d**, **e**) Eosinophilic folliculitis: Monomorphic erythematous and hyperpigmented papules on the (**d**) face and (**e**) upper chest in a patient with HIV.

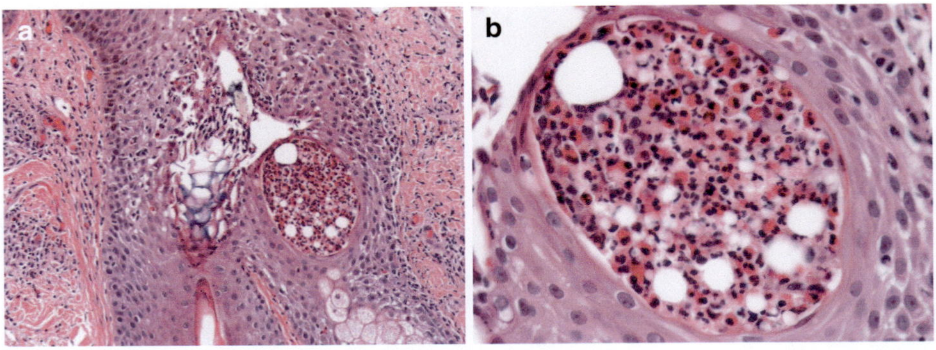

Fig. 35.2 Eosinophilic folliculitis *(10×, 40×; H&E)*: (**a**) Within the hair follicle is a collection of neutrophils and eosinophils with surrounding inflammation in the dermis. (**b**) Higher power highlights the intrafollicular pustule packed with neutrophils and eosinophils.

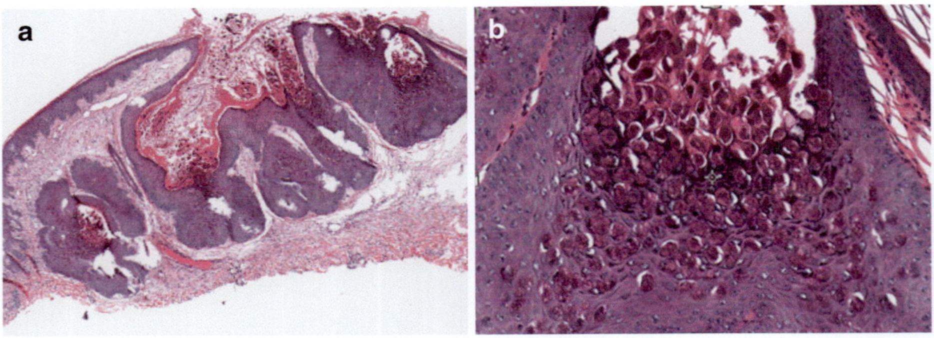

Fig. 35.3 Molluscum contagiosum (*H&E 2.5×, 10×*): Umbilicated dome shaped appearance of lesion evident on low power (**a**) with epidermal hyperplasia with large eosinophilic inclusions known as molluscum bodies (**b**).

Kaposi Sarcoma

36

Nkanyezi N. Ferguson

Overview

- Endothelial proliferative disorder strongly linked to human herpesvirus-8 (HHV-8) with variable presentation from indolent cutaneous-limited lesions to a rapidly progressive course with extensive mucocutaneous and visceral involvement
- Four clinical variants of Kaposi sarcoma (KS):
  - Classic KS is an uncommon typically indolent disease primarily affecting elderly men of Mediterranean or Jewish descent characterized by the development of angiomatous lesions on the lower distal extremities typically in the absence of visceral involvement
  - AIDS-associated/epidemic KS: an AIDS defining illness, affects the upper body, head and neck, and mucosa, with rapidly progressive course, with common visceral involvement, more frequently seen in men who have sex with men, improvement can be seen with CD4 count recovery with HAART
  - Iatrogenic or transplantation-associated KS: classily seen following immunosuppressive therapy and in transplant patients; often improves with decreased/adjusted immunosuppression
  - African/endemic KS: encompasses several subtypes, the lymphadenopathic subtype most commonly affects children and is characterized by an aggressive often fatal course with cutaneous and widespread lymph node involvement

Clinical Presentation

- Violaceous to red-brown macules, patches, plaques or nodules which bleed easily and may ulcerate (Fig. 36.1)
- Mucosal involvement can be seen with conjunctival, oral and genital forms
  - Oral KS commonly presents on the palate as violaceous patches, plaques or nodules and may be the first and only sign of KS
- Extracutaneous visceral involvement can involve the gastrointestinal tract, lymph nodes, lungs, liver, and heart (more commonly seen in the setting of AIDS-associated KS)
- Uncommon morphologic variants include: telangiectatic, ecchymotic, keloidal, cavernous, and lymphangioma-like

N. N. Ferguson, MD
University of Iowa Hospital and Clinics, Iowa City, IA, USA
e-mail: nkanyezi-ferguson@uiowa.edu

M. Rosenbach et al. (eds.), *Inpatient Dermatology*,
https://doi.org/10.1007/978-3-319-18449-4_36

- Potential complications include:
  - Edema for obstructed lymphatic flow, secondary localized skin infections, upper airway obstruction and gastrointestinal obstruction

Histopathology

- Characterized by a proliferation of spindled endothelial cells which form abnormal vascular 'slit-like' spaces and later fascicles of streaming tumor cells (Fig. 36.2)
  - Small vessels or normal adnexa protruding into an abnormal vascular space has been termed "promontory sign" and is not specific to KS
- Extravasated erythrocytes, hemosiderin-laden macrophages, and plasma cells often are present
- Positive for expression of HHV-8 and CD31 antigen (endothelial marker)

	Patch stage	Late Patch/Plaque stage	Nodular stage
Clinical	Flat red-brown sometimes scaly patches	Larger violaceous plaques with red-brown areas, variable surface change	Subcutaneous or dermal-based nodules which can be heaped up and appear bright red or purple
Pathology	Small "slit like" vascular structures infiltrate between collagen bundles in the superficial dermis(can be very subtle and missed in early lesions) If perivascular infiltrate is present it is sparse	Process spreads into the deeper dermis with increasing aggregates of ectatic vessels and spindled endothelial cells Brisk lymphoplasmacytic perivascular infiltrate	Process expands into subcutaneous tissue with increased fascicles of spindled cells forming a circumscribed lesion

Differential Diagnosis

- Hemangiomas (lobular capillary, tufted, non-involuting): History may be helpful, and hemangiomas may be less widespread, but biopsy is may be necessary to distinguish
- Bacillary angiomatosis: clinically can be quite similar (though BA is markedly rarer), and biopsy may be necessary
- Angiosarcoma: Also frequently on the head and neck, angiosarcoma is usually more localized, but again biopsy may be necessary to distinguish the two
- Pseudo-kaposi sarcoma (e.g. arteriovenous malformation or stasis dermatitis): as the name implies this can be clinically similar, and biopsy should be considered if in doubt
- Dermatofibroma: usually smaller lesions which are brown and "dimple" inwards when squeezed from both sides, often on the shoulders or lower legs

Work-Up

- A thorough history, physical exam and review of systems to evaluate for cutaneous and potentially associated visceral disease
  - Several modalities can be used to evaluate extracutaneous KS as clinically indicated including: ultrasound, computed tomography, and various endoscopic techniques
  - Pulmonary KS must be distinguished from lymphoma and opportunistic infections
- Punch biopsy of a representative lesion; HHV8 staining in endothelial cells confirms diagnosis
- HIV status of the patient should be determined

Treatment

- Rate of recurrence of KS can be high despite therapy
- Therapy selection is based on disease severity, progression, distribution and clinical type
- Skin directed therapy can range from clinical monitoring to surgical excision, laser therapy (585-nm pulsed dye laser, high energy pulsed carbon dioxide laser), cryotherapy, radiotherapy, or intralesional chemotherapy
- Classic type:
  - Systemic chemotherapy for disseminated disease
  - Retinoids
  - Localized radiation can be performed
  - Intralesional chemotherapy also can be used
- Iatrogenic or transplantation-associated KS
  - Cessation or modification of immunosuppressive agents
- AIDS-associated KS
  - Institution of highly active antiretroviral therapy (HAART)
  - Flares in KS may paradoxically occur due to the immune reconstitution inflammatory syndrome (IRIS)
  - Patients with severe or progressive AIDS-associated KS may benefit from combination HAART treatment with chemotherapy

Suggested Readings

1. Schwartz RA, Micali G, Nasca MR, Scuderi L. Kaposi sarcoma: a continuing conundrum. J Am Acad Dermatol. 2008;59(2):179–206.
2. Ruocco E, Ruocco V, Tornesello ML, Gambardella A, Wolf R, Buonaguro FM. Kaposi's sarcoma: etiology and pathogenesis, inducing factors, causal associations, and treatments: facts and controversies. Clin Dermatol. 2013;31(4):413–22.
3. Gbabe OF, Okwundu CI, Dedicoat M, Freeman EE. Treatment of severe or progressive Kaposi's sarcoma in HIV-infected adults. Cochrane Database Syst Rev. 2014;8:CD003256.

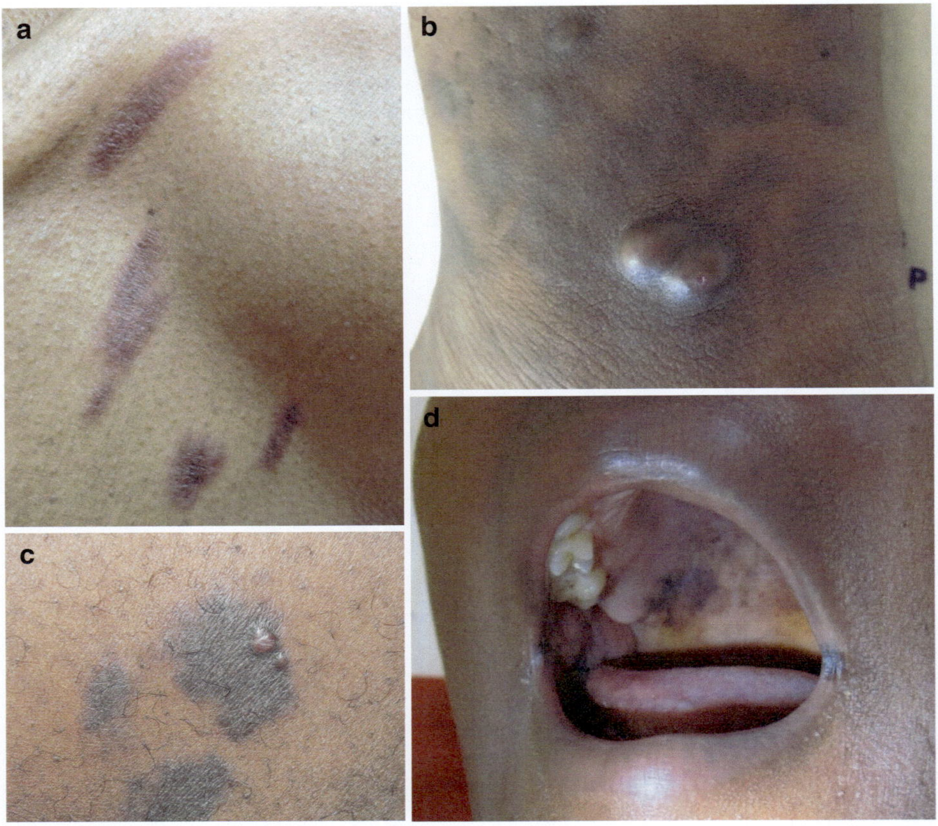

Fig. 36.1 Kaposi sarcoma: (**a**) Violaceous patches oriented along skin tension lines. (**b**) Nodular KS on a background of violaceous patches. (**c**) Violaceous patches with small vascular-appearing papules on the lower leg; the patient had striking edema due to KS involvement of the regional lymphatics. (**d**) KS will frequently involve the oral mucosa and GI tract, and it is important to examine the oropharynx; this is a palatal plaque of KS.

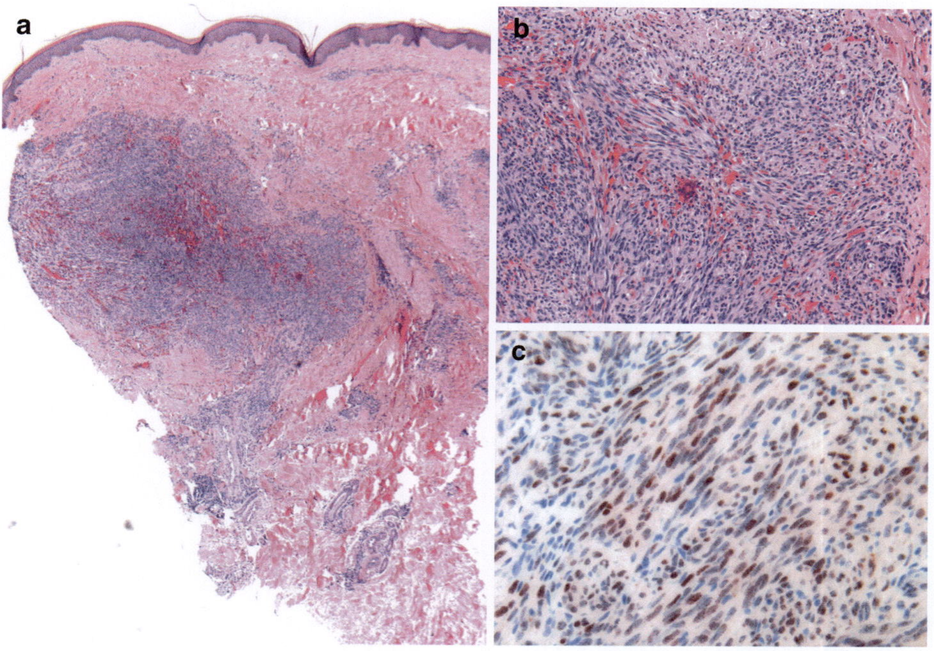

Fig. 36.2 Kaposi sarcoma (*1×, 10× H&E, 20× HHV8 IHC*): (**a**) Low power will demonstrate hemorrhage and increased cells within the dermis. (**b**) Higher power highlights spindled cells with increased blood vessel proliferation and red blood cell extravasation. The sandwich sign of having red blood cells between spindled cells is characteristic. (**c**) HHV8 is a specific immunohistochemical stain that can confirm the diagnosis.

Part VI

Infections: Fungal

Superficial Dermatophyte/Tinea

37

Amanda J. Tschetter

Overview

- Among the most common infectious diseases world-wide
- *Microsporum*, *Trichophyton* and *Epidermophyton*, the 'dermatophytes', comprise the three genera of fungi able to invade and thrive in keratinized tissue (hair, skin, and nails)
- Inflammation caused by dermatophyte invasion leads to considerable morbidity (pruritus, discomfort, and potentially secondary skin and soft-tissue infections)
- Regardless of causative species, dermtophytoses are named "tinea" followed by the Latin word for the affected site (e.g. tinea capitis, tinea corporis, tinea pedis)

Clinical Presentation

- Typically pruritic with varied appearance depending on causative organism and site infected
- **Tinea capitis** (scalp): mainly affects children with varying appearances
  - Mild, diffuse flaking
  - Black dot alopecia (broken-off hairs)
  - Circular alopecic patches with scale
  - Kerion (inflamed, boggy plaque)
  - Diffuse pustules
  - Tender occipital lymphadenopathy may occur and can be a useful clinical diagnostic clue
- **Tinea faciei** (face) & **barbae** (beard): disease of postpubertal boys & men
  - Appearance ranging from annular scaly patches to an erythematous pustular crusted eruption with potential kerion formation
- **Tinea corporis** (body, extremities to dorsal hands/feet): most common in children & young adults
  - Asymmetrically distributed annular, expanding, scaly erythematous patches (Fig. 37.1a)
  - Perifollicular papulopustules (**Majocchi's granuloma)** (Fig. 37.1b)
  - Vesicles and concentric rings (**tinea imbricata**) may be seen
- **Tinea cruris** (groin): "Jock itch", typically seen in adult men
  - Similar in presentation to tinea corporis, but scaling may be masked due to moisture.

A. J. Tschetter, MD
University of Minnesota Health, Minneapolis, MN, USA
e-mail: tschette@umn.edu

M. Rosenbach et al. (eds.), *Inpatient Dermatology*,
https://doi.org/10.1007/978-3-319-18449-4_37

- **Tinea manuum** (hand): most commonly a unilateral palmar infection
  - Typically seen on the dominant hand and seen in conjunction with tinea pedis ("one hand, two foot syndrome")
  - Palms appear xerotic with dry scale accentuating the creases
- **Tinea pedis** (foot): "Athlete's foot", typically affects adults, especially those wearing occlusive footwear (Fig. 37.1a)
  - Most commonly appears as maceration, scaling and fissures of the lateral interdigital webspaces extending medially as disease progresses
  - Moccasin (dry, diffuse scaling, erythema and plantar hyperkeratosis with fissures)
  - Inflammatory (vesicles and bullae of plantar insteps) and ulcerative patterns may be observed
- **Tinea unguium** (nails): onychomycosis caused by a dermatophyte, affects adult men more frequently than women
  - Toe nails significantly more frequently affected than finger nails (Fig. 37.1a)
  - 4 patterns: distal/lateral subungual (most common), proximal subungual (immunocompromised host), superficial white, and total dystrophic
  - Nail plate may be yellow or white, brittle or thickened with onycholysis, subungual hyperkeratosis, and ridging
- **Tinea incognito**: dermatophyte infection inadvertently treated with topical corticosteroids may lose the classic morphology complicating the clinical picture; face and trunk are common sites.
- **Majocchi granuloma:** when superficial dermatophyte infections are unrecognized and treated with topical steroids, local immunosuppression can allow the dermatophyte to penetrate deeper into the dermis,
  - Papules, pustules, and nodules
  - Often requires systemic medication to eradicate as not responsive to topical therapy (see below)
- **Dermatophytid** ("id") reaction: a diffuse, auto-eczematization reaction classically incited by inflammatory tinea pedis, but now known to occur with flares of other dermatididies; this manifests with an exuberant, often monomorphic, papular eczematous eruption which can be widespread due to circulating systemic inflammatory mediators in response to a localized, severe tinea infection

Histopathology

- Biopsy may be avoided if KOH exam/culture is positive (Fig. 37.2a)
- Histopathology demonstrating the characteristic organisms is the definitive diagnosis (Fig. 37.2b)
- Neutrophils within the stratum corneum are frequently seen; high power H&E examination of the narrow, compact eosinophilic layer of stratum corneum just above the granular layer may reveal round hyphae cut on end
- Periodic acid-Schiff (PAS) and silver stains (Grocott-methamine silver, GMS) highlight fungi

Differential Diagnosis

Based on site/pattern, the differential diagnosis may change; clinical morphology of annular erythematous patches with scale is suspicious for tinea, and generally KOH scraping demonstrating organisms is the preferred method to confirm dermatophyte infection in most cases

- Tinea capitis: Langerhans cell histiocytosis, folliculitis decalvans, central centrifugal cicatricial alopecia, alopecia areata
- Tinea corporis: Mycosis fungoides, secondary syphilis, erythema annulare centrifugum, cutaneous lupus erythematous (subacute and chronic), dermatitis (atopic, nummular, stasis, contact, seborrheic, dyshidrotic), psoriasis, lichen planus
- Tinea cruris: irritant dermatitis, Langerhans cell histiocytosis, Hailey-Hailey disease, candida infection, inverse psoriasis
- Tinea pedis: psoriasis, dermatitis
- Tinea unguium/Onychomycosis: pachyonychia congenita, trauma, Darier disease

Work-Up

- Tinea cruris, pedis, unguium and manuum frequently occur in conjunction so a total skin exam must be performed
- Potassium hydroxide (KOH) preparation: branching hyphae extending across keratinocytes (Fig. 37.2a)
- Chlorazol black E stain highlights fungal elements in KOH preps
- Wood lamp exam of tinea capitis will fluoresce yellow (*Microsporum* spp.) or blue-white (*Trichophyton schoenleinii*)
- Nail clipping with PAS stain for histopathologic examination or use of Calcofluor white
- Briskly brushing a disposable toothbrush over affected scalp and submitting the brush in a sterile container (urine cup) is an effective collection method for culture

Treatment

- Treatment is important as an active dermatophyte infection can lead to skin barrier dysfunction thus predisposing to bacterial superinfection and cellulitis or, if immunocompromised, systemic infections
- Simple tinea pedis/manuum/cruris/corporis may be treated topically
  - No difference in effectiveness between azoles and allylamines (terbinafine, naftifine)
  - Apply twice daily for 2–6 weeks, continuing for 2 weeks after clinical cure
  - With significant inflammation a low to moderate-potency corticosteroid may be added to aid clinical cure
- Dermatophytoses involving an extensive surface area, hairy skin, or with extensive inflammation will require systemic therapy for 2–4 weeks
- Tinea capitis must be treated systemically until culture is negative
  - Griseofulvin is more effective against *Microsporum* spp. infections
  - Terbinafine is more effective against *T. tonsurans,* the most common cause of tinea capitis in the US
  - Kerions may require an anti-inflammatory agent (prednisone) to prevent scarring and permanent alopecia
- Tinea unguium, aside from superficial white onychomycosis, necessitates systemic therapy. Duration depends upon finger vs. toe involvement and the agent used (terbinafine, fluconazole, griseofulvin, itraconazole)
- Majocchi granuloma may require systemic antifungal therapy
- Controlling predisposing factors helps prevent repeat infection (breathable shoes/socks, frequent replacement of footwear, avoiding exposures/trauma, treating underlying disease)

Suggested Readings

1. van Zuuren EJ, Fedorowicz Z, El-Gohary M. Evidence-based topical treatments for tinea cruris and tinea corporis: a summary of a Cochrane systematic review. Br J Dermatol. 2015;172(3):616–41.
2. Moriarty B, Hay R, Morris-Jones R. The diagnosis and management of tinea. BMJ. 2012;345:e4380.

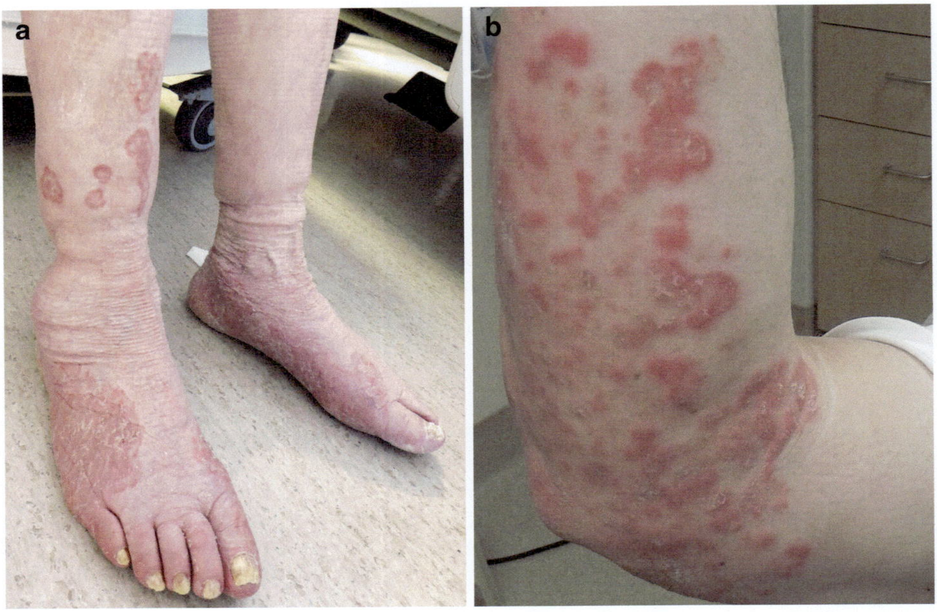

Fig. 37.1 Tinea skin infections/dermatophytosis. (**a**) Yellow, dystrophic nails (due to onychomycosis, or fungal infection of the nail plate) and erythematous, scaling, annular patches with serpiginous borders. (**b**) Inflammatory erythematous serpiginous plaques of superficial tinea corporis with indurated papules with rare pustules of Majocchi granuloma (deeper dermatophyte infection extending down hair follicles due to inappropriate treatment with topical corticosteroids).

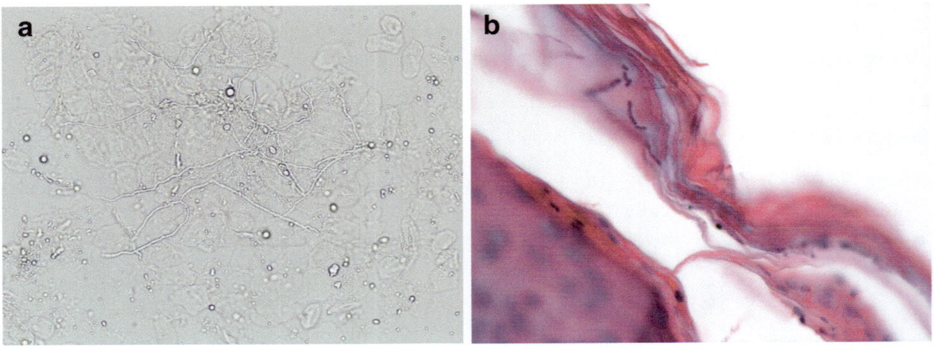

Fig. 37.2 Tinea corporis (KOH, *H&E 40×*). (**a**) Potassium hydroxide preparation demonstrates refractile, often branching hyphae. (**b**) On histopathology, collections of neutrophils with parakeratosis within the stratum can be a diagnostic clue. A superficial lymphocytic and neutrophilic infiltrate in the dermis with exocytosis can also be seen. Hyphae within the stratum corneum on H&E or highlighted on PAS stain is diagnostic.

Candidiasis

38

Badri Modi

Overview

- Opportunistic fungal infection most commonly associated with *Candida albicans*
  - *Candida albicans* commonly colonizes the skin, gastrointestinal and genitourinary tracts; can become pathogenic leading to superficial candidiasis in the setting of fungal overgrowth in a favorable environment (warm, moist, alkaline) or disseminated in an immunocompromised host
- **Superficial candidiasis** favors intertriginous areas (skin folds, axillae, inframammary, perianal, etc.—*see Intertrigo section);* can involve mucosal surfaces as is seen in oropharyngeal candidiasis (thrush)
- **Disseminated candidiasis** and sepsis can present in an immunosuppressed host including patients with HIV, malignancies (mainly leukemia or lymphoma), or patients on chronic immunosuppressive therapy
  - Risk factors for developing disseminated candidiasis include broad-spectrum antibacterial agents, central venous catheter, parenteral nutrition, renal replacement therapy, prolonged neutropenia, implantable prosthetic devices, immunosuppressive agents, prior surgery, IV drug use
- Rates of disseminated disease are decreasing because of widespread use of fungal prophylaxis in immunocompromised patients. However, this has also led to development of azole-resistant *Candida* species and other opportunistic fungal infections

Clinical Presentation

- **Superficial candidiasis:**
  - Oropharyngeal candidiasis (thrush): Gray to white plaques develop on an erythematous mucosal surface
  - Can be seen in a variety of settings:
    - Neonates exposed to candida during vaginal birth
    - Following the use of inhalers or antibiotics in otherwise healthy individuals
    - Immunocompromised patients
  - Vulvovaginal candidiasis: Pruritis and white thick discharge; vulvar swelling and erythema may be present and patients may experience dysuria

B. Modi, MD
Division of Dermatology, City of Hope, Duarte, CA, USA

M. Rosenbach et al. (eds.), *Inpatient Dermatology*,
https://doi.org/10.1007/978-3-319-18449-4_38

Increased risk with diabetes, antibiotic, steroid use, HIV, and elevated estrogen states (pregnancy, oral contraceptive pill (OCP) use)
  - Balanitis: Candidial plaques with associated pruritus involving the penis; may extend to the scrotum, thigh, or buttocks (Fig. 38.1)
- **Disseminated candidiasis:**
  - Often identified in patients who are febrile or deteriorating with an unidentified source and failing to respond to broad spectrum antibacterial coverage
  - Skin lesions may be single or multiple, localized or disseminated but are present in <20% of cases
    They range from erythematous papules to translucent pseudovesicles, frank pustules, papulonodules, and necrotic eschars; pink-red dermal papules are frequently seen
    In patients unable to mount an immune response, skin lesions may take the form of macular erythema or cellulitis, occasionally with skip areas
  - Meningitis, endocarditis, pericarditis, renal failure, and pneumonia are among the complications associated with visceral invasion
    Diffuse muscle tenderness may occur due to candidal abscesses and pyomyositis
  - Endophthalmitis may present as blurred vision and is a distinct complication of candidemia (Fig. 38.2)

Histopathology

- KOH touch prep may be useful for rapid diagnosis: may demonstrate pseudohyphae and spores
- Biopsy the center of a lesion, pustule, or necrotic area to increase the yield
  - **Superficial:** Candida can be visualized in the stratum corneum as round to ovoid spores and typically vertically oriented pseudo-hyphae (tinea tends to run horizontally)
  - **Disseminated:** Organisms may be seen as septic emboli within blood vessels and may invade perivascular dermal tissue with or without associated vasculitis
- PAS or Grocott (GMS) stain will aid in visualization of the organisms

Differential Diagnosis

- Disseminated varicella zoster or herpes infection: often clusters of true vesicles or punched out erosions, sometimes in a single region or dermatome
- Miliaria rubra: often more pruritic, excoriated lesions, limited to the back in immobilized patients
- Morbilliform drug eruption: demonstrate blanchable erythema, versus the fixed pink-red deeper papular lesions of disseminated candidiasis
- Bacterial cellulitis: candida cellulitis can be hard to distinguish, but is often a duller-brown color with deeper induration, but the differences can be subtle and biopsy is important (Fig. 38.3)

Work-Up

- **Superficial candidiasis:**
  - Clinical diagnosis is often sufficient; KOH preps or rarely superficial cultures can confirm the diagnosis
- **Disseminated Candidiasis:**
  - Blood cultures from peripheral veins and central venous catheters
  - Urinalysis and urine culture may reveal dissemination to the kidneys
  - Various imaging modalities to look for other sites of involvement as indicated by clinical symptomatology: i.e. echocardiogram, brain MRI
  - Ophthalmologic examination to rule out endophthalmitis, which may additional treatment and longer duration of antifungal therapy
    Exam should occur when candidemia is identified and after the blood-stream infection has been controlled, particularly as the patient's white blood cell counts recover
    Neutropenic patients may not manifest symptoms of endophthalmitis until after counts recover

Table 38.1 General pattern of candida species susceptibility[a]

Species	Fluconazole	Itraconazole	Voriconazole	Posaconazole	Flucytosine	Amp-B	Candins
C. albicans	S	S	S	S	S	S	S
C. tropicalis	S	S	S	S	S	S	S
C. parapsilosis	S	S	S	S	S	S	S to R
C. glabrata	S-DD to R	S-DD to R	S-DD to R	S-DD to R	S	S to I	S
C. krusei	R	S-DD to R	S	S	I to R	S to I	S
C. lusitaniae	S	S	S	S	S	S to R	S

[a]Adapted from IDSA 2009 guidelines for management of candidiasis
S sensitive, *R* resistant, *S-DD* susceptible dose-dependent, *I* intermediately susceptible

Treatment

- **Superficial candidiasis:**
  - While topical nystatin is effective, generally the authors recommend a topical—azole antifungal to treat for both yeast and dermatophytes, which are frequent co-infectors
  - Mucosal involvement may require special formulations, such as troches for the mouth
- **Disseminated candidiasis:**
  - Generally, fluconazole is an effective option, but it depends on the immune status of the patient and prior anti-fungal exposures (Table 38.1)

Suggested Readings

1. Pappas PG, et al. Clinical practice guidelines for the management of candidiasis: 2009 update by the infectious disease society of America. Clin Infect Dis. 2009;48:503–35.
2. Grossman ME, et al. Candidiasis. In: Cutaneous manifestations of infections in the immunocompromised host. 2nd ed. New York: Springer; 2012. p. 12–9.

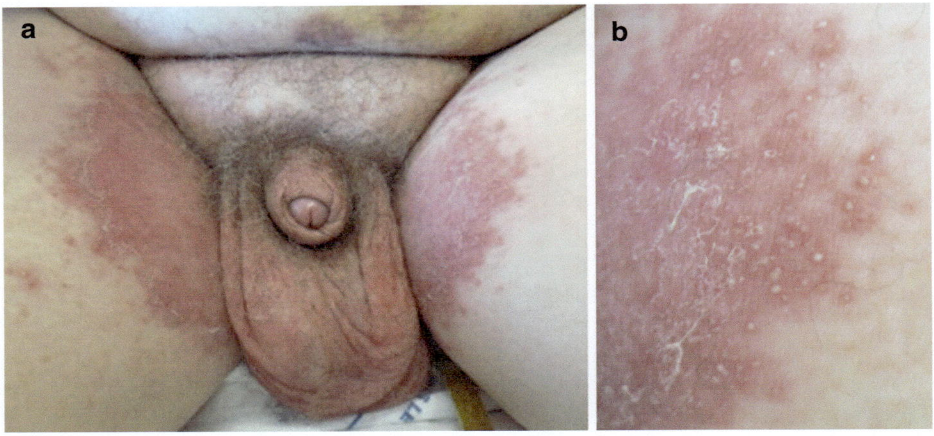

Fig. 38.1 Candida skin infection: (**a**) Candidal intertrigo: Bright red inguinal erythema with satellite papules and pustules consistent with candida intertrigo. Involvement of the scrotum is characteristic of candida but not dermatophyte infection. (**b**) The edges of candidal infections often show "satellite pustules" from lesions just beyond the edge of the main infection.

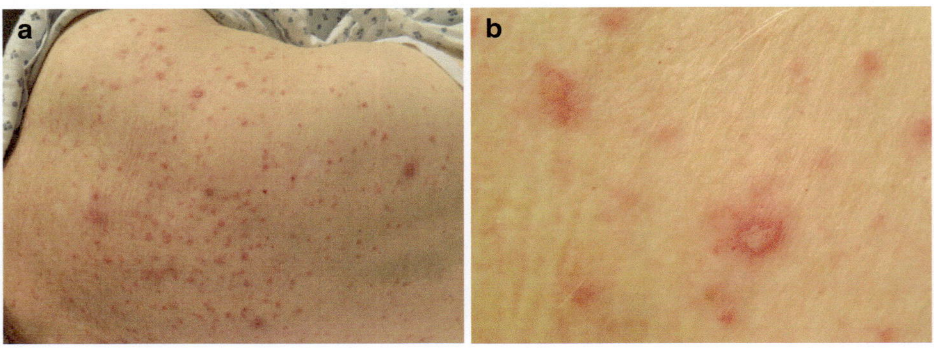

Fig. 38.2 Disseminated candidiasis: (**a**) Disseminated red dermal-based papules, with scattered pustules and incipient, pseudopustules. (**b**) Close-up of a red papule with incipient pustule, or pseudovesicle.

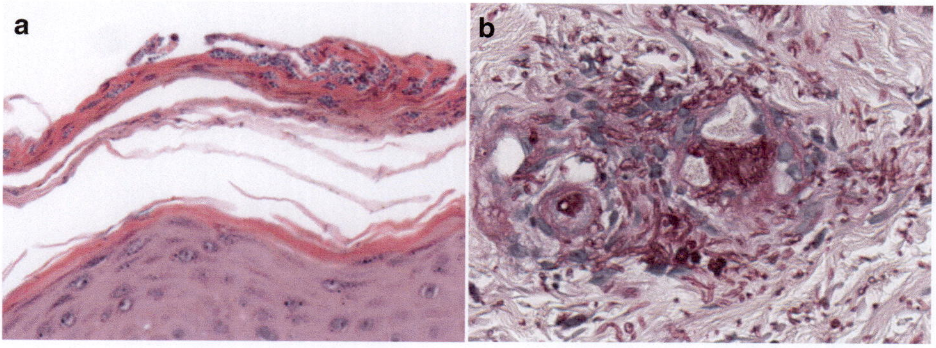

Fig. 38.3 Candidiasis (*20×; H&E; 40×; periodic acid–Schiff*): The first image (H&E, 20x) is of superficial candidiasis. Neutrophils in the upper region of the epidermis including the stratum corneum, sometimes forming spongiotic pustules, can be a clue to the presence of Candida. Spores are easily seen on H&E, but PAS and Grocott/GMS stains may be used to better visualize fungal elements (not shown here). (**a**) In disseminated candidiasis, there are dense dermal neutrophilic microabscesses, often focused around blood vessels (not shown). Yeast forms are best seen on special stains such as GMS or PAS. This high power PAS image demonstrates aggregates of hyphae/pseudophyphae and spores within vessels and infiltrating the dermis (**b**).

Angioinvasive Fungal Infections

39

Sasha Stephen

Overview

- Acute, rapidly evolving, often fatal infections due to vasculotropic invasive mycoses, such as *Aspergillus* (*flavus, fumigatus, niger*), *Fusarium (solani, oxysporum, verticilioides)*, and Zygomycetes (*Mucor, Rhizopus, Rhizomucor,* and more)
- The causal organisms are ubiquitous molds common in soil, decomposing plant and animal matter, as well as air
- Primary cutaneous infections are caused by direct inoculation and secondary cutaneous infections are due to hematogenous dissemination of systemic infection
- **Primary inoculation** has been reported as a result of contaminated bandages or nosocomial infection, such as at sites of intravenous cannulas/tape, and can occur following colonization of burns, surgical sites, or other areas of skin disruption
  - It is more often seen in children and immunocompetent adults
- **Disseminated disease** is usually seen in the immunosuppressed setting, such as: bone marrow or solid organ transplant, prolonged neutropenia, GVHD, HIV/AIDS, iatrogenic immunosuppression, poorly controlled diabetes mellitus, burns, chronic renal failure, severe malnutrition, hematologic malignancies (especially AML), and immune reconstitution syndrome

Clinical Presentation

- Lesions typically present as tender rapidly enlarging bright red to purple papulonodules which rapidly develop areas of ischemic necrosis, ulcers, and/or hemorrhagic bullae, which may be accompanied by purpura, erythema, warmth, and induration (Fig. 39.1)
- Tissue infarction can occur from trauma associated with an inoculation injury or ischemic damage from septic fungal emboli
  - Palatal or sinus necrosis may manifest as black eschars with facial pain and swelling

S. Stephen, MD
Department of Dermatology, Perelman School of Medicine at the University of Pennsylvania, Philadelphia, PA, USA
e-mail: sasha.stephen@uphs.upenn.edu

M. Rosenbach et al. (eds.), *Inpatient Dermatology*,
https://doi.org/10.1007/978-3-319-18449-4_39

- *Aspergillus* may present with a pulmonary "fungus ball" and sinusitis; it may colonize an eschar in severe burns or surgical sites and invade surrounding tissue
  - May see dispersed cutaneous lesions in the setting of invasive pulmonary disease secondary to embolic spread; these can present with angulated dusky purpuric papules with dark centers at distal sites
- Zygomycosis infections can present with a targetoid "bull's eye" lesion with central ulcer or hemorrhagic bulla surrounded by a necrotic or violaceous border; the violaceous/purpuric rim is often studded with black, necrotic flecks from tissue ischemia
  - Mucormycosis presents with 5 clinical forms: (1) rhinocerebral, (2) pulmonary, (3) cutaneous, (4) gastrointestinal and (5) disseminated

    Sinus invasion is most common followed by pulmonary and cutaneous infection; cutaneous and gastrointestinal involvement are more common in children

Histopathology

- Touch preps or frozen biopsy specimens may be rapidly performed to visualize the characteristic hyphae
- Biopsy should be performed near the edge of the necrotic ulcer
- Hyphal elements may be best visualized within blood vessel lumens
- *Aspergillus* and *Fusarium* display septate hyphae with 45° acute-angle branching (Fig. 39.2)
- Zygomycetes display non-septate thick walled hyphae with 90° right angle branching and a hollow, circular-tubular ("ribbon-like") appearance on cross section (Fig. 39.3)
- Tissue culture is required for definitive species identification

Differential Diagnosis

- Ecthyma gangrenosum: can be clinically similar and both entities represent emergencies which need empiric treatment and rapid diagnostic testing
- Cellulitis: more broad, pink-red inflammation usually without the black/necrotic findings of angioinvasive infections
- Calciphylaxis: more chronic, thus often forms a thick eschar, though the angulated purpuric edges of calciphylaxis can resemble endovascular infection
- Vasculitis/vasculopathy: embolic fungal infection within vessels can resemble both a small vessel vasculitis or a vasculopathic process; these findings in a suppressed host warrant rapid diagnostic testing
- Sweet syndrome: typical lesions are rounder, more well-demarcated, and more edematous than those of angioinvasive fungus
- Leukemia cutis: typically purple dermal-based papules usually without dusky necrosis

Work-Up

- Concern for angioinvasive fungal infection represents a true medical emergency, and expedited diagnosis is critical
- Touch prep or biopsy for frozen section with fungal staining
- A biopsy for histopathologic examination and for tissue culture, which is imperative for identification of fungal species, should be performed
  - Deep biopsies should be performed to aid in differentiation of superficial and invasive infection
- Evaluation for intravascular dissemination with blood cultures and measurement of biologic markers, such as the galactomannan *Aspergillus* antigen and the fungal wall component (1–3)-β-D-glucan, if available, should be performed
- Chest, sinus, and brain imaging with CT scans should be considered if there is no evidence of systemic infection to direct treatment

Treatment

- Mortality remains high; patients require rapid, coordinated, multidisciplinary care, including immediately consultation with an infectious disease expert
- Treatment is dependent on primary cutaneous or disseminated nature of disease and the specific organism; it is important to be aware of potential co-fungal infections
- Primary cutaneous inoculations have the highest chance of cure with rapid, wide surgical debridement and broad spectrum antifungal therapy, usually with amphotericin B
  - Intraoperative frozen-sections during surgery may be used to assure clear excision margins
- Amphotericin B should be used for initial treatment of disseminated infections
  - Other antifungal agents include: Voriconazole, which is effective for *Aspergillus* species, itraconazole, posaconazole, and caspofungin also may be used, but not effective against all Zygomycetes
- Colony stimulating factors and other forms of aggressive supportive care have limited evidence but may be used to augment the immune response in appropriate clinical settings
- All patients should be managed in concert with an experienced infectious disease physician

Suggested Readings

1. Galimberti R, et al. Emerging systemic fungal infections. Clin Dermatol. 2012;30(6):633–50.
2. Skiada A, et al. Diagnosis and treatment of mucormycosis in patients with hematological malignancies: guidelines from the 3rd European Conference on Infections in Leukemia (ECIL 3). Haematologica. 2013;98(4):492–504.
3. Perfect JR. The impact of the host on fungal infections. Am J Med. 2012;125(1 Suppl):S39–51.
4. Rubin AI, Grossman ME. Bull's-eye cutaneous infarct of zygomycosis: a bedside diagnosis confirmed by touch preparation. J Am Acad Dermatol. 2004;51(6):996–1001.
5. Petrikkos G, et al. Epidemiology and clinical manifestations of mucormycosis. Clin Infect Dis. 2012;54:S23–34.

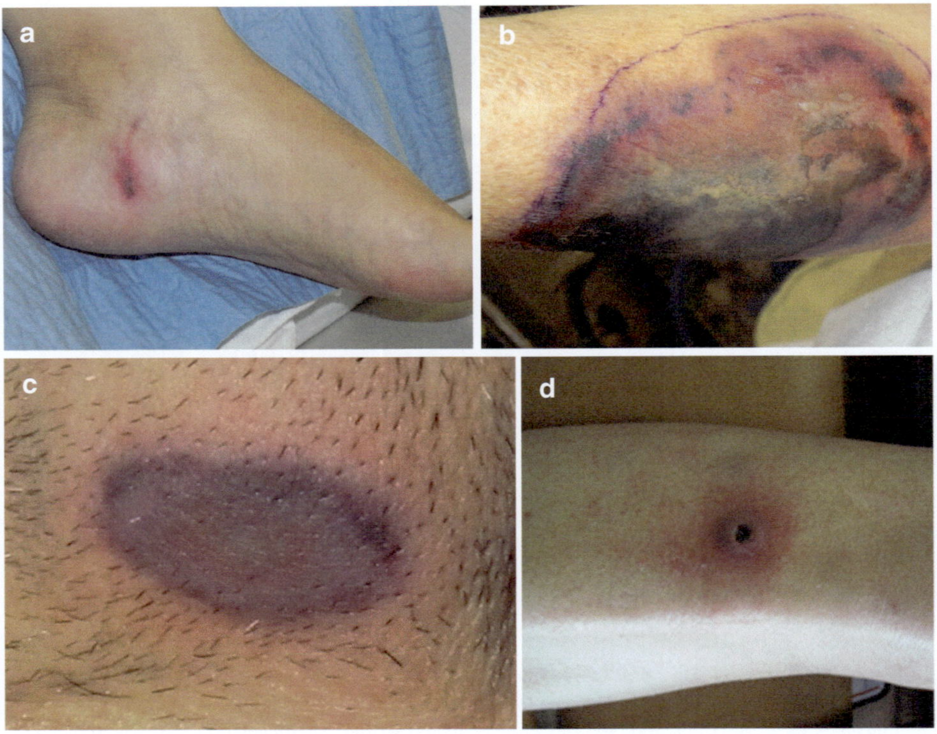

Fig. 39.1 Angioinvasive fungal infections: (**a**) Violaceous angulated purpuric and centrally necrotic plaque of embolic angioinvasive fungus in a patient with an intraaortic abscess. (**b**) "Bull's eye" lesion of zygomycosis (mucormycosis). The center is necrotic gray tissue, rimmed by violaceous discoloration studded with necrotic patches due to tissue ischemia from intravascular occlusion by spreading mold. (**c**) Bull's eye lesion of mucormycosis in a patient with acute myelogenous leukemia; the intravascular growth leads to downstream ischemia and tissue necrosis. (**d**) Violaceous nodule with necrotic center due to angioinvasive fungal infection.

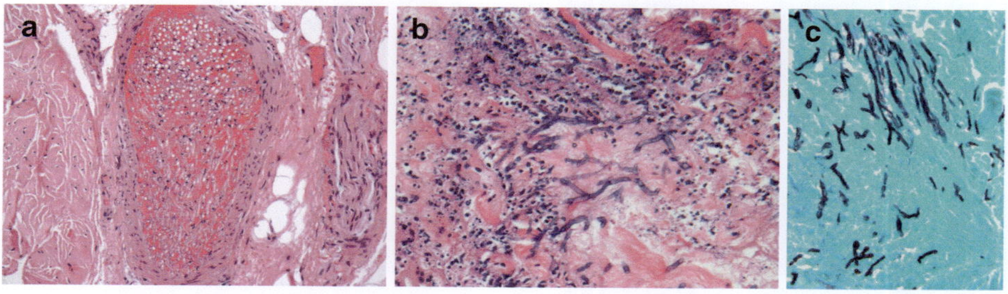

Fig. 39.2 Aspergillosis (*10×, 40×: H&E; 20× GMS*): (**a**) On lower power, histopathology often demonstrates dermal hemorrhage with a pauci-inflammatory infiltrate. (**b**) On higher power, organisms within and surrounding vessels is diagnostic. (**c**) For aspergillus, septate, narrow hyphae with acute angle (45°) branching is diagnostic and organisms can be better visualized with GMS. Histopathology alone generally should not be used to speciate fungal organisms; culture is essential to identify the species.

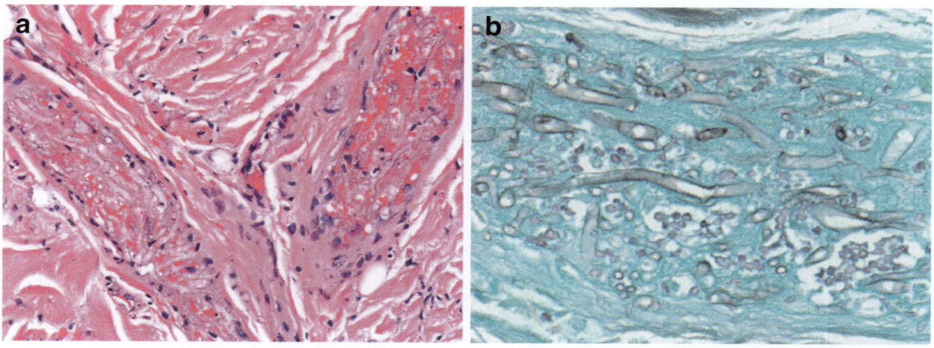

Fig. 39.3 Mucormycosis (*10×; H&E; 40×; grocott*): (**a**) On low power, there are prominent fungal elements within blood vessels. (**b**) A GMS was performed to highlight and better characerize the fungal forms (shown on the right). Note the broad "ribbon-like" non-septate hyphae with wide-angle branching. Tissue cultures speciated the fungus as Zygomycetes.

Histoplasmosis

40

Nkanyezi N. Ferguson

Overview

- Granulomatous infection caused by the dimorphic fungus, *Histoplasma capsulatum* var. *capsulatum*
- Worldwide distribution with prevalence in the Mississippi and Ohio River Valleys in the United States
- Found in soil and vegetal detritus contaminated by bird and bat droppings with acquisition via aerosol inhalation or less commonly via direct innoculation
- Risk factors include immunocompromised host and occupations with exposure to high risk environments
- Immunocompromised individuals are more likely to develop disseminated disease to various extrapulmonary locations (e.g. liver, spleen, lymph nodes, bone marrow, skin, CNS, adrenal glands)
  - Fever, malaise, loss of appetite and fatigue are common nonspecific presenting symptoms
  - Cutaneous involvement is uncommon (~5% of cases, may be higher in severely immunosuppressed hosts) but is a helpful diagnostic clue when present

Clinical Presentation

- In the majority of cases the infection is asymptomatic or mild with a self-limited course
- Characterized by three different forms—namely pulmonary, primary cutaneous, and disseminated disease, the latter of which is severe
- Primary cutaneous histoplasmosis due to direct inoculation is uncommon and presents as an isolated ulcer with regional lymphadenopathy that self-resolves
- Secondary cutaneous histoplasmosis seen in disseminated disease is due to hematogenous spread and is characterized by diverse skin morphology including papules, plaques, nodules, umbilicated papules, acneiform, abscess, cellulitis, pyoderma gangrenosum-like lesions or painful mucocutaneous ulcers (Fig. 40.1)
  - Areas of involvement include the face, extremities, trunk, and mucosa (especially oral)

N. N. Ferguson, MD
University of Iowa Hospital and Clinics, Iowa City, IA, USA
e-mail: nkanyezi-ferguson@uiowa.edu

M. Rosenbach et al. (eds.), *Inpatient Dermatology*,
https://doi.org/10.1007/978-3-319-18449-4_40

- Depending on organ involvement in disseminated disease symptomatology will vary but may include: petechiae, easy bruising, fatigue, weakness (thrombocytopenia and anemia from bone marrow involvement), hepatomegaly, splenomegaly, lymphadenopathy, altered mental status, photophobia, headache (CNS involvement)

Histopathology

- A varying degree of inflammation is seen characterized by a granulomatous, lymphocytic and/or a mononuclear infiltrate (Fig. 40.2)
- Yeast forms are 2–4 microns in size, often elongated, may demonstrate narrow budding, can have a peripheral rim of clearing
- Organisms are often parasitized by macrophages
- Yeast forms are highlighted by periodic acid-Schiff (PAS), Gomori-Grocott, or silver methenamine (GMS) stains

Differential Diagnosis

In all cases, travel history and exposure history is essential in narrowing the diagnosis; pathologic findings are often diagnostic and biopsy should be considered if any of these entities are suspected.

- Blastomycosis: may see larger lesions with a raised, crusted border with or without ulceration
- Coccidioidomycosis: there may be clinical overlap, but pathology is different and diagnostic
- Cryptococcosis: may have varied clinical presentations and can overlap with histoplasmosis skin findings; biopsy, culture, and serologic testing are helpful
- Paracoccidioidomycosis: lesions may be larger crusted nodules, but biopsy is diagnostic
- Leishmaniasis: bite-site crusted ulcers, which may be grouped, and frequently involve the ear can be helpful; be cautious with pathology as both leish and histo can look similar
- Tuberculosis: can be varied depending on if primary cutaneous involvement or a tuberculid response; pathologic findings are diagnostic

Work-Up

- A thorough history and physical exam should be obtained including evaluation of mucosal sites (oral and perianal)
- Histopathologic evaluation of a punch biopsy from a representative skin lesion should be performed
- Culture is considered the gold standard with an incubation time of 3–6 weeks
- Antigen testing of urine, serum, bronchial lavage or CSF is sensitive for acute disseminated and pulmonary histoplamsosis, but there is cross-reactivity with Paracoccidioides and Blastomyces
- Hypercalcemia has been described, which may be nonspecific (present in many granulomatous diseases)
- Evaluation for disseminated disease should be targeted based on potential organs of involvement
  - CBC: leukopenia, thrombocytopenia, anemia (bone marrow/spleen involvement)
  - Peripheral blood smear review to visualize the organism (Wright's stain)
  - CMP: abnormal AST, ALT, bilirubin
  - Chest x-ray: typically will show diffuse interstitial or reticulonodular pulmonary infiltrates
  - Abdominal CT (assess for enlarged liver, spleen, lymph node)
  - Brain CT/MRI, lumbar puncture (CNS involvement)
  - Endoscopy: Visualize GI lesions

Treatment

- Treatment choice is based on disease severity and underlying comorbidities
- Amphotericin B is the agent of choice for induction therapy for severe disease
- Itraconazole is preferred for mild to moderate disease and is commonly used for maintenance therapy
- If conventional treatment fails additional options include voriconazole or posaconazole
- Patients with HIV/AIDS may require additional management and infectious disease experts should be consulted

Suggested Readings

1. Chang P, Rodas C. Skin lesions in histoplasmosis. Clin Dermatol. 2012;30(6):592–8.
2. Fernandez-Flores A, Saeb-Lima M, Arenas-Guzman R. Morphological findings of deep cutaneous fungal infections. Am J Dermatopathol. 2014;36(7):531–53.
3. Gupta V, Singhal V, Singh MK, Xess I, Ramam M. Disseminated histoplasmosis with hypercalcemia. J Am Acad Dermatol. 2013;69(5):e250–1.

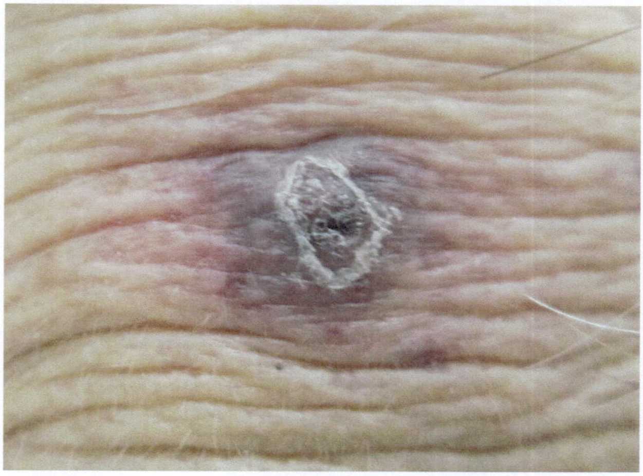

Fig. 40.1 Cutaneous histoplasmosis: Necrotic verrucous violaceous plaque on the forehead.

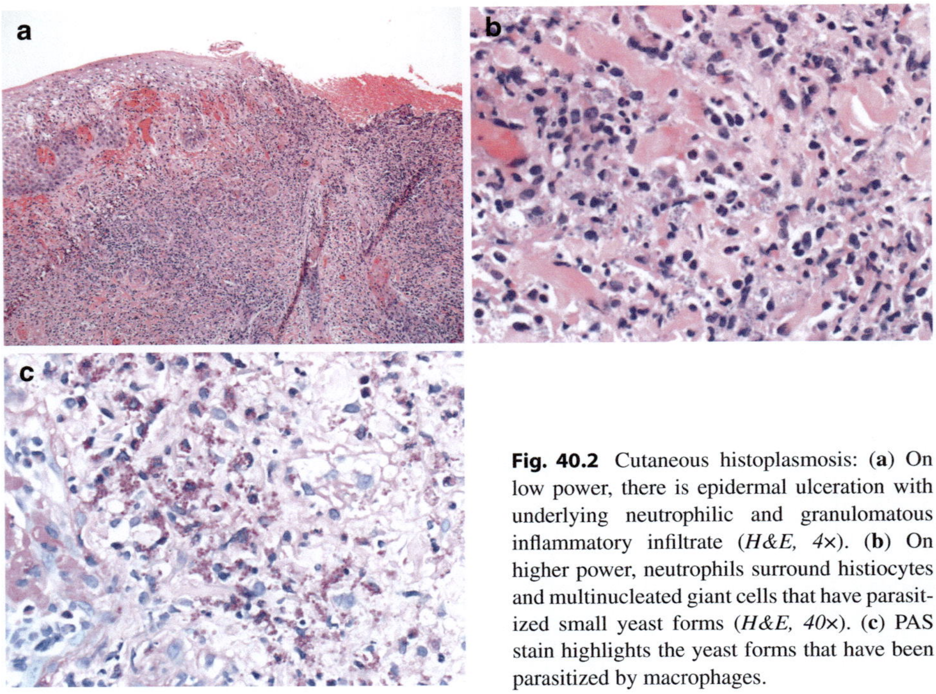

Fig. 40.2 Cutaneous histoplasmosis: (**a**) On low power, there is epidermal ulceration with underlying neutrophilic and granulomatous inflammatory infiltrate (*H&E, 4*×). (**b**) On higher power, neutrophils surround histiocytes and multinucleated giant cells that have parasitized small yeast forms (*H&E, 40*×). (**c**) PAS stain highlights the yeast forms that have been parasitized by macrophages.

Coccidioidomycosis

41

Katherine T. Steele

Overview

- Caused by the dimorphic fungus *Coccidioides (C. immitis* and *C. posadasii*), which is endemic to the Southwestern United States ("San Joaquin Valley fever"), Mexico, and Central and South America
- Inhalation of fungal spores causes a primary pulmonary infection in the majority of individuals living in endemic areas; although typically asymptomatic, approximately 40% will develop flu-like symptoms
- Dissemination following primary pulmonary infection occurs in less than 1% of cases and typically in an immunocompromised host
  - The most commonly involved sites in disseminated disease are the skin, bones and meninges

Clinical Presentation

- Primary pulmonary infection is asymptomatic in the majority of affected individuals, but flu-like symptoms, including fevers, chills, night sweats, fatigue, myalgias, headache, cough and pleuritic pain, may occur within several weeks of exposure
- Cutaneous manifestations of disseminated coccidioidomycosis are highly variable and include papules, pustules, plaques, abscesses or ulcerations (Fig. 41.1)
  - Scalp and face involvement, classically on the nasolabial folds is common, but may occur anywhere on the body
  - A nonspecific diffuse macular eruption may be seen early in the disease
- Associated erythema nodosum on the lower extremities has been reported
- Primary cutaneous coccidioidomycosis rarely can occur as a result of direct inoculation
  - These lesions may appear as a firm painless papulonodule with or without ulceration and may develop sporotrichoid lymphangitic nodules

K. T. Steele, MD
Department of Dermatology, Perelman School of Medicine at the University of Pennsylvania, Philadelphia, PA, USA
e-mail: katherine.steele2@uphs.upenn.edu

M. Rosenbach et al. (eds.), *Inpatient Dermatology*,
https://doi.org/10.1007/978-3-319-18449-4_41

Histopathology

- Key histopathologic features include a mixed suppurative granulomatous reaction with histiocytes, lymphocytes, neutrophils and giant cells; eosinophils also can be seen (Fig. 41.2)
  - Endospore-containing spherules measuring 5–75 μm, usually in the papillary dermis but can be found throughout the dermis (Fig. 41.2)
  - Sporangia, containing numerous endospores and measuring up to 300 μm, can also be seen
- Special stains: Periodic acid Schiff (PAS), Grocott's methenamine silver (GMS) can highlight the organisms

Differential Diagnosis

In all cases, travel history and exposure history is essential in narrowing the diagnosis; pathologic findings are often diagnostic and biopsy should be considered if any of these entities are suspected.

- Blastomycosis: may see larger lesions with a raised, crusted border with or without ulceration
- Histoplasmosis: variable and nonspecific; histopathology may be diagnostic
- Cutaneous tuberculosis: can be varied depending on if primary cutaneous involvement or a tuberculid response; pathologic findings are diagnostic
- Cryptococcosis: may have varied clinical presentations; biopsy, culture, and serologic testing are helpful
- Leishmaniasis: bite-site crusted ulcers, which may be grouped, and frequently involve the ear can be helpful
- Sarcoidosis: violaceous indurated papules and plaques clustered around the nares, perioral/periorbital region, scars, and tattoos

Essential Work-Up

- Biopsy for histology and tissue culture
- Bloodwork:
  - CBC with differential (assess for leukocytosis, eosinophils)
  - CMP (baseline LFTs before starting Fluconazole)
  - *Coccidioides* antibody titers (IgG and IgM) by complement fixation (IgG and IgM) at diagnosis and serially to monitor response to treatment
  - Consider HIV screening testing, T-cell panel to assess for immunodeficiency
- Imaging:
  - Chest radiograph may demonstrate hilar adenopathy or pulmonary infiltrates consistent with pneumonia
  - Consider bone scan if high *Coccidioides* antibody titers, given propensity for dissemination to bone
- If neurologic symptoms or vertebral lesions on bone scan, consider brain imaging and lumbar puncture

Treatment

- Primary cutaneous lesions typically heal without treatment
- Disseminated disease requires prolonged systemic antifungal therapy
  - First line therapy: Fluconazole
  - Other azoles may also be used: Itraconazole, Voriconazole, Posaconazole
- For severe, progressive or meningeal disease: combination of Amphotericin B and Fluconazole

Prolonged antifungal therapy may be required and differs based on host factors (HIV, comorbidities) and should be determined in conjunction with an infectious disease physician.

Suggested Reading

1. Carpenter JB, Feldman JS, Leyva WH, DiCaudo DJ. Clinical and pathologic characteristics of disseminated coccidioidomycosis. J Am Acad Dermatol. 2010;62(5):831–7.
2. Galgiani JN, Ampel NM, Blair JE, et al. Coccidioidomycosis. Clin Infect Dis. 2005;41:1217.
3. Welsh O, Vera-Cabrera L, Rendon A, et al. Coccidiodomycosis. Clin Dermatol. 2012;30:573–91.

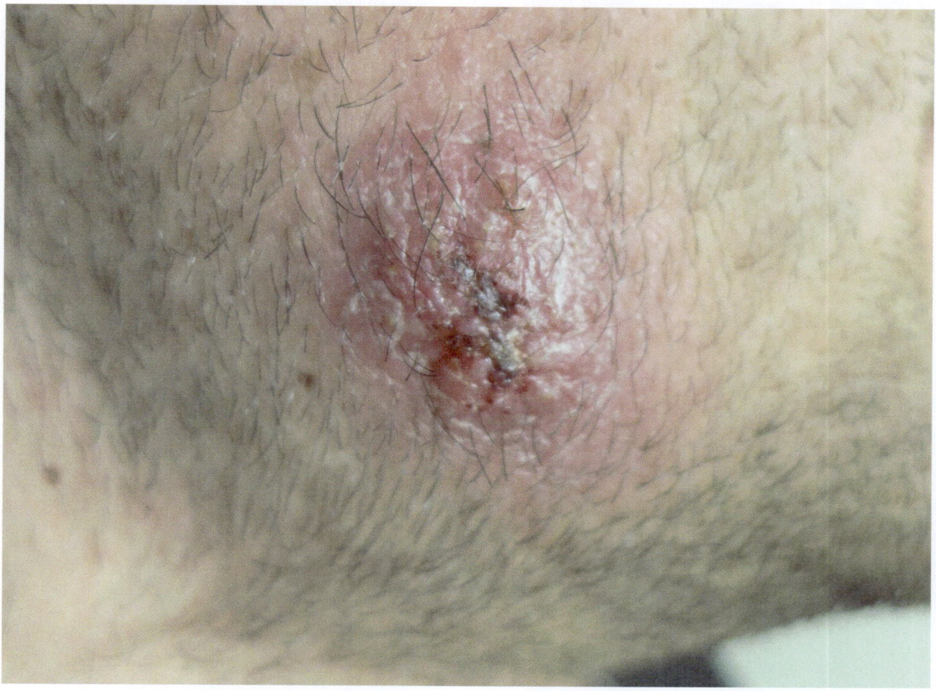

Fig. 41.1 Coccidiodomycosis: Crusted erythematous plaque of disseminated coccidioidomycosis after travel to the Southwest US.

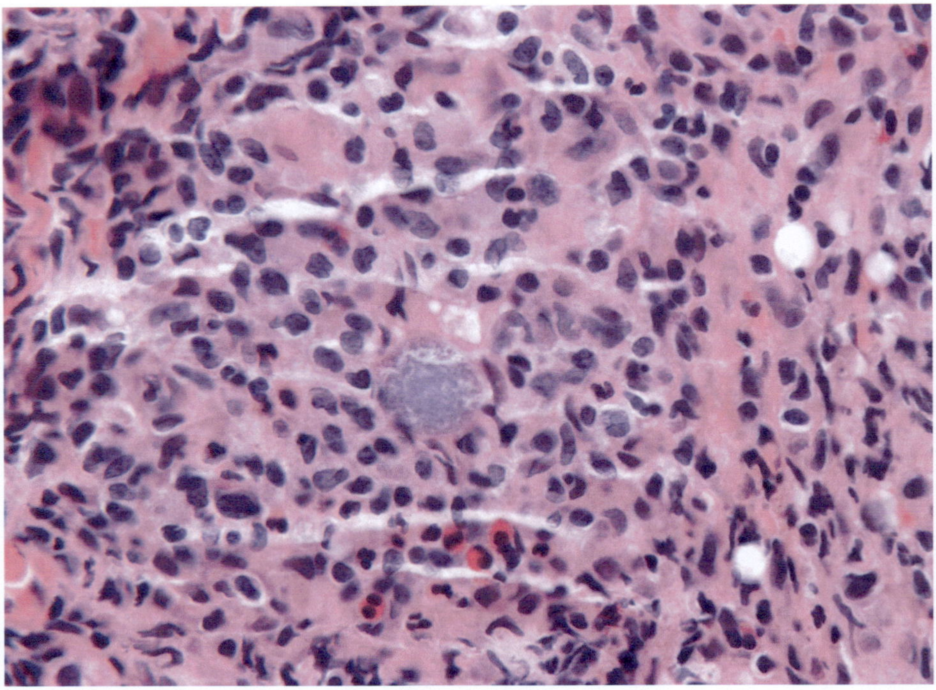

Fig. 41.2 Coccidiodomycosis (*20×, H&E*): Histopathology demonstrates both acute and chronic inflammation with neutrophils, eosinophils, and histiocytes. *Coccidioides immitis* is a variably sized organism with spherules that range in size from 10 to 70 μm in diameter with endospores. PAS and GMS stains highlight these organisms.

Blastomycosis

42

Amanda J. Tschetter

Overview

- Caused by the dimorphic fungus, *Blastomyces dermatitidis* which inhabits the soil
- Infections are endemic to U.S. Southern and Southeastern states bordering the Mississippi River and Ohio River valleys, the Midwestern states and Canadian provinces bordering the Great Lakes, and areas of South Africa and Zimbabwe
- Male gender, low socioeconomic status, outdoor occupations/recreations, and diabetes are risk factors for pulmonary and disseminated disease
- Immunocompromised patients (AIDS, sarcoidosis, organ transplantation, long-term corticosteroid therapy, etc) are at risk for severe, progressive disease with early systemic dissemination, CNS involvement, relapses, and an increased mortality despite therapy
- Skin is the most common organ affected by extrapulmonary blastomycosis and lesions occur via dissemination or through primary inoculation

Clinical Presentation

- Primary pulmonary blastomycosis is the most frequent form, as most infections are acquired via inhalation, with presentations ranging from asymptomatic infection to frank pneumonia, high fevers, weight loss, chest pain, fevers and acute respiratory distress syndrome (ARDS)
- Self-resolving papules, pustules and regional lymphadenopathy can be seen in primary cutaneous blastomycosis following direct inoculation (penetrating injury with contaminated soil, laboratory accident, dog bite); multiple nodules may develop overlying infected lymphatic channels (Fig. 42.1)
- Skin lesions more frequently occur from systemic dissemination than from primary cutaneous inoculation, are present in up to 80% of cases, and may be the presenting symptom
  - Cutaneous manifestations vary greatly and include scaly papules and pustules (Fig. 42.1), ulcerated verrucous and vegetative plaques, and fungating tumors
  - Oral and nasal mucosa involvement presents with ulcers or friable lesions
  - Lesions often expand peripherally and heal with central atrophy or cribiform scarring

A. J. Tschetter, MD
University of Minnesota Health, Minneapolis, MN, USA
e-mail: tschette@umn.edu

M. Rosenbach et al. (eds.), *Inpatient Dermatology*,
https://doi.org/10.1007/978-3-319-18449-4_42

- Bone involvement (long bones, vertebrae, ribs, cranium, sacrum) is variable and may present as osteomyelitis and, rarely, septic arthritis; subcutaneous abscesses may develop from direct extension from infected bone
- Central nervous system dissemination (meningitis, abscess, granuloma) occurs in 5–10% of cases
- Genitourinary disease (10–30% of cases) most commonly involves the prostate, testicles and epididymis with organisms found in prostatic fluid; sexual transmission has been reported

Histopathology

- Large punch biopsy or incisional biopsy is often necessary
- *B. dermatitidis* yeasts are 8–15 µm round to oval organisms with thick, refractile double-walls that demonstrate broad-based budding (Fig. 42.2)
- Prominent pseudoepitheliomatous hyperplasia and intraepidermal pustules (Fig. 42.2) are characteristic
- Histopathologic findings depend on the time course and immune status of the patient
  - Early lesions/low immunity: neutrophils and many organisms
  - Late lesions/strong immunity: noncaseating granulomas, epithelioid histiocytes and giant cells with few organisms
- Stains: periodic acid-Schiff (PAS) and Grocott-Gomori methanamine silver (GMS) allow better visualization of organisms

Differential Diagnosis

In all cases, a travel and exposure history is essential in narrowing the diagnosis; pathologic findings are often diagnostic and biopsy should be considered if any of these entities are suspected.

- Dimorphic fungal infections (coccidioidomycosis, histoplasmosis, paracoccidioidomycosis): specific travel history is helpful, but with clinical overlap a biopsy is often necessary
- Tuberculosis: verrucous lesions of cutaneous TB can share some overlap, but biopsy will be diagnostic
- Mycobacterial infection: morphology may vary by type, but crusted nodules and plaques can clinically resemble some lesions of blastomycosis; biopsy can be helpful
- Chronic herpes simplex infection: often crusted or eroded vegetative plaques which still maintain some scalloped edging; biopsy again is often diagnostic
- Pyoderma gangrenosum: classically more of an actively inflamed, violaceous, edematous border; vegetative PG can clinically resemble blasto, but pathologic features can differentiate the two

Work-Up

- Chest radiography must be obtained in all forms to evaluate for pulmonary involvement
- Further approach and specimen collection depends on the affected organ system
  - Pulmonary: sputum or bronchial washings, biopsy
  - Bone: joint fluid, synovial tissue biopsy (imaging not specific)
  - CNS: cerebrospinal fluid (ventricular puncture more sensitive than lumbar puncture)
  - Genitourinary: urine collection (FNA for prostate)
- If there is suspicion for blastomyocosis infection the mycobacteria laboratory should be informed as there are specific culture requirements
- Visualization of characteristic yeasts forms via direct smear or histopathologic exam
- *In situ* hybridization is accurate, but not widely available

Treatment

- Primary cutaneous disease tends to resolve spontaneously without treatment
- Itraconazole, posaconazole, or voriconazole, continued for months, are appropriate treatments options
- Immunocompromised patients and those with chronic pulmonary or disseminated extrapulmonary blastomycosis: amphotericin B for 1–2 weeks followed by itraconazole for 12 months
- CNS involvement requires lipid amphotericin B for 4–8 weeks followed by an oral azole antifungal for 1+ year

Suggested Readings

1. López-Martínez R, Méndéz-Tovar LJ. Blastomycosis. Clin Dermatol. 2012;30(6):565–72.
2. Motswaledi HM, Monyemangene FM, Maloba BR, Nemutavhanani DL. Blastomycosis: a case report and review of the literature. Int J Dermatol. 2012;51(9):1090–3.
3. Saccente M, Woods GL. Clinical and laboratory update on blastomycosis. Clin Microbiol Rev. 2010;23(2):367–81.

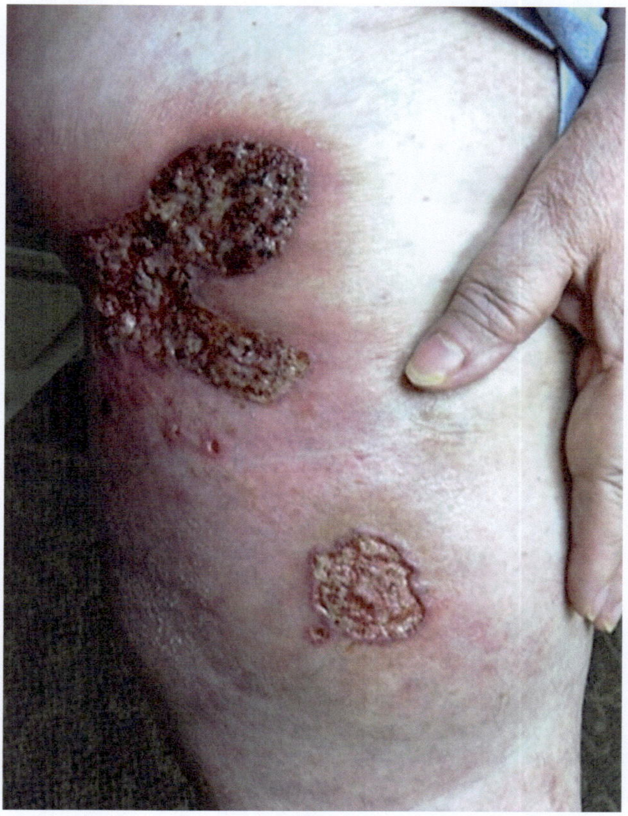

Fig. 42.1 Blastomycosis: ulcerative and verrucous plaques of blastomycosis with sporotrichoid spread along cutaneous lymphatics. Courtesy of Diane Thaler MD and Robert Rudolph MD.

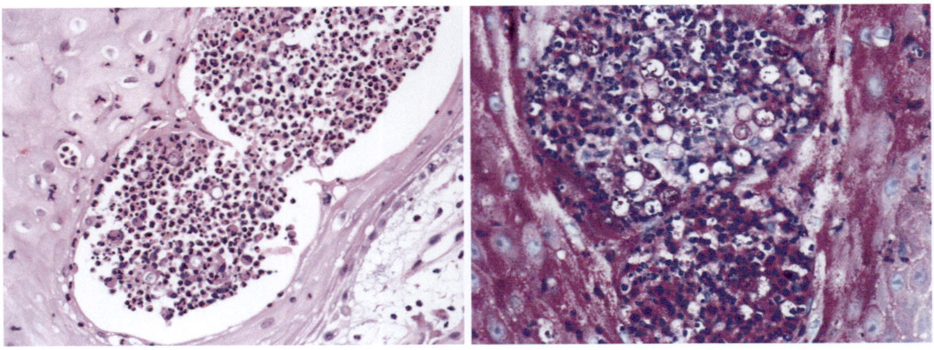

Fig. 42.2 Acute and chronic inflammation with neutrophils and histiocytes can be seen on low power. Overlying pseudoepitheliomatous hyperplasia often can be seen. *Blastomycosis dermatides* have a doubly refractile wall, broad based budding, and are approximately 10–15 µm. PAS and GMS stains highlight these organisms. Photos courtesy of Brian Swick, MD.

Cryptococcosis

43

Amy K. Forrestel

Overview

- Infection with encapsulated yeast *Cryptococcus neoformans* or *gattii*
  - *C. neoformans* is found in bird and bat droppings and contaminated soil/dust; *C. gattii* colonizes trees/wood debris
- Infection typically occurs following inhalation leading to variable pulmonary manifestations (ranging from asymptomatic mild pneumonitis to acute respiratory distress syndrome (ARDS))
  - The majority of cases will remain contained within the lungs
  - Reactivation can occur when immunosuppression prevents continued proper containment of a latent infection
- Cutaneous lesions almost always result from embolic hematogenous spread in disseminated disease
  - Approximately 10% of cryptococcal infections will become disseminated, typically occurring in immunocompromised patients (HIV/AIDS, chemotherapy, organ transplant, chronic steroid use); dissemination rates may reach up to 50% in AIDS patients, often occurring when CD4 counts are below 50–100/μL
  - In patients with disseminated disease, hematogenous spread leads to CNS (70–90%) and skin (10–15%) involvement most commonly
- Primary cutaneous cryptococcosis is very rare following direct innoculation; skin involvement should lead one to suspect and evaluate for systemic disease in all cases

Clinical Presentation

- Severe mengingo-encephalitis in immunocompromised patients is the most common clinical presentation of disseminated disease; most mycotic meningitis cases are secondary to cryptococcosis
  - Patients commonly experience fever, headache, and meningeal signs
  - Fatal if untreated; so a high index of suspicion is necessary
- Symptomatology is based on the distribution of disseminated disease and can include lymph nodes, skin, eye, kidney, bones, etc.

A. K. Forrestel, MD
Department of Dermatology, Perelman School of Medicine, University of Pennsylvania, Philadelphia, PA, USA
e-mail: amy.forrestel@uphs.upenn.edu

M. Rosenbach et al. (eds.), *Inpatient Dermatology*,
https://doi.org/10.1007/978-3-319-18449-4_43

- In disseminated disease cutaneous lesions are most commonly found on the head and neck and may present as umbilicated or crateriform nodules, indurated or soft plaques, ulcers, blisters, tumor-like masses, or draining sinuses
  - Molluscum-like papules with central umbilication, acneiform pustules, and Kaposi sarcoma-like lesions can be seen in AIDS patients.
- Cyrptococcal cellulitis is seen in severely immunocompromised hosts and has an abrupt onset of red-brown erythema with rapid progression
- In primary cryptococcosis lesions may be ulcers, nodules, abscesses, or plaques favoring exposed areas at the site of prior skin trauma with local adenopathy (Fig. 43.1)

Histopathology

- Pseudoepitheliomatous hyperplasia, acanthosis, or ulceration with gelatinous and/or granulomatous tissue reactions are typical (Fig. 43.2)
  - Gelatinous reactions are associated with an impaired immune response and consist of a high concentration of organisms free in the tissue with minimal associated inflammation/tissue reaction
  - Granulomatous reactions consist of fewer organisms which are mostly located within multinucleated giant cells with a surrounding dense dermal lymphohistiocytic infiltrate
- Organisms are round to ovoid yeasts (5–15 μm) with a thick-walled spherule with a polysaccharide capsule
- The capsule can be highlighted with mucicarmine (red), methylene blue (purple), alcian blue (purple), or Fontana-Masson/Melanin (dark brown to black) staining

Differential Diagnosis

- Molluscum contagiosum: can resemble the umbilicated papular type of crypto; bedside diagnostic testing can show characteristic Hendersson Patterson bodies of the pox-virus, and pathology can distinguish the two
- Acne: most patients with acne will have some comedonal lesions
- Histoplasmosis: varied morphologies and hard to distinguish clinically, biopsy is diagnostic
- Coccidioidomycosis: travel history and biopsy can be helpful
- Herpes simplex virus: clustered vesicles and uniform punched out erosions should prompt evaluation for HSV
- Cellulitis: bacterial cellulitis may be more rapidly developing than cryptococcal cellulitis, and should improve on antibiotics; persistent refractory cellulitis, or deeper indurated red-brown cellulitis may prompt evaluation for cryptococcal infection

Important Work-Up

- Thorough history should elicit potential exposures and immune status (e.g. HIV, chemotherapy use, transplant, etc); physical exam should assess for cutaneous lesions and other symptoms of systemic involvement
- In cases of disseminated disease without a known cause of immunosuppression an HIV test should be performed; in patients with known HIV/AIDS a current CD4 count should be obtained
- *If suspected pulmonary involvement*:
  - Chest X-ray or CT: infiltrates, nodules, pleural effusions
  - Sputum: culture often negative, may need bronchial lavage sent for cryptococcal antigen or open lung or bronchoscopic biopsy
- *If suspected CNS involvement*:
  - Head CT/MRI: perform prior to lumbar puncture; nodular lesions in basal ganglia, masses

  - Lumbar puncture: elevated intracranial pressure, normal cell count or mild pleocytosis (less than 20 cells/μL with 100% lymphocytes); cryptococcal antigen (CrAg) test on CSF—either latex agglutination (LA), ELISA, or lateral flow assay (LFA) tests
  - If no access to CrAg testing: India ink smear of CSF, and fungal culture of CSF
- *Evaluate for other systemic involvement, as appropriate*:
  - Serum, urine, pleural fluid, sputum: culture and/or CrAg
  - Tissue samples: skin, lung, lymph node, bone marrow
  - Other tests include ESR, CBC, BMP, LFTs, urinalysis

Treatment

- Consult infectious disease specialist
- Please refer to full protocol recommendations from the Infectious Diseases Society of America and WHO, as dosing and duration of treatment depend on burden of disease, sites of infection, and immune status of patient
- CNS Involvement:
  - Induction therapy: Amphotericin B + flucytosine for at least 2 weeks
  - Consolidation therapy: fluconazole for minimum 8 weeks
  - Maintenance therapy: fluconazole for at least 6–12 months; in HIV at least 12 months and with undetectable viral load and CD4 > 100 cells/μL (on two separate tests 6 months apart)
- No CNS Involvement:
  - If cryptococcemia or severe pulmonary disease: Same as CNS disease
  - Moderate pulmonary disease or single site infection in non-immunosuppressed patient: fluconazole for 6–12 months
- Antiretroviral Therapy (ART) in HIV-positive patients
  - Current recommendations from the WHO recommend deferring ART initiation in patients with cryptococcal meningitis due to the high risk of IRIS until there is evidence of sustained clinical response to anti-fungal therapy following 2–4 weeks of induction and consolidation treatment

Suggested Readings

1. Perfect JR, Dismukes WE, Dromer F, et al. Clinical practice guidelines for the management of cryptoccal disease: 2010 update by the Infectious Diseases Society of America. Clin Infect Dis. 2010;50(3):291–322.
2. Negroni R. Cryptococcosis. Clin Dermatol. 2012;30(6):599–609.
3. WHO HIV/AIDS Programme Rapid Advice. Diagnosis, prevention, and management of cryptococcal disease in HIV-infected adults, adolescents, and children. Geneva: WHO; 2011.

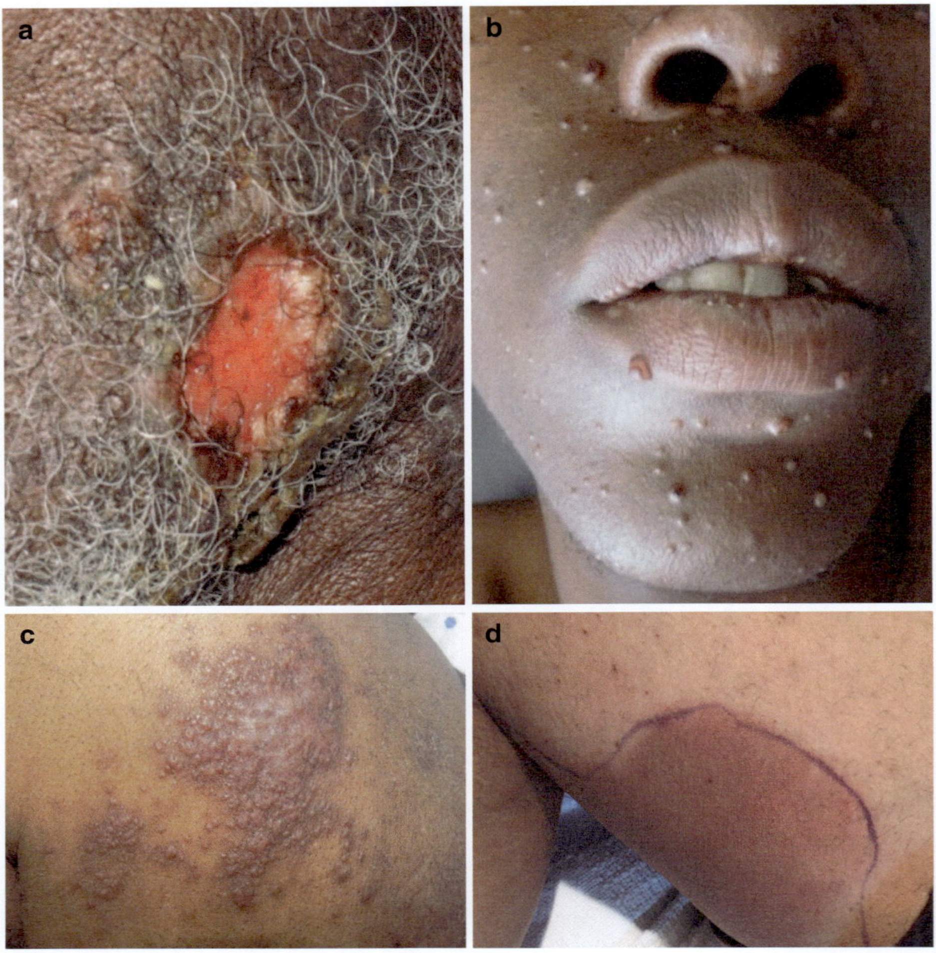

Fig. 43.1 Cryptococcal skin infection: (**a**) Ulcerated plaque of *Cryptococcus* with verrucous border in a patient with newly diagnosed HIV/AIDS. (**b**) Umbilicated papules on the face. (**c**) Cobblestoned plaque on the shoulder of a patient with disseminated Cryptococcus. (**d**) Cryptococcus is a rare cause of atypical recalcitrant cellulitis. This tends to be a deeper red-brown with indurated skin, as shown here in a heart transplant recipient who developed cryptococcal cellulitis with disseminated infection.

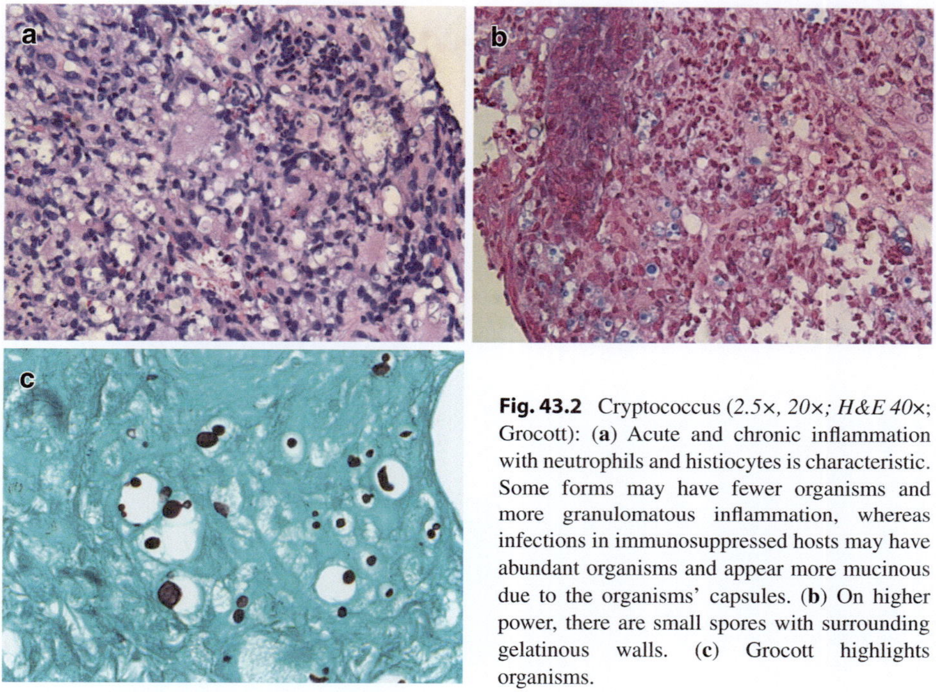

Fig. 43.2 Cryptococcus (*2.5×, 20×; H&E 40×*; Grocott): (**a**) Acute and chronic inflammation with neutrophils and histiocytes is characteristic. Some forms may have fewer organisms and more granulomatous inflammation, whereas infections in immunosuppressed hosts may have abundant organisms and appear more mucinous due to the organisms' capsules. (**b**) On higher power, there are small spores with surrounding gelatinous walls. (**c**) Grocott highlights organisms.

Part VII

Infections: Ectoparasitic Infestations

Scabies

44

Evan Piette

Overview

- Scabies is caused by an infestation of the mite *Sarcoptes scabiei* var. *hominis*. It typically presents with intense pruritus with skin lesions, and is spread by close contact
- Crusted scabies ("Norwegian scabies") occurs most often in immunosuppressed patients or those with neurologic disorders, and results from hyper-infestation with mites
- It is very important to correctly identify the condition as it is extremely contagious, especially in the setting of crusted scabies, which can lead to ward or hospital-wide outbreaks if unrecognized

Clinical Presentation

- Intense pruritus, often worse at night, and frequently accompanied by a history of pruritic contacts, recent exposure to hospitals, nursing homes, or homeless shelters, and/or an immunocompromised state
- Cutaneous findings are typically characterized by pruritic pink and red small papules, often with prominent scaling and evidence of excoriation
  - Classic locations of involvement include the finger web spaces (Fig. 44.1d), wrists, waistband area and umbilicus, nipples in women and groin in men (including red papules on the glans (Fig. 44.1e) or crusted scrotal papules)
  - Scalp and face are typically spared in adults, even in crusted scabies, but these areas can be involved in infants
- Burrows of mites typically appear as elevated, tortuous, often gray-colored lines in the skin (Figs. 44.1b and 44.1c)
- Nodular lesions can appear during active infestation, and may be persistent after clearance, commonly involving the scrotum and thighs
  - More common in children, the nodules may be confused with a neoplastic process even on biopsy due to intense reactive inflammation
- In patients with crusted scabies, thick, hyperkeratotic sandpaper-like crusts and scales develop, which are teeming with mites and highly contagious (Fig. 44.1)

Histopathology

- Skin scrapings can be done to identify the ova, feces, and mites under direct light microscopy (Fig. 44.2c)

E. Piette, MD
University of Pennsylvania, Philadelphia, PA, USA

M. Rosenbach et al. (eds.), *Inpatient Dermatology*,
https://doi.org/10.1007/978-3-319-18449-4_44

- In atypical or difficult cases, skin biopsy may be performed and demonstrates a patchy or diffuse inflammatory infiltrate with prominent eosinophilia; mites are sometimes visualized attached to the stratum corneum. Additionally, small curly eosinophilic strands (likely ovum remnants) and foreign material consistent with feces (scybala) may be seen (Figs. 44.2a and 44.2b)
  - Intact mites have round bodies containing striated muscle and dorsal spines
  - Visualization of the mite, ovum, or feces is sufficient for diagnosis
- In nodular lesions, inflammation is more prominent and mites are less frequently visualized
- In crusted scabies there is pronounced orthokeratosis/parakeratosis housing numerous mites in various stages of development and underlying epidermal psoriasiform hyperplasia

Differential Diagnosis

Burrows are an important clue to the diagnosis but may not always be evident; the differential of the pruritic papules is broad, and can include:

- Atopic dermatitis: Patient history is helpful; eczematous patches in the antecubital and popliteal fossae are more common than web-space scaling and crusted papules
- Auto-eczematization (id) reactions: Can be a challenge as scabies itself can result in an id reaction, which is a widespread, monomorphic, often fine papular eruption due to a robust immune response
- Arthropod bites (such as bed bugs): Usually fewer, more discrete lesions clumped in groups of 2–4 ("breakfast, lunch, dinner"), with visible puncta
- Dermatitis herpetiformis: Intensely pruritic condition, typically presents with crusted papules on the elbows, knees, and buttocks; finger involvement is rare
- Bullous pemphigoid: Can be intensely pruritic, but scabies should not show the same tense bullae

Work-Up

- The diagnosis can be made clinically with confirmation by direct visualization using light microscopy of skin scrapings
  - This can be done by gently scraping the skin in an area where a mite is suspected by using a scalpel or curette; a drop of mineral oil or other viscous liquid on a glass slide helps trap the mite
- If there is strong clinical suspicion, treatment is generally benign and can be considered even in the absence of definitive visualization of the organism
- Patients with crusted scabies should be evaluated for an underlying immunosuppressed state

Treatment

- Patients should be placed on contact precautions
- First line treatment includes topical application of an antiscabietic medication twice, one week apart
  - The medication should be applied at night from the neck down in adults, and whole body in infants. After leaving the medication on overnight, the entire body should be washed
  - Additionally, all household contacts should be simultaneously treated, and all clothing/linens should be washed in hot water; this should be repeated one week later
- Topical antiscabietic medications include:
  - Permethrin cream: Safety data not available in infants less than 2 months
  - Lindane lotion or cream: Not recommended for infants, children, or breastfeeding mothers.
  - Compounded sulfur ointment: Recommended formulation for infants less than 2 months
- Oral Ivermectin in one or two doses is a systemic therapeutic option, though caution must be exercised in the elderly; no safety data is available in pregnant women and children less than 15 kg
- There are no well-defined guidelines for treatment of crusted scabies, but a combination of ivermectin (typical systemic agent of choice) coupled with aggressive use of topicals is typically used (see the CDC webpage for up to date dosing interval recommendation)
  - Repeat skin scrapings must be obtained weekly to document clearance
  - Treatment should be repeated until scrapings return negative
  - Due to the high burden of mites, these patients are considered extremely infectious until they are cleared completely of the infestation

Suggested Readings

1. Mounsey KD, McCarthy JS. Treatment and control of scabies. Curr Opin Infect Dis. 2013;26(2):133–9.
2. Tijoe M, Vissers W. Scabies outbreaks in nursing homes for the elderly: recognition, treatment options and control of reinfestation. Drugs Aging. 2008;25(4):299–305.

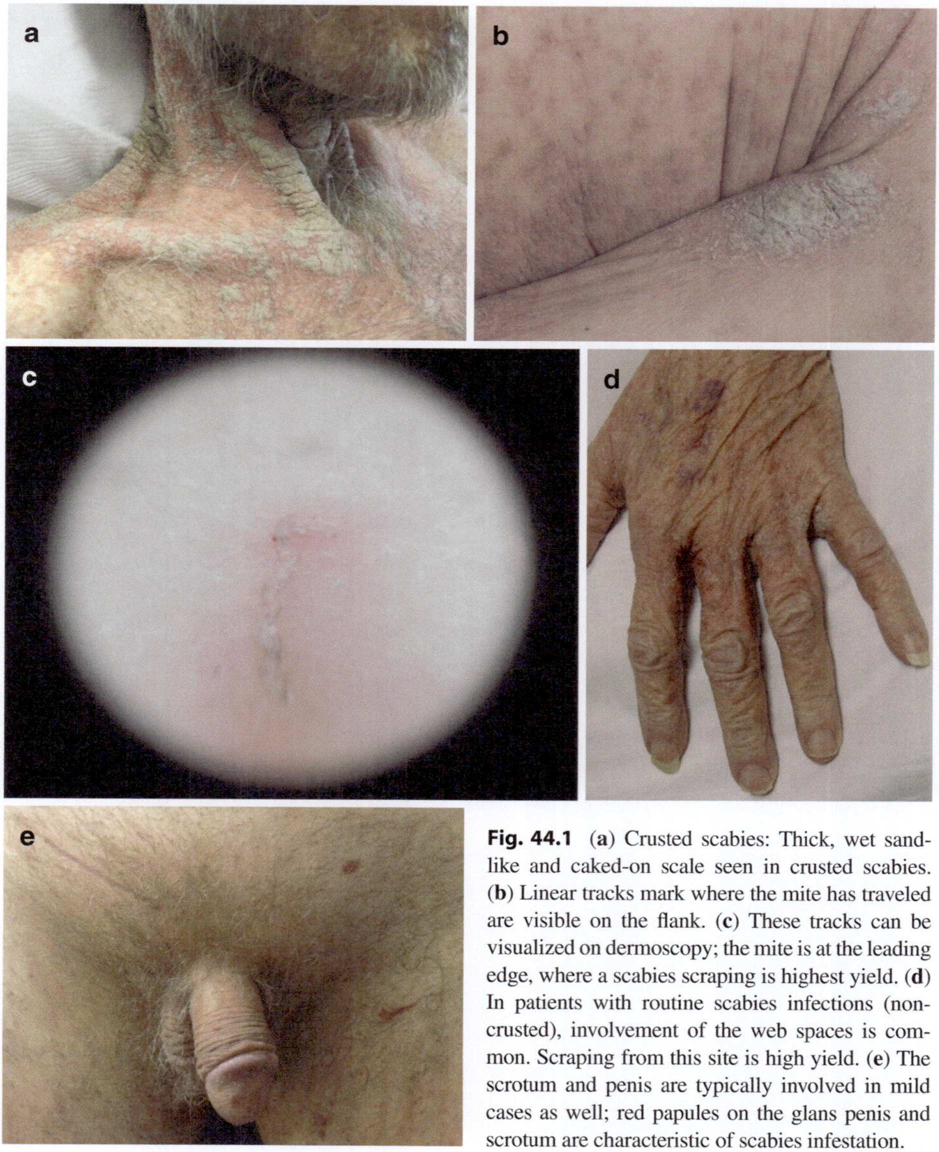

Fig. 44.1 (**a**) Crusted scabies: Thick, wet sand-like and caked-on scale seen in crusted scabies. (**b**) Linear tracks mark where the mite has traveled are visible on the flank. (**c**) These tracks can be visualized on dermoscopy; the mite is at the leading edge, where a scabies scraping is highest yield. (**d**) In patients with routine scabies infections (non-crusted), involvement of the web spaces is common. Scraping from this site is high yield. (**e**) The scrotum and penis are typically involved in mild cases as well; red papules on the glans penis and scrotum are characteristic of scabies infestation.

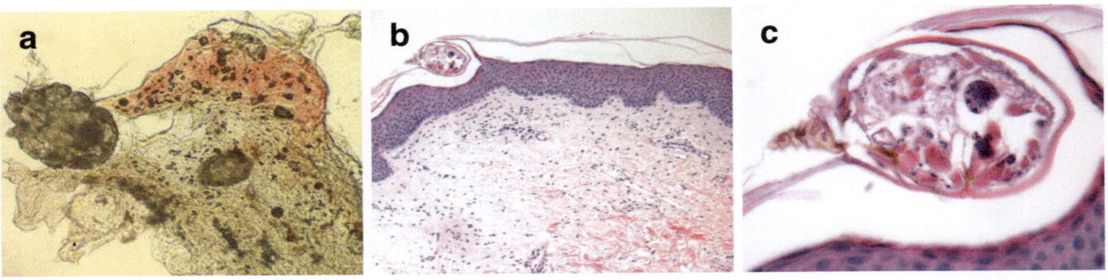

Fig. 44.2 Scabies (*mineral oil 40×; 10×, 40× H&E*): (**a**) Mineral oil or potassium hydroxide preparation demonstrates the mite, egg (large oval structure) and scybala (feces; small black dots). (**b, c**) Histopathology highlights the organism or parts of the organism within the stratum corneum (small pigtails or curly Q's are often seen at sites the mite has traversed the epidermis) often with spongiosis and an eosinophilic dermal infiltrate. In the absence of a mite, spongiotic epidermis with neutrophils in the stratum corneum and a superficial and deep eosinophilic infiltrate may be seen.

Lice

45

Rachel Klein

Overview

- Human infestation is caused by three different subtypes, which are site-specific, including:
  - *Pediculus humanus capitis* (head louse)
  - *Pediculus humanus humanus* (body louse)
  - *Pthirus pubis* (crab/pubic louse)
- Transmission only occurs through direct contact with an infected individual or fomites (infested clothing)
  - Crab lice, in particular, tend to be sexually transmitted
- Body lice are vectors for certain infections, including:
  - *Borrelia recurrentis* (relapsing fever)
  - *Bartonella quintana* (trench fever, bacillary angiomatosis)
  - *Rickettsia prowazekii* (epidemic typhus)

Clinical Presentation

- Mild cases, particularly of head lice, may be asymptomatic; more widespread involvement is often pruritic
  - Hypersensitivity reaction associated with saliva from the lice introduced during feeding leads to pruritus and secondary excoriations
  - Regional lymphadenopathy may variably be present
- Visible lice and nits (eggs) in the hair (head and crab lice) or seams of clothing (body louse) evident on physical exam with sites of predilection including (Fig. 45.1):
  - Head lice: bilateral temples, posterior auricular, and the neck
  - Crab lice: although classily associated with pubic hair any hair-bearing skin can be involved including eyelashes, axilla, beard, eyebrows, etc.
    In most cases there will be two or more sites of involvement
  - Body lice: inhabit and lay eggs in clothing, only moving to the skin for feeding, so lesions typically on skin in direct contact with infested clothing
- Secondary impetiginization can occur on excoriated skin characterized by pustules, yellow crust
- Auto-eczematization (Id) reaction also can occur depending on the extent of infection

R. Klein, MD
Accent Dermatology, Medford, NJ, USA
e-mail: rachel@accentderma.com

M. Rosenbach et al. (eds.), *Inpatient Dermatology*,
https://doi.org/10.1007/978-3-319-18449-4_45

- Maculae ceruleae: blue-gray macules on the thighs, buttocks, and genitals secondary to hemosiderin deposition by crab lice; rare finding but highly specific for crab lice when identified
- Pediculosis ciliaris: Conjunctivitis, crusting, and edema of the eyelid from infestation of the eyelashes

Histopathology

- Biopsy is typically unnecessary since the louse is visible to the naked eye and direct microscopy can help differentiate pubic lice from other types

Differential Diagnosis

- Scabies: not grossly visible, often finger web space crusting, and involves the trunk (axilla to groin) more than hair bearing areas
- Black or white piedra: usually elongated tube-like shapes coating numerous hairs, not discrete nits
- Seborrheic dermatitis: greasy scale and flaking on scalp more than small nits adhering to hair shafts

Work-Up

- Patients with crab lice should be tested for other sexually transmitted infections
- Consider a complete blood count or HIV testing in patients with a heavy, chronic infestation
- Close contacts also should be evaluated

Treatment

- Mechanical
  - Shaving can be helpful for many forms but crab lice may persist
  - Wet combing: must be repeated every 2–3 days for several weeks
- Topical
  - Neurotoxic compounds were first line therapies for many years, as such, resistance to these agents is now common; this class of agents includes:
    - Permethrin; requires nit-combing
    - Malathion; should be avoided in lactating women due to concern for respiratory depression of the infant
  - Spinosad does not require nit-combing, more effective than permethrin
  - Lindane is contraindicated in children less than 3 years of age due to concern for neurotoxicity
  - Benzyl alcohol
  - Topical ivermectin
  - Plant-based essential oils
- Systemic
  - Ivermectin orally once, and then repeated in one week if needed; safety data is not available for pregnant women and children less than 15 kg
- Wash all clothing, bed sheets in hot water and dry on high heat; objects that cannot be put in a washing machine should be dry-cleaned or placed in an airtight bag for 2–4 weeks

Suggested Readings

1. Feldmeier H. Pediculosis capitis: new insights into epidemiology, diagnosis and treatment. Eur J Clin Microbiol Infect Dis. 2012;31:2105–10.
2. Madke B. Pediculosis capitis an update. Indian J Dermatol Venereol Leprol. 2012;78(4):429–38.
3. Markova A, et al. Common cutaneous parasites. Ann Intern Med. 2014;161(5):ITC1–16.

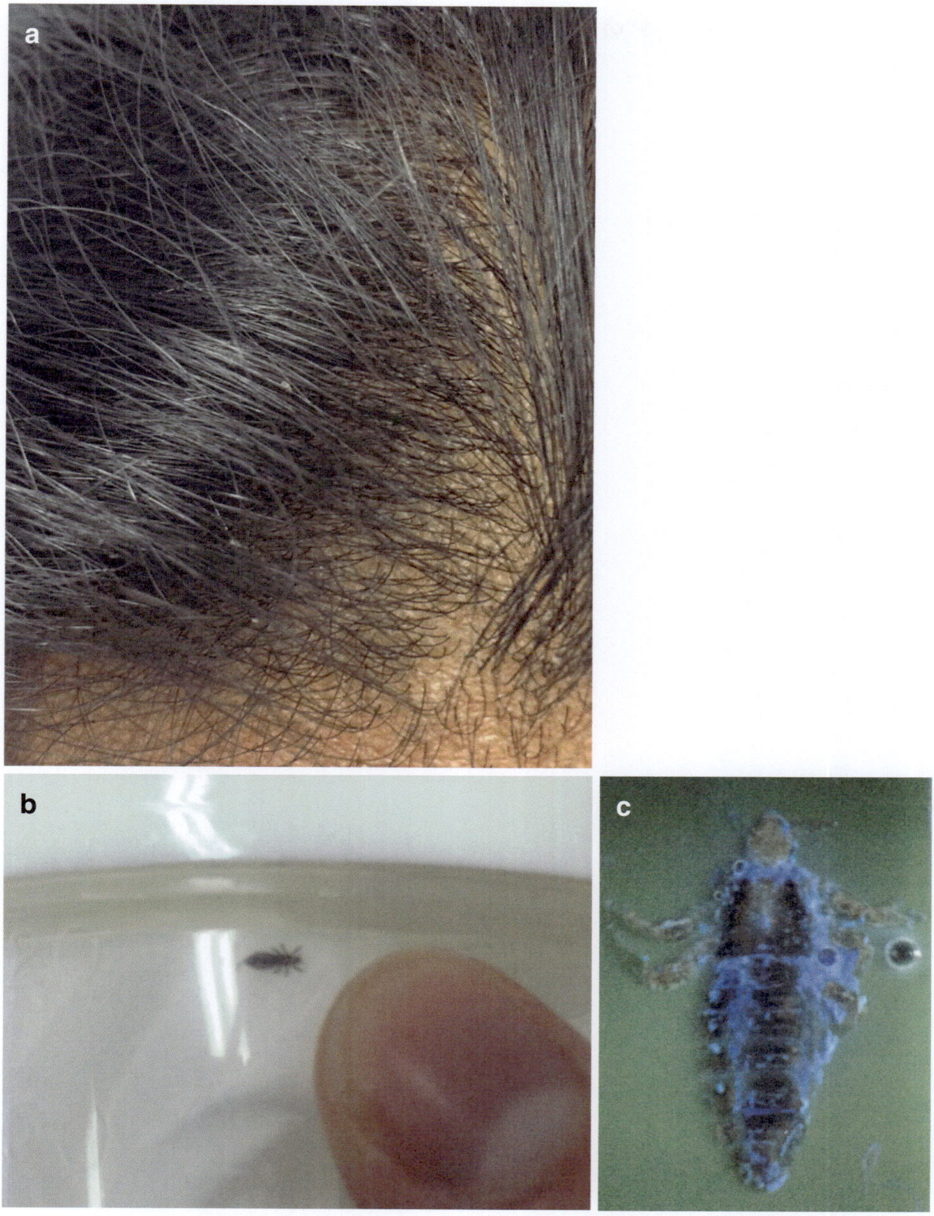

Fig. 45.1 Lice infestation. (**a**) White adherent louse eggs (nits) attached at right angles to hair shafts. There may be excoriations on the scalp and neck. (**b**) Head louse (*Pediculus humanus capitis*). (**c**) Head and body lice have elongated bodies with six legs.

Bed Bugs

46

Karolyn A. Wanat

Overview

- Bed bugs (*Cimex lectularius*) infestations are rapidly increasing worldwide
- Bed bugs have painless bites and feed on human blood every 3–5 days. They are hearty insects and can survive up to 1 year without a bloodmeal, making infestations difficult to control and eradicate
- Hypersensitivity reaction to bites may represent an IgE-mediated immune response to bed bug salivary antigen nitrophorin
- No diseases have been reported to be transmitted by bed bugs, although they can cause extreme pruritus and emotional distress for patients

Clinical Presentation

- Some individuals have no reaction to bites
- Most common cutaneous manifestations include groupings of lesions ranging from barely visible puncta to grouped urticarial eruptions. The grouping is characteristic, with 3–4 clustered lesions ("breakfast, lunch, dinner" sign) (Fig. 46.1)
- Exposed areas are affected. Head, neck, and upper extremities are common locations as bed bugs are attracted to carbon dioxide, though the pattern of bites may depend on patients' garments, with clusters around the waist also a common presentation
- Rare exuberant reactions can mimic erythema multiforme or eosinophilic cellulitis
- Secondary infections can occur due to scratching and manipulation

Histopathology

- Histopathology demonstrates a hypersensitivity reaction including spongiosis, papillary dermal edema, and a dense superficial and deep perivascular and interstitial inflammatory cell infiltrate, including lymphocytes, numerous eosinophils, and variable number of neutrophils (Fig. 46.2)

K. A. Wanat, MD
Department of Dermatology, Medical College of Wisconsin, Milwaukee, WI, USA
e-mail: karolyn-wanat@uiowa.edu

M. Rosenbach et al. (eds.), *Inpatient Dermatology*,
https://doi.org/10.1007/978-3-319-18449-4_46

Differential Diagnosis

- Other arthropod bites (mosquitoes, gnats, fleas, spider bites, scabies): the pattern of lesions, sites affected, and exposure history can be helpful clues
- Cellulitis: exuberant reactions leading to eosinophilic cellulitis can mimic true cellulitis, but even so the grouped puncta at bite-sites are often visible
- Urticaria: simple urticarial usually lacks the central puncta characteristic of bites, and bed bug bites are frequently grouped in collections of 3–4 lesions

Work-Up

- A thorough history and physical exam should be obtained including recent travel to hotels, other affected family members, and when bites occur (most often noticed in the morning on exposed skin)
- Diagnostic clues to bed bug bites include new lesions in the morning, or presence of blood or feces on the linen or identification of the bugs under the mattress, in headboard or baseboards
- If characteristic grouped lesions consistent with arthropod bites are observed, then no additional laboratory work-up or histology is necessary but referral to a respected exterminator is important
- If atypical lesions or exuberant reactions occur, then biopsy can be performed for histopathology

Treatment

- Supportive and symptomatic treatments: High potency topical steroids for individual bites and oral antihistamines for symptomatic relief from bites
- In cases of severe or generalized bites, a short course of oral corticosteroids can be used
- Eradication from experienced exterminator including methods of heating and/or fumigation with insecticides

Suggested Readings

1. Vasievich MP, Villarreal JD, Tomecki KJ. Got the travel bug? A review of common infections, infestations, bites, and stings among returning travelers. Am J Clin Dermatol. 2016;17(5):451–62.
2. Foulke GT, Anderson BE. Bed bugs. Semin Cutan Med Surg. 2014;33(3):119–22.

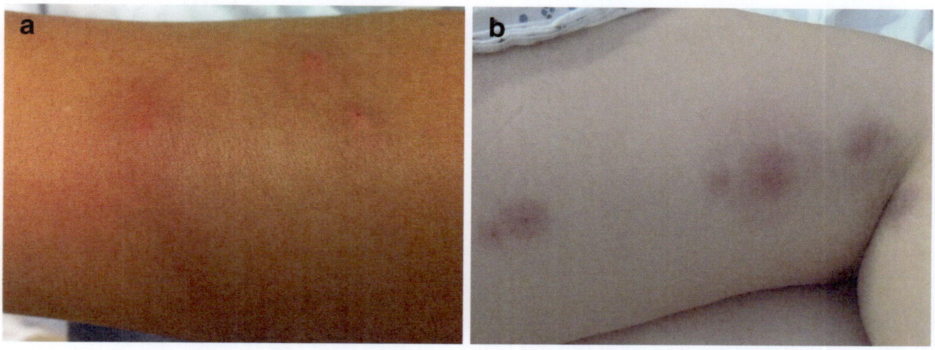

Fig. 46.1 (**a**) There are grouped erythematous papules with a central punctum at the bite site. These are often described as clustered in a linear array, the "breakfast, lunch, dinner" sign of multiple bites and blood meals. (**b**) Exuberant bite reactions can occur de novo, or in the setting of CLL. This patient has bed bugs and an EM-like reaction to the bites.

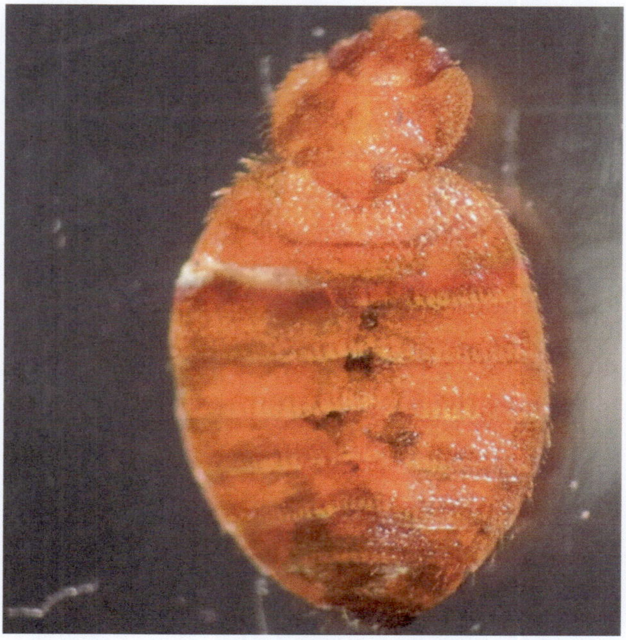

Fig. 46.2 A *Cimex lectularius* (bed bug) up close (life-sized organisms are about the size of a sesame seed), demonstrating characteristic horizontal segments across the back (similar to the slats under a mattress).

Part VIII

Purpura: Vasculitis and Vasculopathy

The various causes of vasculitis and vasculopathy can present dramatically in the skin but are even more important for what such presentations can signify for overall health and systemic disease. Few diseases engender more confusion from non-dermatologists and dermatologists alike, but a systematic approach can lead to successful diagnosis and management. This chapter aims to detail the clinical and pathologic findings and serologic work-up for patients presenting with cutaneous manifestations of vascular injury.

Vasculitis is the overarching term for the presence of vascular inflammation, in contrast to vasculopathy, which signifies vessel "sickness." Vasculitis is generally categorized by the size of the affected vessel, which organs are affected, and what inflammatory cells are most predominant. Vasculopathy typically results from coagulopathy and/or embolic disease which is generally categorized by the intraluminal substance contributing to damage. This can range from fibrin clots (which can form centrally and embolize, as in valvular heart disease or atrial fibrillation, or form de novo in the distal small vessels, as in cryoglobulinemia or anti-phospholipid antibody syndrome) to alternate substances (such as calcium and resultant secondary clots as in calciphylaxis, or cholesterol or fat emboli depositing within the vascular lumens). One source of confusion is that both entities can coexist; when there is vasculitis damaged vessels become a nidus for clot formation and fibrin thrombi, resulting in findings of vasculopathy. Similarly, when there is vascular injury from a primary thrombotic process, a resultant inflammatory host response develops to try to resolve the clot, often causing a secondary vasculitis. Some entities can in fact present with a mixed vasculitic and vasculopathic picture, such as inflammatory cryoglobulins (type II and III) or levamisole-related purpura. Making an accurate diagnosis often requires a thorough history, detailed physical exam, clinical-pathologic correlation, and serologic testing to rule in or rule out entities on the differential diagnosis.

Clinical clues to vasculitis may include palpable purpura, nodules, livedoid erythema, or inflammatory purpura with a blanchable component. Signs of vasculopathy may include angulated purpura with areas of dusky central necrosis. There is no definitive diagnostic sign of vascular inflammation which excludes vasculopathy, and vice versa. In all cases, an appreciation for lesion morphology (e.g. palpable purpura or retiform purpura) and location (e.g. lower extremities or distal sites) opens a window onto the underlying disease state and pathophysiology. One important distinction is between livedo reticularis and livedo racemosa. Livedo reticularis is the faint purple appearance of the dermal vascular network appears as a fence-work, lattice-like violaceous erythema and can be visible in slow flow states, such as in the presence of extrinsic pressure on proximal vessels, or hyperviscous states such as cryoglobulins or antiphospholipid antibodies, or as a nonspecific sign in some forms of vascular injury. Livedo racemosa is jagged, incomplete links and suggests a more acute and severe intravascular process, such as frank thrombi. In all cases of suspected vasculitis/vasculopathy, the history, clinical exam, and review of systems should be tied in with skin biopsy and judicious use of symptom-based laboratory work-up to ensure accurate diagnosis and appropriate treatment.

Careful collaboration with other subspecialties is often important in these cases. While the skin contains clinically visible superficial vessels, frequently vasculitis or vasculopathic processes are multisystem diseases. It is essential in all cases to not only evaluate the skin, but to examine patients for multiorgan disease.

Leukocytoclastic Vasculitis/Cutaneous Small Vessel Vasculitis

47

Aileen Y. Chang

Overview

- Cutaneous small vessel vasculitis (CSVV) is typically caused by inflammation of postcapillary venules in the superficial and mid dermis classically presenting as palpable purpura in dependent areas
  - Inflammatory response leads to the palpability of the lesions and the purpuric, non-blanching red color is secondary to RBC extravasaion
- Overall etiology: 50% idiopathic, 15–20% infection, 15–20% autoimmune connective tissue disease, 10–15% drug, 5% neoplasm
  - In the inpatient setting, drug-induced and infection-associated small vessel vasculitides are by far the most common
- Usually skin-limited, but it is important to rule out renal and other systemic involvement
- Pathogenesis is thought to be secondary to deposition of circulating immune complexes resulting in compliment activation leading to an inflammatory response, including neutrophil and mast cell recruitment with subsequent degranulation, resulting in vessel wall damage

Clinical Presentation

- Cutaneous lesions develop 7–10 days following the inciting event and are typically self-limited, resolving within 4 weeks, but may be chronic/recurrent in 10%
- Patients may experience arthralgia, malaise, low grade fevers, or dull muscle pains
- Palpable purpura, purpuric macules, or urticarial lesions develop in dependent areas (Fig. 47.1)
  - Often the lower extremities are involved with associated edema, but in bed-ridden/hospitalized patients involvement of the buttock and posterior thigh are typical

Histopathology

- Termed "leukocytoclastic vasculitis"

A. Y. Chang, MD
Department of Dermatology, University of California,
San Francisco, CA, USA
e-mail: aileen.chang@ucsf.edu

M. Rosenbach et al. (eds.), *Inpatient Dermatology*,
https://doi.org/10.1007/978-3-319-18449-4_47

- Transmural neutrophilic infiltration with endothelial cell damage and fibrinoid necrosis of small vessel walls, leukocytoclasia (degranulation and fragmentation of neutrophils/nuclear dust), and extravasated RBCs (Fig. 47.2)
- DIF in most cases will demonstrate granular deposition of C3, IgM, IgG, or IgA within vessel walls

Differential Diagnosis

- Arthropod bites: more urticarial, partially blanching, and often with some visible bite-site puncta; may be clustered
- Eythema multiforme: should show multiple zones of different colored inflammation, and acral involvement (palm involvement is common in EM, rare in vasculitis)
- Thromboemboli (infection, hypercoaguable state): may closely mimic and in some cases occur in conjunction with CSVV (e.g., if vasculitis is due to endocarditis); more often angulated, distal digital involvement
- Pigmented purpuric dermatosis (capillaritis): usually more faint, patches of clustered petechiae with individual pinprick-sized Cayenne-pepper like purpuric macules
- Other vasculitis (e.g. cryo vasculitis, ANCA vasculitis): any size vasculitis may present with small vessel skin findings and warrants thorough investigation; distinguishing vasculitides requires clinical, pathologic, and laboratory evaluation
- Other primary rash (e.g. morbilliform drug eruption) with hemorrhage: patients with thrombocytopenia may "bleed into" other rashes and develop nonblanching purpuric macules; these are usually more diffuse and less palpable than typical CSVV

Important Work-Up

- A thorough exam and review of systems should be performed to evaluate for associated systemic diseases; pay particular attention to renal, joint, gastrointestinal, and neurological manifestations
- Punch biopsy for H&E and DIF should be performed to rule out vasculitis mimics and aid in prognostication of the lesion
  - H&E of a fresh but well-formed purpuric papule and DIF of a fresh/new purpuric macule or papule (lesion less than one day old) are ideal
- Laboratory work-up to help determine underlying cause or trigger of vasculitis and rule out extacutaneous involvement: CBC, Creatinine, UA with micro in all cases; stool guaiac, and chest X-ray is often indicated
  - Complement levels may be helpful, as hypocomplementemia may be a sign patients are more likely to have extracutaneous disease
  - Targeted workup to identify possible causes based on symptoms may include: Blood cultures +/– echocardiogram, ASO/anti-DNase B, Hepatitis B/C serologies, ANA, ANCA, cryoglobulins, rheumatoid factor, SPEP/UPEP, malignancy screening

Treatment

- Supportive care (rest, leg elevation, compression stockings), eliminate potential triggers
  - NSAIDs may help with arthritis
  - Topical steroids for symptomatic relief from itching or burning
- Colchicine or dapsone can be used for chronic or symptomatic cutaneous disease
- If skin disease severe/progressive, or systemic organ involvement, consider oral steroids, other steroid-sparing agents

Suggested Reading

1. Micheletti RG, Werth VP. Small vessel vasculitis of the skin. Rheum Dis Clin N Am. 2015;41(1):21–32.

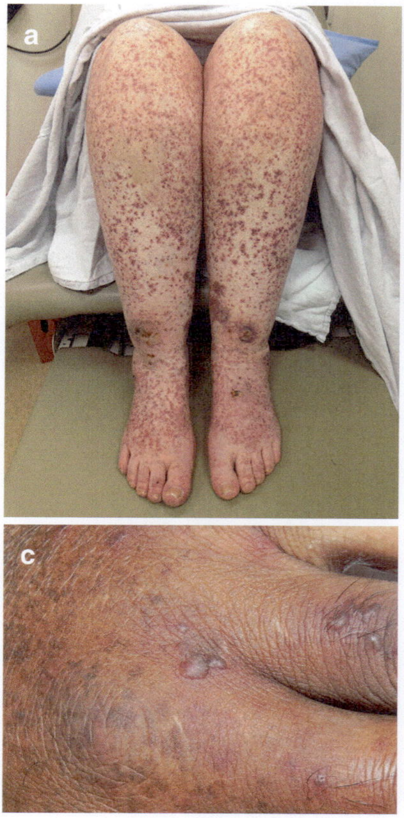

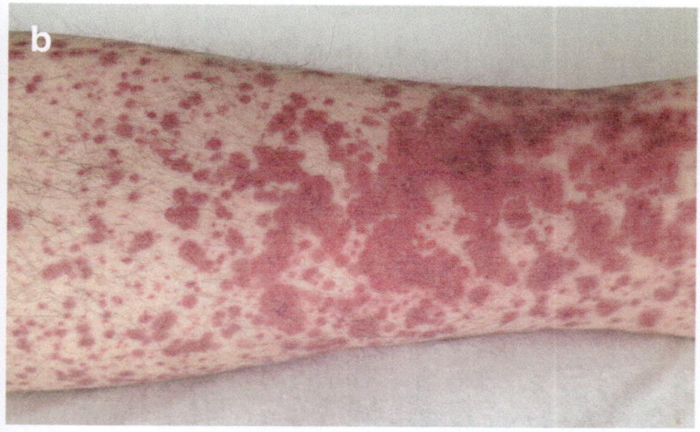

Fig. 47.1 Cutaneous small vessel vasculitis (leukocytoclastic vasculitis). (**a**) Innumerable purpuric macules and papules on the lower legs consistent with small vessel vasculitis. (**b**) Coalescing purpuric macules and papules ("palpable purpura") on the lower leg due to small vessel vasculitis. (**c**) Purpuric macules also can result in vesicles and pustule formation.

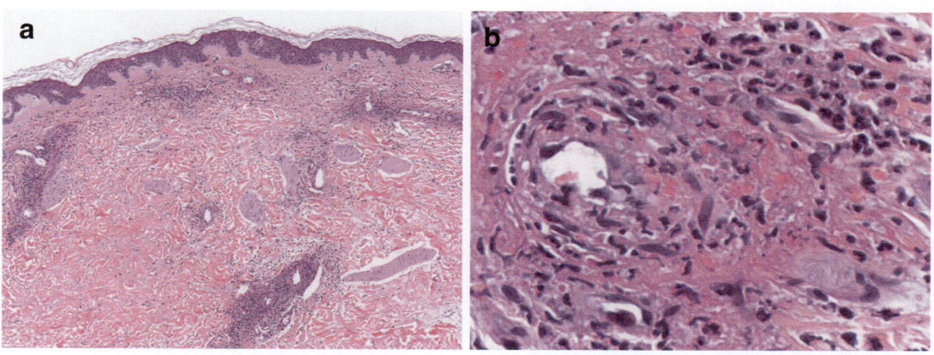

Fig. 47.2 LCV (*5×,40×; H&E*): (**a**) There is acute neutrophil-rich inflammation centered around blood vessels in the superficial to mid dermis. (**b**) On higher power, neutrophils within vessel ways with leukocytoclasia and nuclear debris, fibrinoid necrosis, and extravasated red blood cells are diagnostic of LCV.

Granulomatosis with Polyangiitis

48

Douglas J. Pugliese

Overview

- Granulomatosis with polyangiitis (GPA), formerly known as Wegener's granulomatosis, is a rare multisystem autoimmune disease of unknown etiology causing necrotizing granulomatous inflammation and pauci-immune, classically c-ANCA positive, vasculitis in small and medium sized blood vessels
- Typically affects the upper and lower respiratory tract and kidneys, but can have diffuse involvement more commonly including the eyes, ears, skin, nerves, joints, and heart
  - The limited form primarily involves the respiratory tract with renal sparing and is associated with a better prognosis
- Affects both sexes almost equally with most cases occurring in 40–65 year old caucasians
- In the absence of treatment GPA patients survive on average only 5 months, with infection, pulmonary and renal failure being the most common causes of mortality

Clinical Presentation

- 90% of patients present with symptoms associated with involvement of the respiratory tract but fever, weight loss, malaise in addition to a wide range of clinical manifestations can develop over days to months
- Mucocutaneous findings occur in 45% of patients and can manifest as palpable purpura, petechiae, nodules, mucocutaneous ulcers, hypertrophic gingivitis (strawberry gums), or saddle-nose deformity (Fig. 48.1)
  - Purpura and ulcerations are common. Cutaneous nodules are firm, flesh or violet colored, and tend to favor extensor extremity surfaces
    Intra-nasal nodules can lead to sinusitis or epistaxis from ulceration and bleeding
    Pulmonary nodules can lead to pneumonia, hemoptysis, and cavitation
- Secondary infections are common including post-obstructive pneumonia, recurrent sinusitis, and secondary infections with *S. aureus*

D. J. Pugliese, MD
Department of Dermatology, Perelman School of Medicine, Penn Presbyterian Medical Center, University of Pennsylvania, Philadelphia, PA, USA
e-mail: douglas.pugliese@uphs.upenn.edu

M. Rosenbach et al. (eds.), *Inpatient Dermatology*,
https://doi.org/10.1007/978-3-319-18449-4_48

Clinical Manifestations of GPA

Upper respiratory tract	Nasal congestion, epistaxis, purulent nasal discharge, sinusitis (acute or chronic/recurrent), sinus mucoceles, oral/nasal ulcers, polychondritis, perforated septum, and saddle nose deformity
Lower respiratory tract	Cough, dyspnea, pleuritic chest pain, hemoptysis, and wheezing
Renal involvement	Ranges from asymptomatic hematuria to rapidly progressive glomerulonephritis
Joint involvement	Arthralgias, myalgias, and typically non-deforming arthritis
Ocular involvement	Conjunctivitis, episcleritis, retro-orbital inflammatory pseudo-tumor with proptosis
Mucocutaneous manifestations	Palpable purpura, petechiae, nodules prone to ulceration, hypertrophic gingivitis "strawberry gums"
Otologic	Otitis media, polychondritis, hearing loss
CNS	Peripheral neuropathy (mononeuritis multiplex), cranial nerve palsies from entrapment
Cardiac	Pericarditis (may be asymptomatic or with chest pain)

Histopathology

- Typically shows leukocytoclastic vasculitis involving small and medium vessels with or without granulomatous inflammation (Fig. 48.2)
  - "Blue" palisading granulomas are classic but rarely seen; they are composed of granulomatous inflammation with multinucleated giant cells surrounding collections of degenerating collagen, neutrophils and basophilic debris
  - The epidermis may be ulcerated or necrotic

Differential Diagnosis

- Infection (bacterial, fungal, viral, mycobacterial, protozoal): GPA can have multiple morphologies, some of which may resemble infections; special stains and tissue cultures can distinguish
- Cocaine abuse (levamisole vasculopathy/vasculitis): may cause nasal septal ulcerations and widespread livedo and purpura; history is important as is a rapid urine drug screen
- Pyoderma gangrenosum: GPA can cause lesions characterized as "malignant pyoderma" which can closely resemble PG, and the two can co-occur; ANCA testing of PG patients is reasonable
- Other types of vasculitis (ANCA positive and negative) especially eosinophilic granulomatosis with polyangiitis (formerly Churg-Strauss) or microscopic polyangiitis: diagnosis is usually made by combining clinical features, distribution of organ involvement, serologies, and pathology
- Malignancy: Ulcerated lesions of aggressive lymphomas (such as NK/Tcell) can mimic some morphologies of GPA; histology can help differentiate

Work-Up

- A thorough history and physical exam is essential
  - Based on symptomology appropriate consultations such as nephrology, rheumatology, pulmonology, otolaryngology should be requested
- CBC, CMP, urinalysis, should be performed:
  - Lab abnormalities may include: positive rheumatoid factor (RF), abnormal renal function (elevated BUN/Cr and proteinuria) and urinalysis (WBCs, casts, dysmorphic RBCs), elevated inflammatory markers (ESR/CRP), and mild anemia or leukocytosis with neutrophil predominance
  - Additional tests can help exclude other entities, such as RF, Cryoglobulins, ANA, and more depending on the clinical presentation

- ANCA testing with indirect immunofluorescence and ELISA confirmation; when using both modalities ANCA detection approaches 100% in active generalized GPA
  - Cytoplasmic antineutrophil cytoplasmic antibody (c-ANCA) are autoantibodies targeting proteinase 3 (PR3); c-ANCAs are most specific for GPA and occur in approximately 90% of patients with classic or severe disease but only 60% with limited disease
- p-ANCA (anti-MPO antibodies) can occur in up to 10% of cases; pulmonary imaging should be performed
  - The most common radiologic finding is diffuse pulmonary nodules often with cavitation as well as diffuse ground glass opacities, atelectasis, and consolidation
- Biopsy can be helpful in the diagnosis of GPA; kidney and pulmonary biopsies typically demonstrate the most specific pathology

Treatment

- Systemic immunosuppression is necessary; rituximab and glucocorticoids have supplanted cyclophosphamide and glucocorticoids as first line therapy in most cases
  - After initial induction therapy promoting remission, then methotrexate, azathioprine, or other agents may be used
- Trimethoprim-sulfamethoxazole is often added to the maintenance immunosuppressive regimen since relapses are often associated with *S. aureus* respiratory infections and nasal carriage

Suggested Readings

1. Finkielman JD, Lee AS, Hummel AM, et al. ANCA are detectable in nearly all patients with active severe Wegener's granulomatosis. Am J Med. 2007;120(7):643. e9–643.14.
2. Stone JH, Merkle PA, Spiera R, et al. Rituximab versus cyclophosphamide for ANCA-associated vasculitis. N Engl J Med. 2010;363(3):221–32.

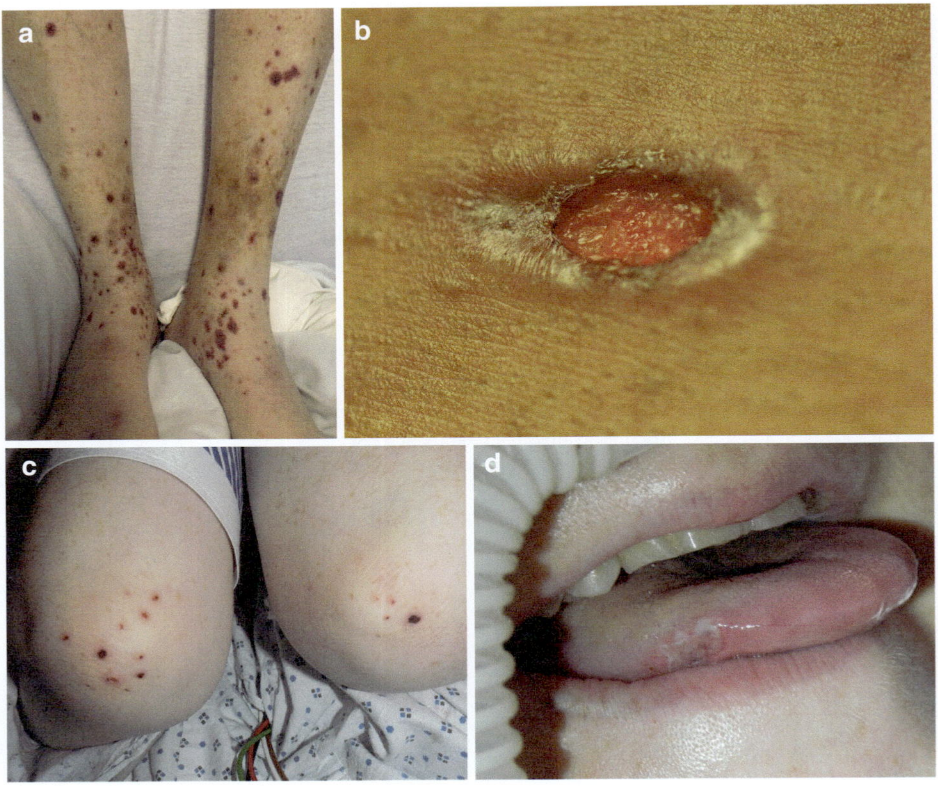

Fig. 48.1 Granulomatosis with polyangiitis: (**a**, **b**) Round and retiform purpuric lesions and ulceration signifying small and medium vessel vasculitis in granulomatosis with polyangiitis. (**c**) Necrotic papules on the extensor elbows commonly seen in patients with granulomatosis with polyangiitis. Such lesions histologically may have features of palisaded neutrophilic and granulomatous dermatitis. (**d**) GPA commonly involves the oral mucosa and upper respiratory tract, resulting in ulceration of the tongue, perforation of the palate, and saddle nose deformity.

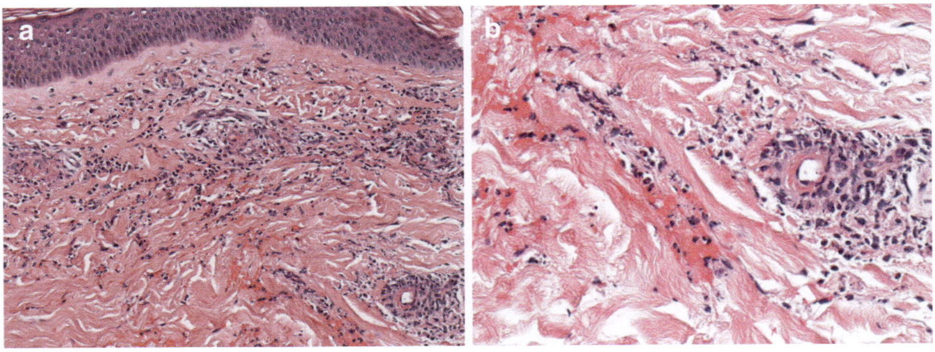

Fig. 48.2 Granulomatosis with polyangiitis (GPA) (*10×, 40×; H&E*): (**a**) GPA is a small to medium vasculitis affecting both post-capillary venules (as shown above) and potentially deeper vessels at the dermal-subcutaneous junction. (**b**) There is a leukoclastic vasculitis with eosinophilic fibrinoid material deposited in the walls of the injured vessels. Leukoclastic vasculitis may progress to "stellate abscesses" with associated palisading granulomas.

Eosinophilic Granulomatosis with Polyangiitis

49

Robert G. Micheletti

Overview

- Eosinophilic granulomatosis with polyangiitis (EGPA), formally known as Churg-Strauss Syndrome, is a rare multisystem autoimmune disease of unknown etiology which manifests as both a hyperesoinophilic syndrome and a small-medium vessel pauci-immune, typically p-ANCA associated, vasculitis
- Classically associated with asthma, allergic rhinitis, and peripheral eosinophilia
- Pulmonary and cutaneous manifestations are most common but patients have a diverse clinical course based on organs of involvement; additionally, patients are at increased risk for thromboembolic disease
- Average age at diagnosis is 40; there is no gender predilection
- Occurs in three phases: prodromal, eosinophilic, and vasculitic
- Often fatal if left untreated with death typically resulting from congestive heart failure due to granulomatous myocardial involvement

Clinical Presentation

- Should be suspected in a patient with a history of refractory asthma and recurrent upper respiratory symptoms with peripheral neuropathy, eosinophilia, and/or evidence of vasculitis
- The clinical syndrome evolves through three phases:
  - **Prodromal phase**: lasting months to years manifests as worsening allergic symptoms, asthma, rhinitis, and constitutional symptoms
    - >90% of patients will develop asthma with an average age of onset of 35 compared to allergic asthma which typically develops in childhood; exacerbations may be worse and/or more frequent in advanced disease phases
  - **Eosinophilic phase:** peripheral eosinophilia, fevers, urticaria and nonspecific dermatitis, eosinophilic infiltration of viscera (lungs, myocardium, GI tract, CNS) with associated symptoms (gastroenteritis, eosinophilic pneumonia, etc.)
  - **Vasculitic phase:** Most commonly affects the lungs, skin, and gastrointestinal organs with sequelae related to small and medium sized vasculitis and extravascular granulomatous inflammation

R. G. Micheletti, MD
Department of Dermatology, Perelman School of Medicine, University of Pennsylvania, Philadelphia, PA, USA
e-mail: robert.micheletti@uphs.upenn.edu

M. Rosenbach et al. (eds.), *Inpatient Dermatology*,
https://doi.org/10.1007/978-3-319-18449-4_49

- Skin manifestations are seen in up to two-thirds of patients, favoring the extremities, and are consistent with both small and medium vessel vasculitis (Figs. 49.1)
  - Palpable purpura is seen in 50% of patients and associated with small vessel vasculitis
  - Medium vessel vasculitis can present as livedo reticularis, retiform purpura, or tender subcutaneous nodules
    - "Churg-Strauss nodules" (a.k.a. palisaded and neutrophilic granulomatous dermatitis) are ulcerated papules on the extensor elbows and scalp which are characteristic but not specific for EGPA and develop in approximately 30% of patients
  - Occasionally diffuse ecchymoses and petechiae may develop

Clinical Manifestations of EGPA

Pulmonary	Asthma, hemoptysis, pleural effusions (may be eosinophilic), pulmonary-renal syndrome
Cutaneous	Palpable purpura, livedo reticularis, urticaria, retiform purpura, subcutaneous nodules (30%), generalized ecchymoses/petechiae
Upper airway	Allergic rhinitis, chronic sinusitis, nasal polyposis, nasal obstruction with secondary infection
Otologic	Otitis media, sensorineural hearing loss
Gastrointestinal	Pain, diarrhea, colitis, bleeding
Renal	Ranging from asymptomatic hematuria to necrotizing glomerulonephritis; pulmonary-renal syndrome
CNS	Peripheral neuropathy (mononeuritis multiplex) with foot or wrist drop
Cardiac	Cardiomyopathy, pericarditis, pericardial effusions, heart failure
MSK	Myalgia, less commonly migratory polyarthralgias and arthritis

Histopathology

- Leuokocytoclastic vasculitis with a marked eosinophilic infiltrate (Fig. 49.2)
- Vasculitis typically involves superficial venules and deeper medium sized vessels with "red" palisading granulomas composed of histiocytes, sometimes with giant cells, arranged around central collections of degenerating collagen, neutrophils and eosinophils
- Biopsy of nonspecific dermatitis or urticaria will often reveal nonspecific histologic findings such as those of a dermal hypersensitivity reaction

Differential Diagnosis: (Varies by Phase of the Disease)

- Other ANCA-associated vasculitides (granulomatosis with polyangiitis and microscopic polyangiitis): may share significant overlap and requires careful clinical, pathologic, and serologic correlation
- Drug-induced vasculitis (levamisole-tainted cocaine, other): may share clinical and histologic features, nad important to exclude with specific testing (urine drug screen) and history
- Chronic urticaria: nonspecific lesions of EGPA can include urticaria—the diagnosis is made by the extracutaneous involvement and serologic testing
- Atopic diathesis: while many patients with EGPA will have antecedent atopy, the vasculitis and eosinophilic phases should be distinguishable based on the constellation of symptoms
- Parasitic infection: persistent peripheral eosinophilia may be a manifestation of infection, and depending on patients' travel and exposure history, it is important to exclude these entities prior to systemic suppression for EGPA

Work-Up

- Due to the varied clinical manifestations a thorough history and physical exam is necessary; additional work up and consultations will be dictated by the associated findings
- Most patients warrant consultation with appropriate specialists (rheumatology, plus others depending on pattern of organ involvement)
- CBC with differential, creatinine, urinalysis with microscopy, ANCA, IgE
  - Lab abnormalities may include: eosinophilia (>1500/μL or >10% of leukocytes) and mild anemia on CBC, elevated IgE, positive rheumatoid factor (low titer), evidence of abnormal renal function (elevated BUN/Cr and proteinuria), elevated inflammatory markers (ESR/CRP)
  - ANCA: ANCA positivity is found in 40–60% of cases, of which 75% demonstrate p-ANCA
    p-ANCAs are antibodies directed at myeloperoxidase and result in perinuclear staining with indirect immunofluorescence which is then confirmed by ELISA testing
    Not that EGPA may be ANCA negative
- Biopsy of skin or other involved organs
- Additional work up may include: EMG for neuropathy, Sinus evaluation, Pulmonary imaging, renal evaluations

Treatment

- EGPA is often exquisitely sensitive to systemic corticosteroids
- Poor prognostic factors include: elevated serum creatinine, proteinuria, GI involvement, cardiomyopathy, CNS involvement
  - Patients without any poor prognostic factors can be treated with corticosteroids alone
  - Patients with a poor prognostic factor are treated with oral steroids and an additional systemic immunosuppressant—either azathioprine or cyclophosphamide.

Suggested Readings

1. Jennette JC. Overview of the 2012 revised international Chapel Hill consensus conference nomenclature of vasculitides. Clin Exp Nephrol. 2013;17(5):603–6.
2. Greco A, Rizzo MI, de Virgillo A, et al. Churg-Strauss syndrome. Autoimmun Rev. 2014;14(4):341–8. https://doi.org/10.1016/j.autrev.2014.12.004.

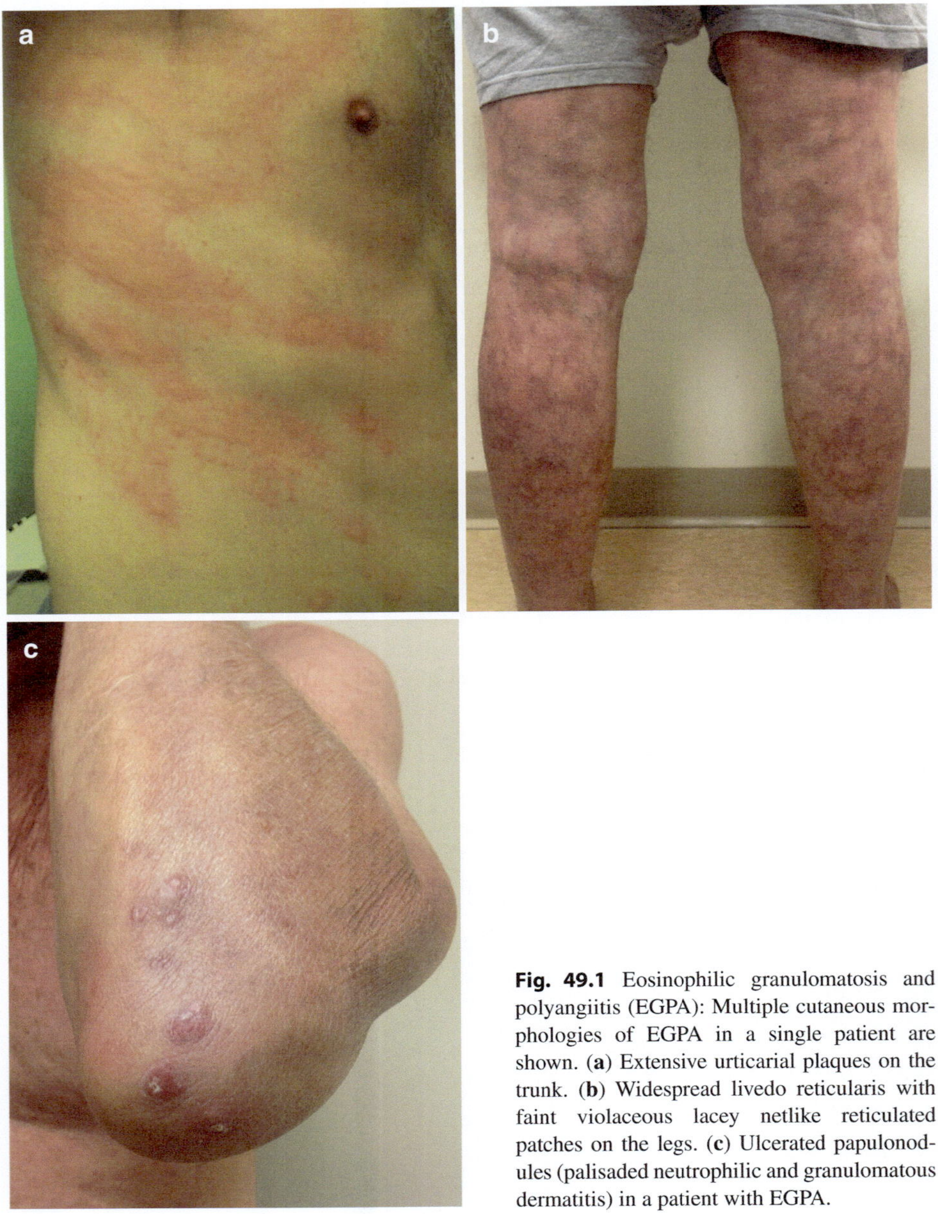

Fig. 49.1 Eosinophilic granulomatosis and polyangiitis (EGPA): Multiple cutaneous morphologies of EGPA in a single patient are shown. (**a**) Extensive urticarial plaques on the trunk. (**b**) Widespread livedo reticularis with faint violaceous lacey netlike reticulated patches on the legs. (**c**) Ulcerated papulonodules (palisaded neutrophilic and granulomatous dermatitis) in a patient with EGPA.

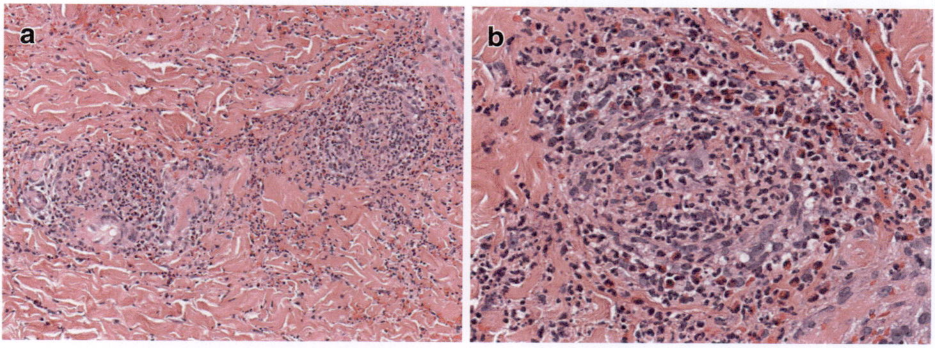

Fig. 49.2 Eosinophilic granulomatosis with polyangiitis (EGPA) *(10×, 40×; H&E):* (**a**) There are eosinophils and palisading necrotizing granulomas with associated vasculitis. This may resemble other forms of small vessel vasculitis, however in EGPA there is often a component of eosinophilic inflammation. (**b**) Higher power demonstrates small vessel destruction with neutrophils and eosinophils.

Microscopic Polyangiitis

50

Robert G. Micheletti

Overview

- A type of ANCA-associated vasculitis, along with granulomatosis with polyangiitis (GPA) and eosinophilic granulomatosis with polyangiitis (EGPA)
- Affects small and medium-sized vessels
- Exists along a clinical spectrum with GPA but lacks granulomatous inflammation and upper respiratory symptoms
- Treatment is similar to that of GPA; 5-year survival is approximately 75%, but disease relapse is common

Clinical Presentation

- Skin findings occur in ~50% and include palpable purpura, livedo reticularis, retiform purpura, urticarial lesions, ulceration, and digital ischemia (Fig. 50.1)
- Common systemic manifestations include constitutional symptoms as a prominent initial finding, glomerulonephritis, mononeuritis multiplex (with possible foot/wrist drop), arthralgia/myalgia, and pulmonary hemorrhage

Histopathology

- Skin biopsy reveals leukocytoclasia and fibrinoid necrosis of small and medium-sized vessels (Fig. 50.2)
- Glomerulonephritis in MPA is characterized by focal pauci-immune crescentic glomerulonephritis

Differential Diagnosis

- Granulomatosis with polyangiitis: may be distinguishable by upper respiratory involvement and histopathology, but considerable overlap as the two are on a spectrum

R. G. Micheletti, MD
Department of Dermatology, Perelman School of Medicine, University of Pennsylvania, Philadelphia, PA, USA
e-mail: robert.micheletti@uphs.upenn.edu

M. Rosenbach et al. (eds.), *Inpatient Dermatology*,
https://doi.org/10.1007/978-3-319-18449-4_50

- Eosinophilic granlomatosis with polyangiitis: peripheral eosinophilia, ANCA serologies, and the pattern of organ involvement can help distinguish
- Polyarteritis nodosa: can be challenging clinically to differentiate, though serologies and the pattern of internal involvement can help distinguish
- Cryoglobulinemic vasculitis: due to clinical overall, serologic testing may be necessary to differentiate the two

Work-Up

- Approximately 60% of patients are p-ANCA/MPO positive, and 30% are c-ANCA/PR-3 positive
- Serum creatinine level and urinalysis with examination of urine sediment (which may require a nephrology consultation) are important to identify renal involvement and should be urgently performed
- Consider EMG for neuropathy, chest imaging, and other work-up dictated by review of systems and exam

Treatment

- Treatment depends on the extent and rate of progression of pulmonary and renal disease
- All patients with MPA should be managed with appropriate consultations with specialists (nephrology, rheumatology) when appropriate, as often the systemic symptoms drive therapy more than cutaneous involvement
- Similar to GPA, patients with MPA receive high-dose steroids plus rituximab or cyclophosphamide, followed by maintenance therapy with azathioprine or methotrexate to help reduce the risk of relapse

Suggested Readings

1. Kallenberg CG. The diagnosis and classification of microscopic polyangiitis. J Autoimmun. 2014;48–49:90–3.

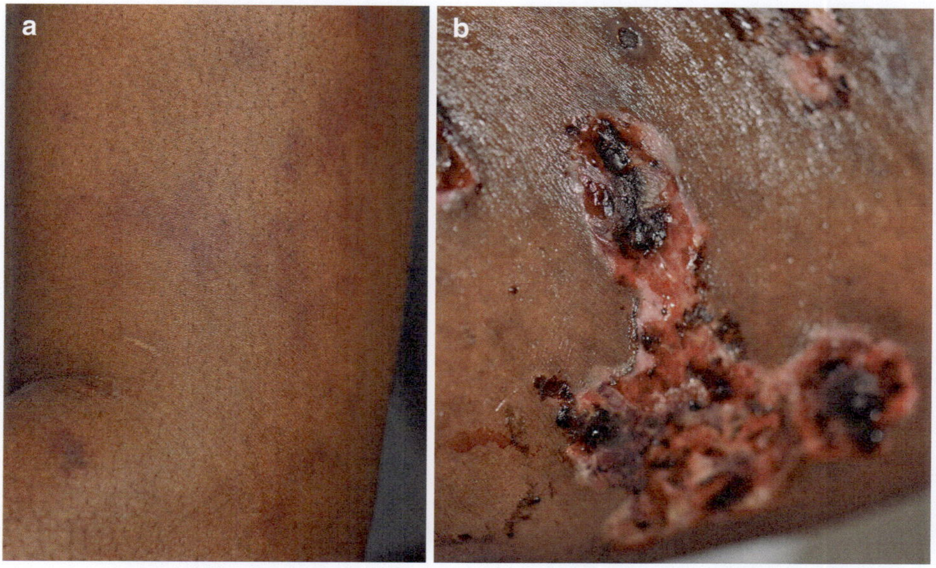

Fig. 50.1 Microscopic polyangiitis (MPA): (**a**) There is angulated incomplete links of livedo with areas of central necrosis. (**b**) Some areas demonstrate ulceration at sites of intense vascular inflammation in this patient with concurrent severe renal involvement.

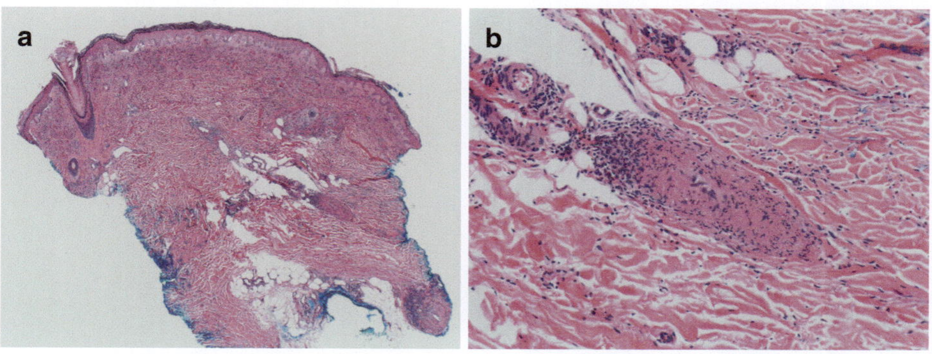

Fig. 50.2 Microscopic polyangiitis (MPA) (*4×, 20×; H&E*): (**a**) While classic features include a necrotizing granulomatous vasculitis, in most cases only a LCV is evident. (**b**) Note the fibrinoid change in the vessel walls which is evident in small vessels in the superficial dermis in addition to deeper medium sized vessels as shown.

Polyarteritis Nodosa

51

Megan H. Noe

Overview

- Polyarteritis nodosa (PAN) is a segmental necrotizing vasculitis of small-to-medium-sized arteries with cutaneous and systemic (classic) variants
  - **Cutaneous PAN** accounts for approximately 10% of cases and is mainly limited to the skin although mild systemic symptoms may occur, including fever, arthralgias and paresthesias. It tends to be chronic but has an overall benign course; rarely progresses to classic PAN
  - **Classic PAN** is a potentially fatal systemic vasculitis commonly involving the skin, peripheral nervous system, gastrointestinal tract, musculoskeletal system, and kidneys, usually lung-sparing
- Classic PAN is more prevalent in men while cutaneous PAN may be more common in women, with an average age of presentation around 45 years old in both; cutaneous PAN is the predominant form in children
- PAN may be associated with infections, medications, inflammatory diseases, and malignancies (Table 51.1)

Table 51.1 Common associations with PAN by subtype

Cutaneous PAN	*Infections*: Streptococcal infection (especially in children), parvovirus B19, tuberculosis
	Medication: minocycline, hydralazine, penicillamine
Classic PAN	*Infection*: HBV, HCV, HIV
	Malignancy: Hairy cell leukemia
Both	*Inflammatory conditions*: IBD, SLE, RA, Sjogren syndrome

M. H. Noe, MD, MPH
Department of Dermatology, University of Pennsylvania, Philadelphia, PA, USA
e-mail: Megan.Noe@uphs.upenn.edu

M. Rosenbach et al. (eds.), *Inpatient Dermatology*,
https://doi.org/10.1007/978-3-319-18449-4_51

Clinical Presentation

- Cutaneous disease presents as palpable purpura, nodules, livedo reticularis, or ulcerations favoring the lower legs (Fig. 51.1)
  - Macular arteritis refers to often pulsatile subcutaneous nodules which may track along blood vessels; the nodules tend to be painful and ulcerate
  - Mixed findings associated with small vessel (palpable purpura) and medium vessel (livedo reticularis) involvement
  - These findings are also present in up to 25–50% of patients with classic PAN
- Individuals also present with fever, weight loss, arthralgias, malaise, and peripheral neuropathy suggestive of mild systemic involvement
- In classic PAN patients have varied clinical courses based on the distribution of their disease (see Table 51.2)
- The ACR diagnostic criteria include: unexplained weight loss, livedo reticularis, testicular pain, myalgias, mono- or polyneuropathy, new-onset diastolic hypertension, elevated BUN or Cr, Hepatitis B, abnormal arteriography, and/or a biopsy demonstrating vasculitis

Histopathology

- Leukocytoclastic vasculitis involving septal small-to-medium sized vessels in the subcutaneous tissue. Leukocytoclastic vasculitis is characterized by neutrophils, nuclear debris, and fibrin deposition in the vessel walls giving a glassy eosinophilic appearance (fibrinoid necrosis), with RBC extravasation (Fig. 51.2)
  - Older lesions may be devoid of neutrophils and appear as a lymphocytic vasculitis
- Superficial biopsies may not capture the arteritis and can show only nonspecific ischemic changes

Differential Diagnosis

- Other small to medium vasculidities: eosinophilic granulomatosis with polyangitis, granulomatosis with polyangiitis, microscopic polyangiitis, rheumatoid vasculitis, leukocytoclastic vasculiitis, cryoglobulinemia, levamisole-tainted cocaine exposure: May have overlapping clinical features, distinguished by history, laboratory evaluation, and biopsy
- Erythema nodosum: usually symmetric red-brown tender nodules on the anterior shins, without livedo reticularis or ulcerations

Table 51.2 Clinical manifestations associated with classic PAN

Renal	Glomerular ischemia and associated variable degrees of renal insufficiency; most patients develop hypertension as a result of their disease
MSK	Myalgias, claudication, arthralgias
Cutaneous	Palpable purpura, nodules, livedo reticularis, ulcerations
GI	Nausea, vomiting, bleeding, mesenteric ischemia with associated postprandial pain and weight loss, rarely causes severe bowel ischemia and perforation
PNS	Peripheral neuropathies, foot or wrist drop is a common manifestation of mononeuritis multiplex
CNS	Transient monocular blindness, TIA, stroke and associated deficits (an uncommon and typically late manifestation)
Ocular	Ischemic retinopathy, retinal detachment, optic neuropathy
Cardiac	Congestive heart failure
Testicular	Orchitis is commonly seen with HBV associated PAN

Work-Up

- Careful history of infections, exposures, and vaccinations (especially recent strep infection in children and HBV, HCV, HIV in adults) in addition to assessing for underlying rheumatologic and inflammatory disease to aid in identifying potential triggers; the diagnostic workup and requested consultations will depend on the physical exam and review of systems
- To evaluate for systemic vasculitis: CBC, Creatinine, UA, ANA, ANCA, RF, complement levels, cyroglobulins
  - High ANA titers, RF positivity, and decreased complement levels can be seen with underlying autoimmune disease and warrants additional work-up
  - ANCA: classically negative in PAN; a positive result strongly favors other vasculitides
- Blood cultures to help exclude an infectious etiology
- Biopsy: a larger sample is preferable including adequate subcutaneous tissue
- Additional workup:
  - Angiography may be used to visualize multiple microaneurysms (a confirmatiory biopsy or imaging study in the appropriate clinical context is necessary for diagnosis)
  - Chest X-ray: typically negative in PAN but pulmonary involvement is prominent in several diseases on the differential so may be warranted
  - EMG studies may indicated to evaluate peripheral neuropathies
- Evaluation for possible triggers should include throat culture/ASO titre (especially in children), hepatitis serology, HIV test

Treatment

- Some mild cases of cutaneous-only disease without systemic symptoms can be treated with NSAIDs and occasionally high potency topical steroids
- Most cases require high-dose oral steroids with a slow taper over weeks to months
- Patients may flare upon steroid taper is common and then other steroid sparing agents may be necessary: NSAIDs, colchicine, hydroxychloroquine, azathioprine, mycophenolate mofetil, methotrexate, cyclophosphamide, pentoxiphylline
- Potential infectious etiologies should be treated

Suggested Readings

1. Fathalla BM, Miller L, Brady S, Schaller JG. Cutaneous polyarteritis nodosa in children. J Am Acad Dermatol. 2005;53:724–8.
2. Fiorentini DF. Cutaneous vasculitis. J Am Acad Dermatol. 2003;48:311–40.
3. Morgan AJ, Schwartz RA. Cutaneous polyarteritis nodosa: a comprehensive review. Int J Dermatol. 2010;49:750–6.

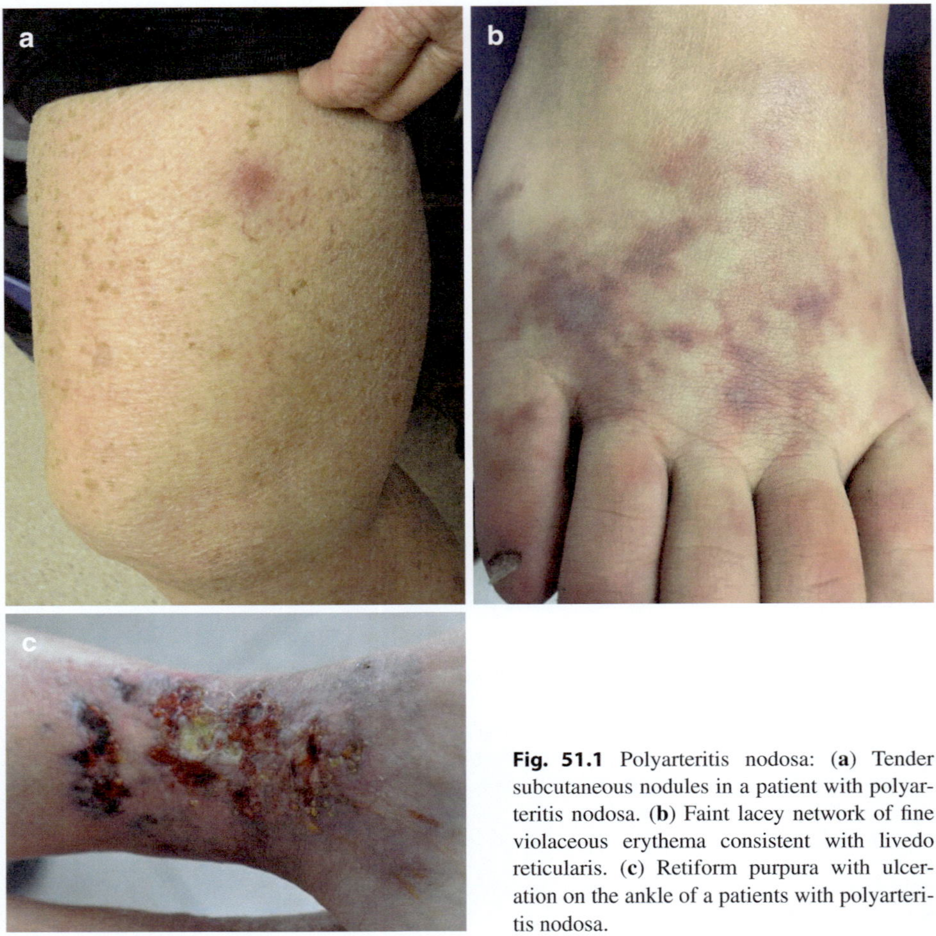

Fig. 51.1 Polyarteritis nodosa: (**a**) Tender subcutaneous nodules in a patient with polyarteritis nodosa. (**b**) Faint lacey network of fine violaceous erythema consistent with livedo reticularis. (**c**) Retiform purpura with ulceration on the ankle of a patients with polyarteritis nodosa.

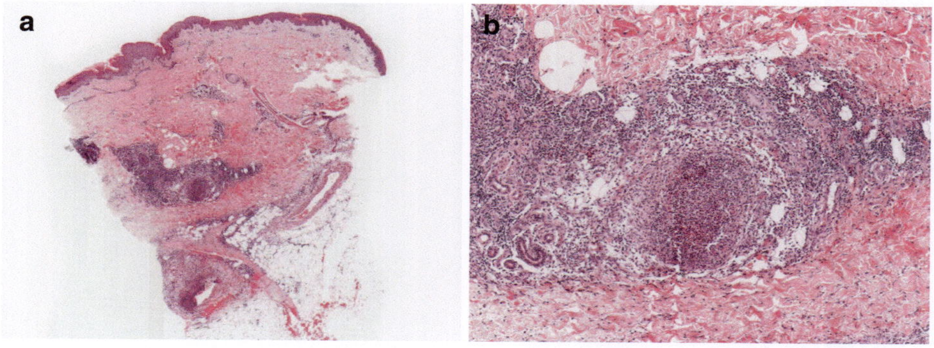

Fig. 51.2 Polyarteritis nodosa (*4×; 10× H&E*): Skip lesions are characteristic, so larger or incisional biopsies are often necessary. (**a**) Medium vessels at the dermal to subcutaneous junction are primarily affected, although overlying small vessels may be involved. Early lesions show infiltration of the vessel with neutrophils, eosinophils, and lymphocytes, with fibrinoid necrosis. There may be occlusion of the vascular lumen and associated leukocytoclasis and dermal hemorrhage. (**b**) Intense vascular inflammation can spill over into the fat lobules and surrounding tissue.

Giant Cell Arteritis

52

Natalie Wright

Overview

- Giant cell arteritis (GCA), also referred to as temporal arteritis, is a medium to large-size vessel vasculitis that usually affects the temporal or occipital branches of the external carotid artery, but can also involve the ophthalmic, vertebral, distal subclavian, and axillary arteries, as well as the thoracic aorta
- Ischemic optic neuropathy is a medical emergency and early steroid treatment is essential to avoid permanent visual loss; a biopsy should be performed but treatment must be prioritized
  - Other complications include scalp necrosis, cerebrovascular events, and aortic dissection and aneurysm
- Can occur concurrently with polymyalgia rheumatica (PMR) in up to 50% of patients
- Most commonly seen in white females over the age of 50, with peak incidence in the seventh and eighth decades

Clinical Presentation

- Classically presents as a unilateral headache unresponsive to analgesics that is associated with exquisite tenderness overlying the temporal or occipital arteries; affected vessel can exhibit decreased or absent pulsation
- Fever, malaise, and jaw claudication are common symptoms
- When a patient has concurrent PMR, symmetric proximal muscle stiffness and arthralgias are also seen
- Cutaneous manifestations are not always present, but the affected vessel can be tender, hard, or tortuous under inflamed, cyanotic, or necrotic skin (Fig. 52.1)
  - Vesicles or bullae may occur and later may evolve into scalp necrosis and gangrene
  - Scalp necrosis is a rare complication that may be associated with optic neuropathy and other severe complications
  - Tender nodules overlying the affected artery or scalp, prurigo nodularis, lingual artery involvement with tongue necrosis, ecchymoses, retiform purpura, urticaria, alopecia, and actinic granuloma have been described

N. Wright, MD
Department of Dermatology, Brigham and Women's Hospital, Harvard University, Boston, MA, USA
e-mail: NAWright@partners.org

M. Rosenbach et al. (eds.), *Inpatient Dermatology*,
https://doi.org/10.1007/978-3-319-18449-4_52

- Visual disturbances include partial or total vision loss and diplopia
  - Vision loss is reported in 10–20% of patients, typically due to anterior ischemic optic neuropathy or less frequently from retinal artery occlusion, which can be irreversible even with treatment
- Other rare and severe complications include extremity claudication, cerebrovascular events, aortic aneurysms and dissections, vascular stenosis, and myocardial infarctions

Histopathology

- A primarily lymphohistiocytic inflammatory infiltrate of the transmural arterial wall is present with interruption of the internal elastic lamina (Fig. 52.2)
  - Multinucleated giant cells may be seen within the inner media, but are not required for diagnosis
  - Elastica van Gieson stain can help highlight elastic lamina fragmentation
- Serial sectioning is helpful as the lesions can be focal, and some patients require bilateral temporal artery biopsies to demonstrate the inflammatory infiltrate

Differential Diagnosis

- ANCA-associated vasculitis, notably granulomatosis with polyangiitis: can often be distinguished by history and physical exam, supplemented with laboratory testing
- Rarely, systemic amyloidosis can present with temporal artery involvement: may have other signs of amyloidosis (pinch purpura, macroglossia), and different histology
- Takayasu's arteritis: can be indistinguishable on histology and imaging, but age of onset and distribution of lesions should preclude this diagnosis

Work-Up

- Temporal artery biopsy is the diagnostic gold standard; however, biopsy can be negative given the focal nature of the arteritis or in those with predominantly subclavian arterial involvement
  - Ideal biopsies consist of a segment at least measuring at least 2 cm
  - Treatment should not be delayed for biopsy if the diagnosis is strongly suspected
- Erythrocyte sedimentation rate (ESR) and C-reactive protein (CRP) are elevated in almost all patients
  - An ESR >50 mm/hr has a sensitivity of 84–86%, albeit low specificity, and is a part of the American College of Rheumatology's diagnostic criteria for GCA
  - Additional criteria include: age $\geq$ 50, new headache, temporal artery symptoms including tenderness and decreased pulsation, and consistent biopsy findings
- As a large vessel vasculitis can occur in up to 25% of patients with GCA, magnetic resonance angiography (MRA) or computed tomographic angiography (CTA) of the aortic arch should be considered
  - These imaging modalities may also be useful in patients in whom GCA is suspected, but not confirmed on biopsy
- Fundoscopy should be performed in patients with visual disturbances in whom GCA is a concern

Treatment

- Systemic corticosteroid monotherapy is effective in the majority of patients
  - Treatment is initiated with prednisone
  - A taper of corticosteroids is usually begun once clinical symptoms and inflammatory markers have normalized with long-term treatment often required
- As ischemic optic neuropathy is a medical emergency, intravenous methylprednisolone should be initiated promptly in patients in whom there is concern for ischemic complications, even if it delays diagnostic biopsy
- The use of steroid-sparing agents has not shown to produce the therapeutic efficacy of steroid monotherapy

Suggested Readings

1. Weyand CM, Goronzy JJ. Clinical Practice giant cell arteritis and polymyalgia rheumatica. N Engl J Med. 2014;371:50–7.
2. Salvarani C, Pipitone N, Versari A, Hunder GG. Clinical features of polymyalgia rheumatica and giant cell arteritis. Nat Rev Rheumatol. 2012;8:509–21.

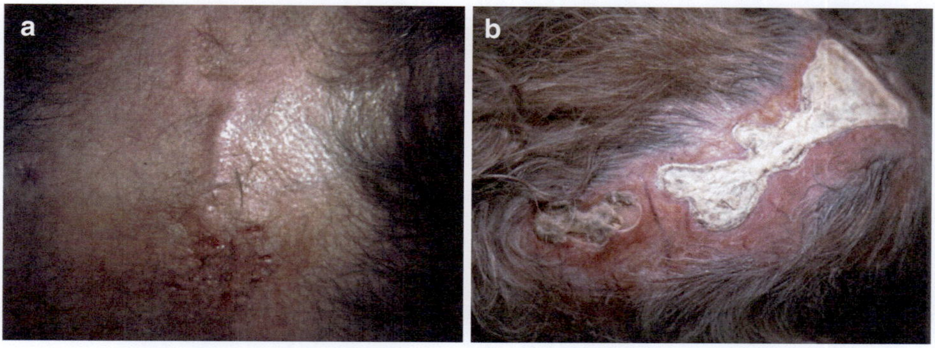

Fig. 52.1 Giant Cell Arteritis: (**a**) Hard, tender, pulsatile temporal artery characteristic of giant cell arteritis. (**b**) Necrosis can result from scalp infarction in giant cell arteritis (Courtesy of Natalie Wright MD & Sam Moschella MD).

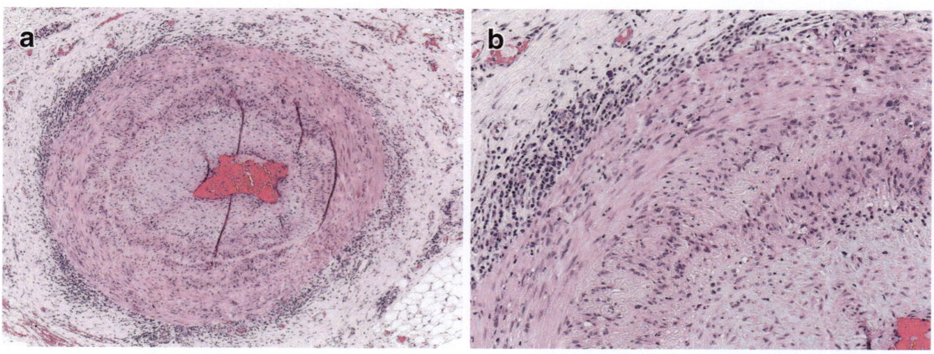

Fig. 52.2 Giant cell arteritis *(10x, 20x; H&E)*: (**a**) Temporal artery demonstrates marked intimal thickening and transmural inflammation with a dense inflammatory infiltrate composed of lymphocytes and histiocytes. (**b**) Multinucleated giant cells also may be seen transversing the arterial wall (Courtesy of Natalie Wright MD & Sam Moschella MD).

Cholesterol Emboli

53

Misha Rosenbach

Overview

- Arterial embolization of cholesterol crystals typically occurring in a patient with severe atherosclerosis following plaque dislodgement secondary to endovascular procedures, thrombolytic therapy or prolonged anticoagulation
  - Symptoms often occur within hours to days of endovascular instrumentation or thrombolytic therapy (may occur 1–2 months into anticoagulant use)
- In patients with multisystem involvement mortality risk is high
- The triad of livedo reticularis, acute renal injury, and eosinophilia should prompt consideration for cholesterol emboli, particularly if observed in a man over 60 years of age with a history of atherosclerotic disease

Clinical Presentation

- Cutaneous findings primarily occur on the distal lower extremities and are characterized by livedo reticularis, nodules, and retiform purpura, often accompanied by evidence of ischemic damage (blue toes, gangrene, cyanosis, ulceration) (Fig. 53.1)
  - Peripheral pulses are usually intact since emboli typically lodge within the arterioles
  - Moderate to severe pain may accompany cutaneous findings
- Visceral organs can also be affected, most commonly the kidneys with resulting renal insufficiency or acute renal failure
  - Additional visceral organs that can be affected include the pancreas, spleen, gastrointestinal tract, liver, brain, and eyes (where a cholesterol embolus may be directly visible on funduscopic exam)

Histopathology

- Presence of needle-shaped cholesterol clefts are seen occluding small arteries and arterioles (Fig. 53.2)
  - Sectioning through the biopsy specimen blocks may be required to find a focus of disease
- Involved vessels may demonstrate intimal hyperplasia and fibrosis
- Variable epidermal changes with ulceration and associated mixed inflammatory infiltrate

M. Rosenbach, MD
Department of Dermatology, Perelman School of Medicine, University of Pennsylvania, Philadelphia, PA, USA
e-mail: Misha.Rosenbach@uphs.upenn.edu

M. Rosenbach et al. (eds.), *Inpatient Dermatology*,
https://doi.org/10.1007/978-3-319-18449-4_53

Differential Diagnosis

- Medium-sized vessel vasculitides: there is overlap in the cutaneous features; vasculitides have distinct histopathology and often serologic tests
- Cryoglobulinemia: cutaneous features may have overlap, though in mixed cryoglobulinemia there is often palpable purpura which is uncommon in cholesterol emboli; lab testing and pathology can distinguish
- Calciphylaxis: usually patients have chronic kidney disease, and larger, more ischemic/necrotic painful skin plaques
- Warfarin necrosis: broad ischemic purpura shortly after initiating warfarin therapy
- APLAS: extensive thrombi can present with livedo and retiform purpura, but histopathology and confirmatory laboratory testing should distinguish

Work-Up

- In classic cases with livedo, eosinophilia, acute kidney injury, and the right demographic (older atherosclerotic patients after endovascular implementation) the diagnosis may be made presumptively, with efforts to exclude entities on the differential diagnosis
- Histopathologic evaluation is important to confirm the diagnosis and obtained biopsies should be deep enough to involve fat
  - The optimal biopsy site is debated, people are tempted to biopsy the purple areas of livedo reticularis but often the pathology is located beneath the blanched area proximal to the necrotic tissue (if present); therefore, the optimal technique is a deep incisional biopsy spanning both the violaceous and blanchable areas of the lesion
- Renal complications can be severe in these patients and creatinine should be monitored closely
- CBC with differential will often demonstrate leukocytosis with eosinophilia
- Work up to exclude underlying vasculitides or other microvascular occlusion syndromes can be considered depending on clinical findings

Treatment

- Prognosis is poor with an overall high mortality rate which may vary depending on patient comorbidities
- Early recognition and aggressive supportive management are key therapeutic elements
- Discontinuation of anticoagulation therapy if possible and avoidance of invasive vascular procedures are important considerations
- Use of systemic corticosteroids is controversial with varied results and may be useful in the setting of significant end organ damage (renal disease in particular)
- Statin drugs may be helpful in some cases
- Visceral disease involving the kidney may require hemodialysis
- Consider role for potential surgical intervention for resection of necrotic symptomatic tissue and for identification and removal of causative atheromatous lesions

Suggested Readings

1. Jucgla A, Moreso F, Muniesa C, Moreno A, Vidaller A. Cholesterol embolism: still an unrecognized entity with a high mortality rate. J Am Acad Dermatol. 2006;55(5):786–93.
2. Pennington M, Yeager J, Skelton H, et al. Cholesterol embolization syndrome: cutaneous histopathological features and the variable onset of symptoms in patients with different risk factors. Br J Dermatol. 2002;146:511–7.

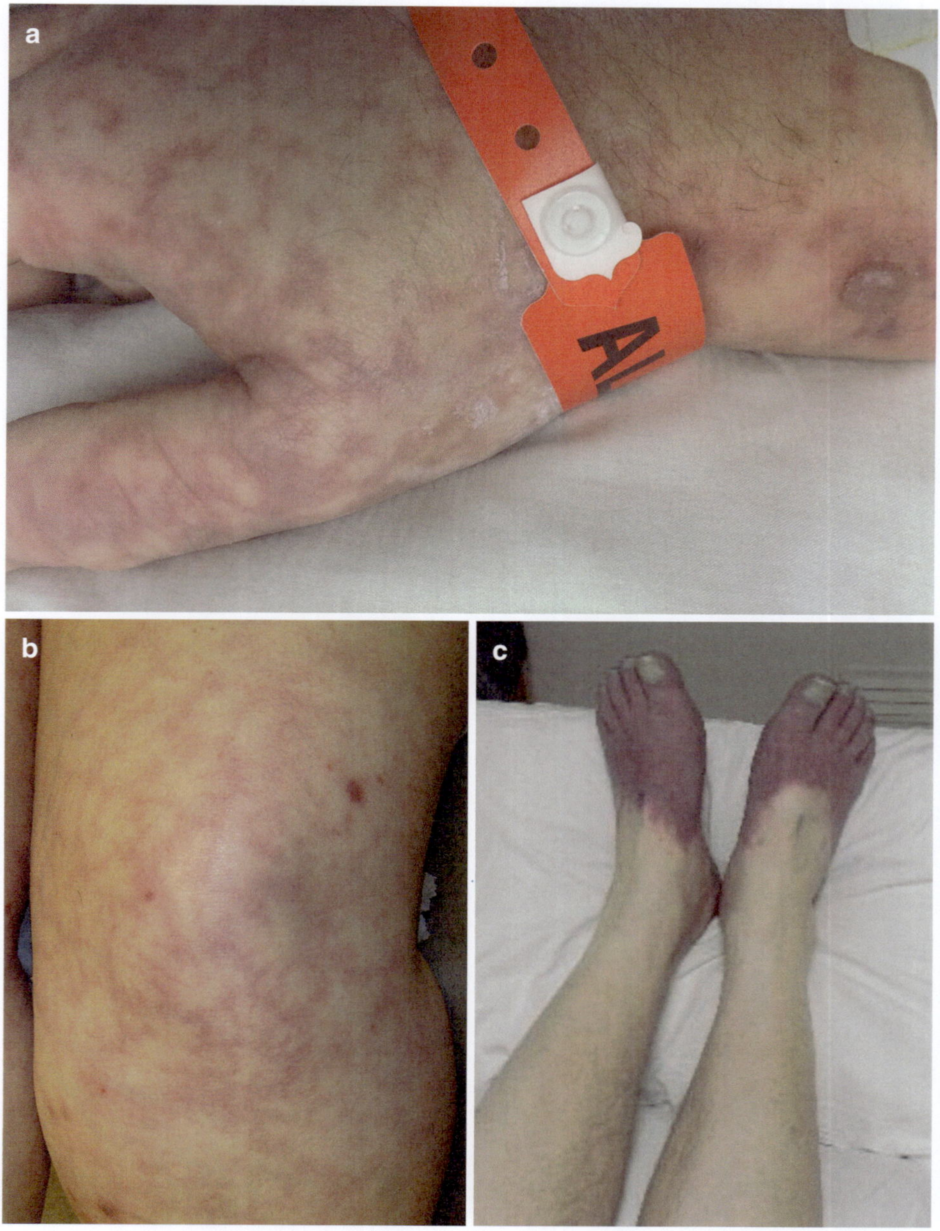

Fig. 53.1 Cholesterol emboli: (**a**) Fixed livedo reticularis of the distal extremities resulting from cholesterol emboli. (**b**) The triad of livedo reticularis, eosinophilia, and acute kidney injury following an intravascular procedure suggests a diagnosis of cholesterol emboli. (**c**) This patient developed striking distal purpura with an angulated, stellate border after abdominal aortic surgery and cholesterol emboli.

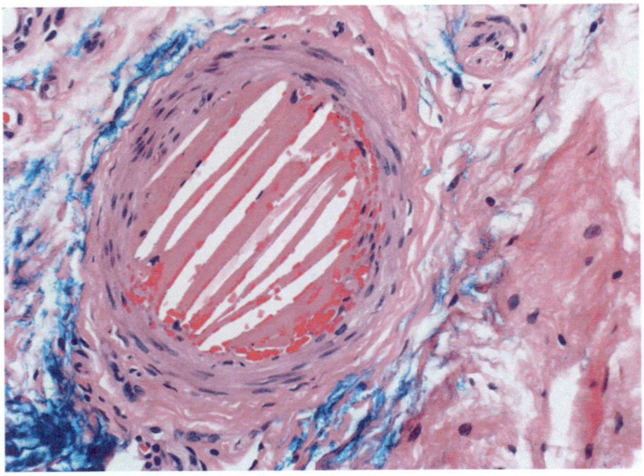

Fig. 53.2 Cholesterol emboli (*40×, H&E*): Histopathologic features including clefts in arterioles and arteries in the dermis and subcutis with associated fibrin thrombi. There may be extensive surrounding necrosis and red blood cell sludging within superficial vessels.

54 Infective Endocarditis

John C. Selby

Overview

- Bacterial infection of native or prosthetic endocardial tissues, primarily the aortic and mitral valves
  - Primarily three forms: (1) native valve endocarditis (NVE), (2) prosthetic valve (PVE), and (3) endocarditis associated with intravenous drug use (IVDU) (Table 54.1)
    Similar findings to PVE can less commonly be seen with implantable cardiac devices such as pacemakers
- *Staphylococcus aureus*, viridans group streptococci, and coagulase-negative staphylococci are the most frequently cultured pathogens
- Clinical diagnosis is based off of the Duke modified criteria (Table 54.2)
- Risk factors include:
  - Age > 60 years, male sex, IV drug use, poor dentition, valvular heart disease, congenital heart disease, presence of an intravascular device or prosthetic heart valve, hemodialysis, diabetes mellitus, HIV infection
- Complications include:
  - Heart failure, perivalvular or intracardiac abscess, and septic emboli that can lead to extra cardiac abscess formation in the brain, kidney, bone, and joint space
- Despite advances in diagnosis, medical therapy, and surgical treatment, in-hospital mortality ranges from 15 to 20% and 1-year mortality approaches 40%

Clinical Presentation

- Most patients present acutely with fever, chills, night sweats, and fatigue with a new heart murmur. However, presentations are diverse and patients may also present with subacute/chronic disease with nonspecific symptoms and a low-grade fever.
- There are four major extracardiac signs: splinter hemorrhages, Osler's nodes, Janeway lesions, Roth spots; these are excellent clinical clues when present but are seen in <10% of cases. Patients may also present with nonspecific petechiae of mucosae/conjunctivae or even a frank leukocytoclastic vasculitis with palpable purpura (Fig. 54.1)
  - Splinter (subungual) hemorrhages: non-specific, non-blanching, longitudinal, linear, red/brown/black streaks in the distal third of the nail bed

J. C. Selby, MD, PhD
University of Iowa Hospitals and Clinics, Iowa City, IA, USA
e-mail: john-selby@uiowa.edu

M. Rosenbach et al. (eds.), *Inpatient Dermatology*,
https://doi.org/10.1007/978-3-319-18449-4_54

Table 54.1 Clinical forms of endocarditis

Native valve endocarditis (NVE)			
Acute	Normal valves	Rapid progressive onset with high grade fevers	Staph, viridans group strepto cocci
Subacute	Abnormal valves	Indolent, nonspecific, low grade fevers	Strep, enterococci
Prosthetic valve endocarditis (PVE)			
Early	Prosthetic valves (mitral > aortic)	<60 days post implantation	Staph, gram-negative co ccobacilli, candida
Late		>60 days post implantation	Staph, strep, entrerococci
Endocarditis associated with intravenousntra venous drug use (IVDU)			
Acute	Often involves previously normal tricuspid valve	Rapid progressive onset with high grade fevers	*Staph*
Subacute	Valvular damage from injected particulates followed by colonization	Indolent, nonspecific, low grade fevers	Less commonly strep and enterococci
Recurrent	Often involves previously normal tricuspid valve	Repeat infection from reintroduction of skin flora may be acute or subacute	

Table 54.2 Modified Duke criteria [1] (2 major *or* 1 major +3 minor *or* 5 minor)

Major criteria	Minor criteria
1. Positive blood cultures	1. Predisposition (e.g. prosthetic heart valve, underlying heart condition, IVDU)
–Typical causative microbial pathogen isolated from two separate blood cultures drawn 12 hours apart	2. Fever >38° C
–If potential skin contaminant need 3 or 4 positive cultures	3. Evidence of septic vasculopathy (mycotic aneurysm, Janeway lesions, intracranial or intraocular hemorrhage/microabscesses, etc.
–Coxiella Burnetii only needs one positive blood culture or IgG phase 1 ELISA antibody titer >1:800	4. Associated immunologic sequelae (immune complex mediated vasculitis and glomerulonephritis)
2. Echocardiographic evidence of valvular vegetations or new regurgitation murmur	5. Positive cultures (that do not meet major criteria)

  - Osler nodes: small (<1.5 cm), painful, erythematous subcutaneous nodules arising on the volar pads of the fingers and toes
  - Janeway lesions: painless, erythematous to hemorrhagic macules arising on the volar surfaces of the hands and feet
  - Roth spots: pale-centered retinal hemorrhages
  - Non-specific petechiae of the oral and ocular mucosae
- Common complications include:
  - Cardiac: Valvular insufficiency and symptoms of heart failure
  - Septic emboli: Commonly involve the kidney and spleen (with possible splenomegaly noted on exam) leading to infectious seeding and infarction

Right-sided endocarditis is common in the setting of IVDU
Septic emboli to the brain can lead to hemorrhagic or ischemic stroke and multiple abscesses with associated neurologic deficits
Valvular abnormality impedes proper blood flow and can also result in sterile embolic disease

Histopathology

- Splinter hemorrhages: non-specific hemorrhage from capillaries of the dermal papillae in the nail bed
- Osler node: sterile leukocytoclastic vasculitis and perivasculitis likely secondary to immune complex deposition
- Janeway lesion: dermal microabscess that is vasculocentric secondary to septic micro embolization, often culture-positive (Fig. 54.2)

Differential Diagnosis

- Cholesterol emboli: distal livedo reticularis with eosinophilia and acute kidney injury, versus the more focal lesions of endocarditis
- Cryoglobulin vasculopathy: endocarditis can be a cause of cryoglobulinemia vasculitis/vasculopathy, and if cryos are found, endocarditis should be considered; thus, the two entities can share extensive overlap
- Antiphospholipid antibody syndrome: causes more broad areas of angulated retiform purpura, and laboratory testing should distinguish the two
- Cutaneous vasculitis: endocarditis can result in a small vessel vasculitis, and thus seeing leukocytoclastic vasculitis should prompt consideration for endocarditis
- Gonococcemia: hemorrhagic pustules over joints with joint pain can occur in both; history, lab testing, and occasional symptoms of genital discharge can help distinguish
- Thrombocytopenia: can result in nonspecific petechiae and even splinter hemorrhages, but should not have positive blood cultures

Work-Up

- Complete blood count with differential: would expect to see a leukocytosis with neutrophilia
- Blood cultures: at least three sets (aerobic and anaerobic) from different sites, >1 hour apart
  - Blood cultures will most commonly grow Staphylococcus aureus, viridans group streptococci, and coagulase-negative staphylococci
  - Less common pathogens include:
    Enterococcus species
    Streptococcus gallolyticus (formally *Streptococcus bovis*)
    Fungi/yeast
    HACEK group organisms: *Haemophilus* species, *Aggregatibacter actinomycetemcomitans*, *Cardiobacterium hominis*, *Eikenella corrodens*, and *Kingella* species
- Echocardiogram: transthoracic if low clinical suspicion, transesophageal if moderate-to-high suspicion
- Electrocardiogram (EKG)
- Urinalysis and urine culture to assess for urosepsis and potential infectious source

Treatment

- Blood cultures should be drawn prior to the initiation of antibiotic therapy
- Intravenous antibiotics with empiric selections dependent on acute versus subacute presentation and native versus prosthetic valve; Infectious Disease consultation often required to guide recommendations

- Indications for surgery: severe valvular dysfunction leading to refractory congestive heart failure, prosthetic valve, uncontrolled infection, systemic embolization leading to or placing patient at risk of severe stroke
- No specific skin-targeted therapies are required but local skin care at sites of necrosis can be useful

References

1. Li JS, Sexton DJ, Mick N, et al. Proposed modifications to the Duke criteria for the diagnosis of infective endocarditis. Clin Infect Dis. 2000;30:633–38. PMID: 10770721.
2. Murdoch DR, et al. Clinical presentation, etiology, and outcome of infective endocarditis in the 21st century: the International Collaboration on Endocarditis-Prospective Cohort Study. Arch Intern Med. 2009;169(5):463–73.
3. Sethi K, Buckley J, de Wolff J. Splinter haemorrhages, Osler's nodes, Janeway lesions and Roth spots: the peripheral stigmata of endocarditis. Br J Hosp Med (Lond). 2013;74(9):C139–42.
4. Baddour LM, et al. Infective endocarditis: diagnosis, antimicrobial therapy, and management of complications: a statement for healthcare professionals from the Committee on Rheumatic Fever, Endocarditis, and Kawasaki Disease, Council on Cardiovascular Disease in the Young, and the Councils on Clinical Cardiology, Stroke, and Cardiovascular Surgery and Anesthesia, American Heart Association: endorsed by the Infectious Diseases Society of America. Circulation. 2005;111:e394–433.

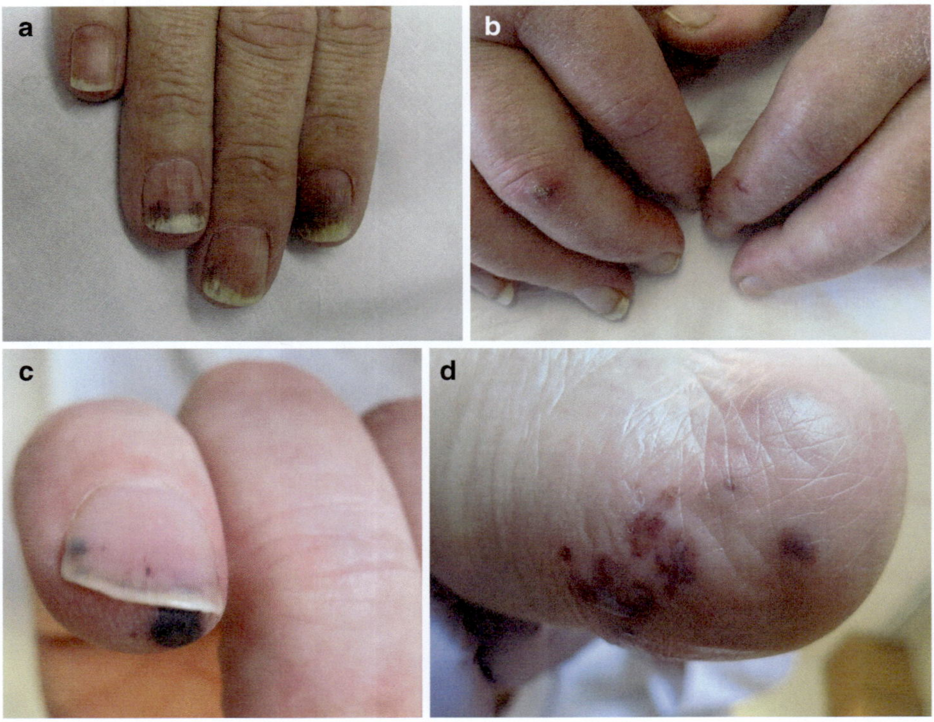

Fig. 54.1 Infective endocarditis: (**a**) Extensive splinter hemorrhages involving more than just the distal nail are common. (**b**) Red tender papules on the dorsal distal extremities due to emboli and immune complex deposition. (**c**) Painless embolic phenomena (Janeway lesions) of the fingertips may be seen with bacterial endocarditis. (**d**) Tender purpuric papules (Osler nodes) on the heel due to bacterial endocarditis.

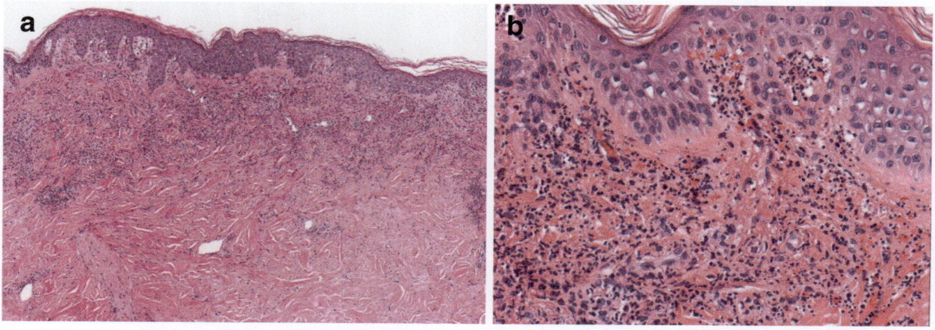

Fig. 54.2 Endocarditis with associated septic vasculitis *(20×, 40×; H&E)*: This biopsy was taken from a patient with endocarditis and *Staphylococcus aureus* sepsis. (**a**, **b**) There is a dense neutrophilic infiltrate spilling out of the vessels into the surrounding tissue with marked red blood cell extravasation.

Cryoglobulinemia

55

Badri Modi

Overview

- Cold-precipitating intravascular proteins (cryoglobulins). Some cryloglobulins (type I) can cause vaso-occlusive "sludging" and small vessel clot formation (vasculopathy); some cryoglobulins (types II and III) may fix complement and cause an inflammatory response as well (vasculitis)
  - A diagnosis of cryoglobulinemia is made based on laboratory confirmation of circulating cryoglobulins in the appropriate clinical context
- Cryoglobulin precipitation often occurs in the skin due to exposure to temperature fluctuations, particularly peripheral cold
- There are three types of cryoglobulinemias, with 80% of cases being type II/III (see Table 55.1)
  - **Type I cryoglobulinemia**, (monoclonal cryoglobulinemia), is due to a monoclonal proliferation secondary to a plasma cell dyscrasia (i.e. Waldenstrom, MGUS, multiple myeloma), frequently with precipitating IgM antibodies resulting in a vasculopathy
  - **Type II/III cryoglobulinemia**, (mixed cryoglobulinemia) occurs in the presence of elevated IgG and IgM antibodies, usually due to a chronic underlying condition (infection, especially hepatitis C or endocarditis, or autoimmune disease) resulting in an immune complex-mediated small to medium vessel vasculitis and concomitant vasculopathy

Clinical Presentation

- Cutaneous findings are evident in essentially all cryoglobulinemia patients and may be the presenting sign of disease (Fig. 55.1)
- Type I Cryoglobulinemia: more often angulated stellate purpura and livedo (vasculopathy), versus Type II/III cryoglobulinemia, which are more likely to demonstrate those findings plus palpable purpura (vasculitis)
  - Primary skin lesions reflect the involvement of both small and medium sized cutaneous vessels, with esions occuring in response to skin hypoxia due to vascular occlusion, with or without an associated vasculitis

B. Modi, MD
Division of Dermatology, City of Hope, Duarte, CA, USA

M. Rosenbach et al. (eds.), *Inpatient Dermatology*,
https://doi.org/10.1007/978-3-319-18449-4_55

Table 55.1 Types of cryoglobulinemia and their associated pathogenesis

Subtype/associated cryoglobins	Underlying etiologies	Vascular disease	Clinicopathologic correlation	RF testing
Type I (monoclonal type)	MGUS Waldenstrom macroglobulinemia Multiple myeloma	Cold-induced immunoglobulin precipitation leads to bland occlusion, without complement activation and inflammation; tissue hypoxia secondary to vaso-occlusion from hyerviscosity from protein accumulation or thrombosis	*Clinical:* angulated stellate purpura and livedo	Negative
Monoclonal IgM > IgG, IgA or light chains	Lymphoma	Over time a secondary vasculitis may develop	*Histology:* Vessels distended by and occluded with eosinophilic amorphous material with little to no associated inflammation	
Type II (mixed type)	Infectious:	Multisystem symptoms related to of small-medium sized vessel vasculitis secondary to circulating immune complexes	*Clinical:* Angulated livedo reticularis plus areas with palpable purpura, particularly distal, cool sites	Positive
Polyclonal IgG +	• Hepatitis C virus			
Monoclonal IgM	• HIV • Endocarditis • Other (osteomyelitis)			
Type III (mixed type)	Non-infectious:	Classically, The IgM antibody functions as a rheumatoid factor by binding to the Fc-moiety of IgG, resulting in activation of complement and an inflammatory vasculitis in addition to the occlusive vasculopathy	*Histology:* Leukocytoclastic vasculitis +/− intravascular eosinophilic amorphous cryopercipitates (less common than in type 1)	
Polyclonal IgG +	Systemic autoimmune disease – Sjogren syndrome – SLE			
Polyclonal IgM	– Rheumatoid arthritis Lymphoproliferative disorders – B cell lymphoma			

  - Petechia, purpura, and livedo reticularis may be seen in mild disease, while cutaneous ulcers, gangrene, digital ischemia, and necrosis are seen in more severe cases
  - There is an acral predominance due to exposure to cooler temperatures; the lower legs, feet, distal toes, and ears are commonly involved.
- Systemic involvement can occur in any organ system with small blood vessels, most commonly the joints and nerves in addition to the skin:
  - General—fevers, malaise, weakness
  - Kidneys—membranoproliferative glomerulonephritis is most common, presenting as proteinuria, microscopic hematuria, RBC casts, hypertension, and renal failure

- Joints—arthralgias, mostly in the hands, wrists, feet and ankles
- Peripheral nerves—sensory paresthesias and motor deficits (mononeuritis multiplex, e.g. foot drop)
- Lungs—interstitial lung fibrosis, diffuse pulmonary infiltrates due to alveolar hemorrhage
- Gastrointestinal—intestinal ischemia presenting as acute abdominal pain and bloody stool
- Cardiac—coronary vasculitis
- CNS—stroke, encephalopathy

Histopathology

- Early lesions of monoclonal cryoglobulinemia demonstrate vascular occlusion by eosinophilic amorphous material without associated vascular damage; older lesions may demonstrate fibrinoid necrosis consistent with a secondary vasculitis (Fig. 55.2)
- In mixed cryoglobulinemia there is a combination of vascular thrombosis and leukocytoclastic small vessel vasculitis composed of transmural neutrophilic infiltrate with karyorrhexis/leukocytoclasis debris and endothelial damage (fibrinoid necrosis)

Differential Diagnosis

- Vasculopathy
  - Anti-phospholipid antibody syndrome: clinically may present similarly, thus workup for peripheral purpuric lesions includes serologic testing for APLAs and cryoglobulins
  - Cholesterol emboli: history of recent endovascular procedure is key, otherwise the clinical features can have substantial overlap; pathology and serologies can often confirm
  - Cocaine (with or without levamisole) abuse: urine drug screen and history are critical, as cocaine can cause vasculitis and addition of levamisole can cause both vasculitis and vasculopathy similar to cryoglobulinemia
  - Thrombo-embolic disease (such as from a cardiac vegetation or atrial thrombus): can also cause peripheral findings, and indeed endocarditis can cause cryoglobulinemia; extensive testing may be necessary to exclude a central embolic source
- Vasculitis
  - Small vessel vasculitis
    - Cutaneous small vessel vasculitis (infectious, autoimmune, drug-induced): some forms of cryoglobulinemia can present with small vessel vasculitis and extensive testing is often needed to distinguish
    - IgA vasculitis (Henoch Schoenlein purpura): clinical overlap means sometimes it will require direct immunofluorescence to demonstrate IgA vasculitis
  - Small to medium vessel vasculitis: the pattern of organ involvement plus serologic testing (and negative cryoglobulins) can help distinguish these entities

Work-Up

- Diagnosis of cryoglobulinemic syndromes requires demonstration of immunoglobulin precipitation, however there is a high rate of false negatives. To minimize this blood should be drawn and kept warm at >37° to avoid premature precipitation
  - Blood can be kept warm by submerging the tube in warm water or carrying it the axilla to the lab
  - Once in the lab, the blood is incubated at 4 °C to facilitate precipitation and the cryoprecipitate is quantified and analyzed for antibody type
- RF to evaluate for the presence of monoclonal or polyclonal IgM targeting the Fc-portion of IgG (rheumatoid factor activity)
  - As cryoglobulin testing is slow and insensitive, RF is a readily available surrogate marker for Type II/III cryoglobulinemia (and will often be a faster test with fewer false negatives)
- C3 and C4 (to evaluate complement consumption); cryoglobulinemia may present with an isolated low C4

- Additional workup will depend on symptomatology and underlying disease:
- SPEP to evaluate for evidence of a monoclonal gammopathy as seen in Type I cryoglobulinemia
- Evaluate for renal involvement using a urinalysis with microscopic examination, urine protein and creatinine, serum creatinine
- Viral hepatitis serologies with HCV testing, viral load should be ordered in the setting of known disease
- Blood cultures in all patients, with echocardiogram if risk factors for endocarditis are present, including new murmur or positive blood cultures
- Additional organ-specific testing should be driven by individual patients' symptomatology

Treatment

- Treatment is determined by extent of involvement (skin limited versus systemic) and underlying illness
- Treatment is directed at the underlying cause in most cases, to reduce cryoglobulin synthesis—this is essential, as without controlling the cause, the immunoglobulin will continue to be produced
- All patients should be educated about core and extremity warming and should avoid excessive cold exposure
- Asymptomatic patients may be monitored with supportive care
- For severe skin only disease leading to ulceration or skin necrosis and/or systemic involvement, more aggressive therapy is indicated:
  - Targeting cryoglobulins: IVIG, plasmapheresis, plasma exchange, rituximab
  - Targeting vasculitis: systemic corticosteroids, colchicine, dapsone, methotrexate

Suggested Readings

1. Motyckova G, Murali M. Laboratory testing for cryoglobulins. Am J Hematol. 2011;86(6):500–2.
2. Retamozo S, Brito-Zerón P, Bosch X, Stone JH, Ramos-Casals M. Cryoglobulinemic disease. Oncology. 2013;27(1098–1105):1110–6.

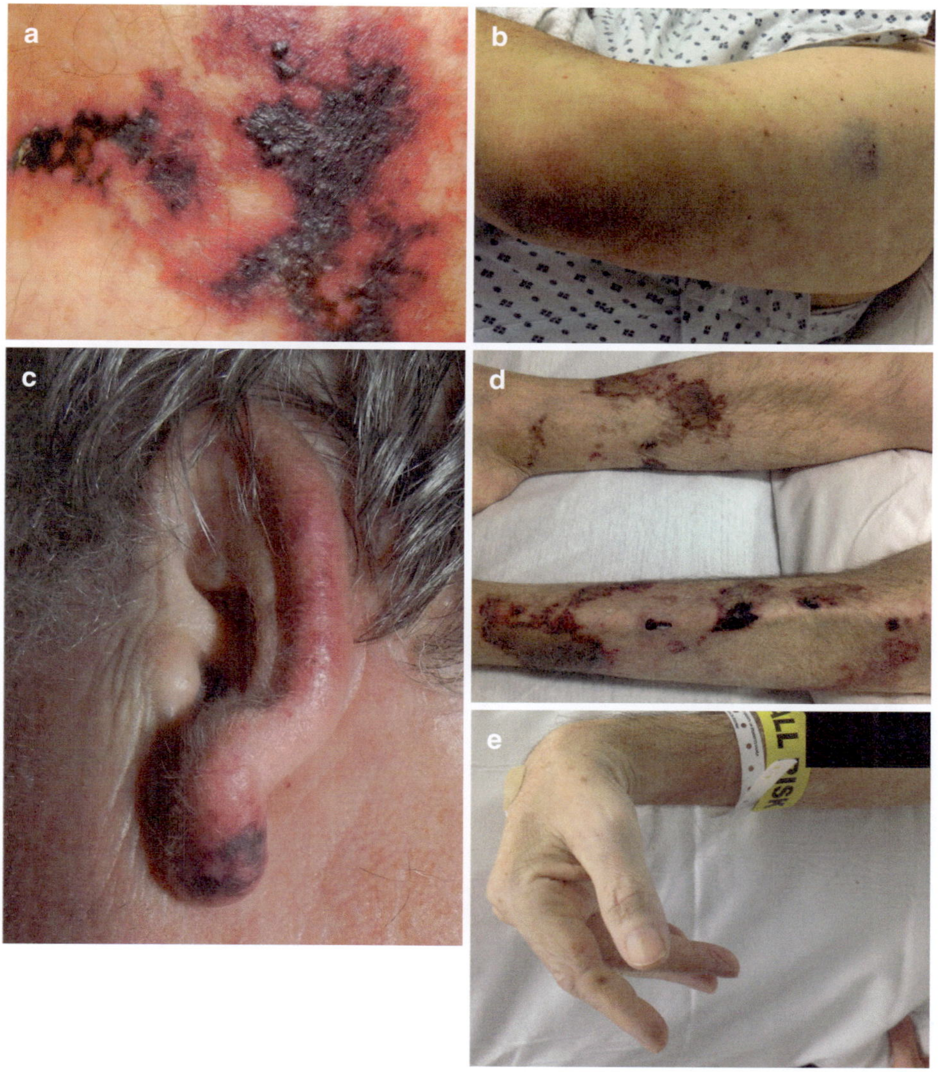

Fig. 55.1 Cryoglobulinemia: (**a**) Jagged angulated non-blanching patchers of retiform purpura. (**b**) Patients may have non-specific signs such as fixed livedo reticularis. (**c**) angulated purpuric macules with acrocyanosis of the earlobe due to type I cryoglobulinemic vasculopathy. (**d**) Retiform purpura and eschar formation on the shins. (**e**) Wrist drop/mononeuritis multiplex due to hepatitis C-related cryoglobulinemic vasculitis.

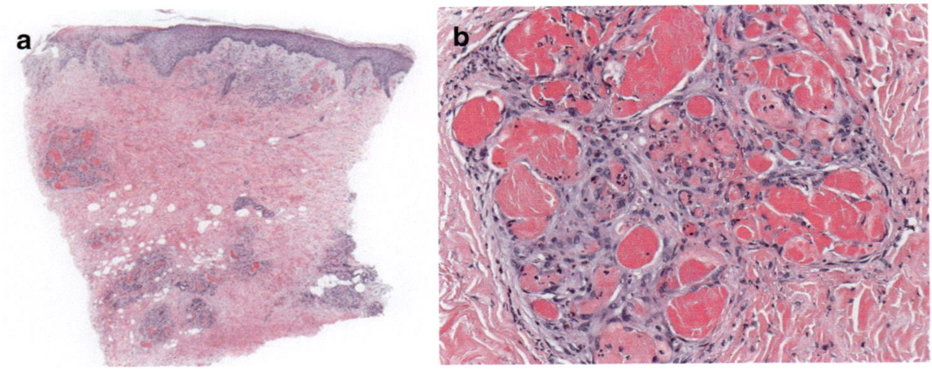

Fig. 55.2 Cryoglobulinemia *(1×, 10×, H&E)*: (**a**) Histopathologic features depend on the type of cryoglobulinemia. Monoclonal cryoglobulinemia (type I) can demonstrate hyaline thrombi that plug the small superficial vessels. In type II and type II, both thrombi and small vessel vasculitis are seen. Here, low power demonstrates the vascular congestion that are hyaline thrombi that plugging the small superficial vessels. (**b**) On higher power, the hyaline thrombi are well-visualized with associated vessel dilation and endothelial swelling. PAS stain highlights the thrombi. This is an example of type I cryoglobulinemia.

Antiphospholipid Antibody Syndrome

56

Molly Moye

Overview

- Antiphospholipid antibody syndrome (APLAS) is an autoimmune condition characterized by venous and/or arterial thrombotic events, including DVTs, PE, TIAs, stroke, and pregnancy complications/miscarriage in the presence of specific antibodies to glycoproteins (see Table 56.1)
  - The most common antibodies include: lupus anticoagulant (LA), anti-cardiolipin antibodies (aCL) and anti-beta-2-glycoprotein I (aGPI)
- APLS typically presents in young women and may be primary or secondary
  - Secondary APLS typically occurs in patients with underlying SLE and less commonly in association with other autoimmune diseases, malignancies, medications or infections
- Stroke (and other neurologic symptoms), nephropathy, thrombocytopenia, deep venous thrombosis (DVT)/pulmonary embolism (PE) and cutaneous manifestations are common presentations of APLS
- Catastrophic antiphospholipid syndrome (CAPS) is the most severe and rare form of the disease and is characterized by multisystem disease with temporally associated thrombotic events in 3+ organs

Table 56.1 Diagnostic criteria for APLS (adapted from the revised Sapporo APS Classification Criteria)

Definite APLS requires at least one laboratory criterion and one clinical criterion	
Cutaneous manifestations are not included in the clinical criteria, patients who solely have cutaneous manifestations and meet laboratory criteria are often diagnosed with "probable APLS"	
Clinical criteria	• Clinical manifestations of venous and/or arterial thrombosis involving any organ with confirmation by imaging and/or histology
	• Pregnancy complications (one of the following):
	– 1+ spontaneous abortion after 10 weeks gestation
	– 3+ spontaneous abortions before the 10th week
	– 1+ premature births before 34 weeks gestation secondary to pre-eclampsia/eclampsia or placental insufficiency
Laboratory criteria	Elevated levels of lupus anticoagulant, anti-cardiolipin and/or anti-beta-2 glycoprotein-I antibodies on 2+ occasions at least 12 weeks apart

M. Moye, MD
Forefront Dermatology, Louisville, KY, USA
e-mail: mollymoye@me.com

M. Rosenbach et al. (eds.), *Inpatient Dermatology*,
https://doi.org/10.1007/978-3-319-18449-4_56

- May occur with infections, drugs (including OCPs and sulfur-containing diuretics), anticoagulant discontinuation and in post-surgical patients
- Mortality is approximately 50% and the vast majority of patients have cutaneous manifestations; purpura fulminans can be the presenting sign, along with renal failure and/or ARDS

Clinical Presentation

- 40–50% of patients have cutaneous manifestations which are often non-specific, so the clinician must have a high index of suspicion (Fig. 56.1)
  - Livedo reticularis is the most common skin finding, livedo racemosa (incomplete, jagged, sometimes non-blanching purpuric links of livedo) can also be seen
  - Retiform purpura that becomes necrotic is common and should be managed as a thrombotic event
  - Other cutaneous manifestations include livedoid vasculopathy, atrophie blanche, palpable purpura (mimicking vasculitis), and digital gangrene
  - Livedoid vasculopathy occurs secondary to medium-sized arteriole vaso-occlusive disease resulting in recurrent painful lesions spanning the lower legs to the dorsal feet with superficial punched-out ulcerations
  - Atrophie blanche refers to the ivory-colored atophic scars which form overlying the healing ulcers
  - Anetoderma can be for a sign of APLS; in patients with systemic lupus erythematosus, it is almost always a sign that the patient has APLS
  - Anetoderma refers to localized oval atrophic cutaneous lesions in areas of decreased to absent elastic fibers allowing subcutaneous tissue herniation which present as soft easily reduced tissue bulges
  - CAPS can present with purpura fulminans
- Pregnancy morbidity is commonly associated with APLS; a history of recurrent spontaneous abortions, severe IUGR and premature birth secondary to severe preeclampsia and or/placental insufficiency should prompt consideration of APLS

Histopathology

- Thrombosis with minimal surrounding inflammation is the characteristic histopathologic finding (Fig. 56.2)
- Newer lesions may have epidermal necrosis, edema, and extravasated red blood cells
- Older lesions may have epidermal atrophy and dermal deposition of hemosiderin, with secondary vasculitis potentially evident in long-standing lesions

Differential Diagnosis

- Other microangiopathic conditions: these are generally all urgent/emergent diagnoses and can share significant overlap in the cutaneous exam findings; differentiating these entities requires rapid serologic testing for specific diagnoses (APLAs, HIT, D-dimer), and often overlapped treatment and intense supportive care while performing evaluation
  - Thrombotic thrombocytopenic purpura (TTP), especially when the patient presents with neurologic findings. Thrombocytopenia in APLS is typically not as severe as in TTP.
  - Hemolytic Uremic Syndrome (HUS)
  - Hemolysis, Elevated Liver Enzymes and Low Platelets (HELLP): especially in a multiparous female in the third trimester. Patients with APLS may experience HELLP, making a definitive diagnosis difficult.
  - Heparin Induced Thrombocytopenia (HIT): recent history of heparin use, precipitous platelet drop, and confirmatory serologic testing is available
  - Disseminated intravascular coagulation (DIC) is in the differential of CAPS as both can present with purpura fulminans. D-dimer is often negative in CAPS. In DIC, patients are thrombocytopenic, have prolonged clotting time and low fibrinogen levels.

- Systemic Lupus Erythematosus (SLE): there is overlap between APLS and SLE, as some patients with SLE will also have APLS; serologies such as ANA, dsDNA, antiSmith, and the other ACR criteria can help diagnose SLE (or a patient with both SLE and APLAs)
- Primary inflammatory vasculitidies: skin biopsy, serologies, and patterns of organ involvement can help differentiate these entities

Work-Up

- Careful history including symptoms related to previous thrombotic events, especially in a young patient, history of or symptoms related to autoimmune disease (notable SLE), and pregnancy history focusing on recurrent pregnancy complications
  - Previous false positive syphilis testing may be a clue since cardiolipin is found in VDRL and RPR tests
- Testing should be performed for lupus anticoagulant, anti-cardiolipin and/or anti-beta-2 glycoprotein-I antibodies; laboratory criteria for diagnosis includes positive testing on two or more tests performed at least 12 weeks apart (see Table 56.1)
- Depending upon the patient presentation, consider laboratory testing to rule out other hypercoagulable states, such as factor V Leiden, glycoprotein G20210A, methyltetrahydrofolate reductase, homocysteine, protein C and S, von Willebrand factor, antithrombin III
- Skin biopsy to demonstrate vascular occlusion or microangiopathy is often essential when patients present with skin findings
- Imaging studies may be necessary to confirm thrombotic disease

Treatment

- Anticoagulation is the primary treatment, often needed life long, so referral to a hematologist is recommended
- Treatment for catastrophic APLS includes anticoagulation, steroids, IVIg, plasmapheresis, cyclophosphamide, and/or rituximab
- For persistent cutaneous disease, such as cutaneous ulcers, aspirin in combination with pentoxifylline or dipyridamol has been used successfully
- For patients with known positive antibodies who have not had a major thrombotic event, aspirin or clopidogrel is typically recommended, although evidence for this is lacking.

Suggested Readings

1. Pinto-Almeida T, Caetano M, Sanches M, Selores M. Cutaneous manifestations of antiphospholipid syndrome: a review of clinical features, diagnosis and management. Acta Reumatol Port. 2013;38:10–8.
2. Thornsberry LA, LoSicco KI, English JC. The skin and hypercoagulable states. J Am Acad Dermatol. 2013;69:450–62.
3. Emmi G, Silvestri E, Squatrito D, et al. An approach to differential diagnosis of antiphospholipid antibody syndrome and related conditions. Sci World J. 2014;2014:1–8.
4. Miyakis S, Lockshin MD, Atsumi T, Branch DW, Brey RL, Cervera R, et al. International consensus statement on an update of the classification criteria for definite antiphospholipid syndrome (APS). J Thromb Haemost. 2006;4:295e–306.

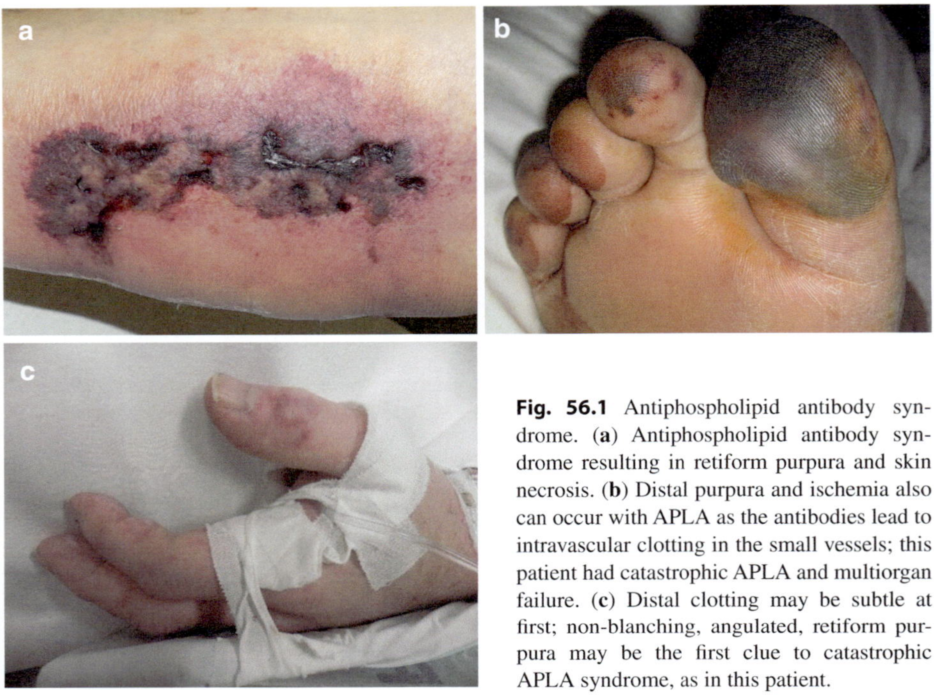

Fig. 56.1 Antiphospholipid antibody syndrome. (**a**) Antiphospholipid antibody syndrome resulting in retiform purpura and skin necrosis. (**b**) Distal purpura and ischemia also can occur with APLA as the antibodies lead to intravascular clotting in the small vessels; this patient had catastrophic APLA and multiorgan failure. (**c**) Distal clotting may be subtle at first; non-blanching, angulated, retiform purpura may be the first clue to catastrophic APLA syndrome, as in this patient.

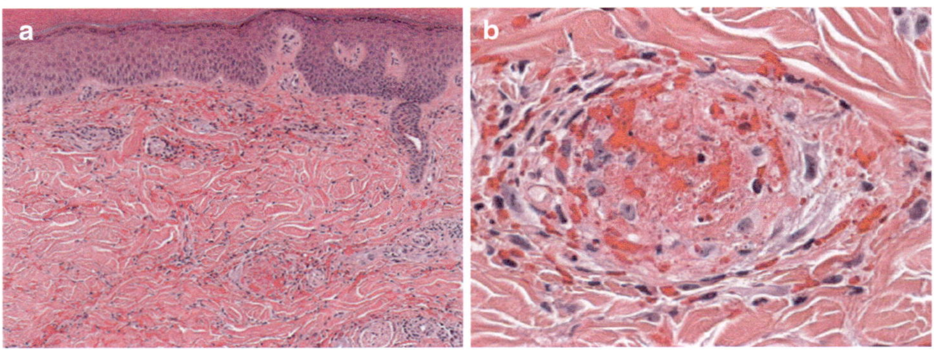

Fig. 56.2 Anti-phospholipid antibody syndrome *(5×, 40×; H&E)*: There biopsy was taken from a patient with APLS. (**a**) Low power demonstrates prominent hemorrhage with relative mild inflammatory infiltrate. (**b**) The presence of an eosinophilic fibrin thrombus without an inflammatory infiltrate is characteristic of a vasculopathy (compared to vasculitis).

Calciphylaxis

57

Karolyn A. Wanat

Overview

- Calciphylaxis (calcific uremic arteriolopathy) is a frequently fatal disorder of progressive vascular calcification with resulting skin and soft tissue necrosis most commonly occurring in patients with end-stage renal disease (ESRD)
  - Nonuremic calciphylaxis also can less commonly occur and has been reported in the setting of primary hyperparathyroidism, malignancy, and warfarin use liver disease
- Medial vessel calcification with resulting vessel damage, intimal fibrosis, thrombosis and downstream tissue ischemia leads to the development of associated sequelae
  - The pathogenesis has not been well defined, but damage secondary to deposition of elevated circulating calcium and phosphate in ESRD patients likely plays a major role
- Calciphylaxis presents with intense pain and jagged, angulated purpura with evolving ischemic, necrotic, ulcerative and bullous features typically concentrated on lower extremities and in areas with increased adiposity (abdomen, buttocks, thighs)
- Risk factors include chronic renal disease, female gender, obesity, diabetes mellitus, and medications including prednisone and warfarin

Clinical Presentation

- Lesions are exquisitely painful, ischemic and likely neuropathic in nature; pain may present prior to the formation of cutaneous lesions
  - Involvement of the glans penis may result in necrotic ulceration necessitating penectomy for pain management
- The appearance of skin findings change over time occurring on the lower extremities in 90% of cases, often with co-existent lesions on the buttocks and abdomen (Fig. 57.1)
  - Livedo racemosa present early as angulated, stellate, jagged erythema with surrounding firmness and induration
  - Lesions can become purpuric, ulcerative, bullous and necrotic with thick black eschar frequently developing in longstanding lesions

K. A. Wanat, MD
Department of Dermatology, Medical College of Wisconsin, Milwaukee, WI, USA
e-mail: karolyn-wanat@uiowa.edu

M. Rosenbach et al. (eds.), *Inpatient Dermatology*,
https://doi.org/10.1007/978-3-319-18449-4_57

  - Regions with eschar are at particular risk for secondary bacterial infections with consequent sepsis, a leading cause of mortality
  - The subcutaneous tissue around the lesions is often firm and tender, sometimes with palpable subcutaneous nodules and plaques

Histopathology

- Classically vessels in the subcutis or near the dermal-subcutaneous junction contain medial calcifications with intimal fibroplasia with resultant luminal narrowing with fibrin thrombi and associated ischemic damage/necrosis (Fig. 57.2)
  - Often there is scattered calcium in subcutaneous tissue
- Findings can be sparse and numerous deeper levels may be required to visualize calcium deposition
  - Special stains including Van-Kossa or Alizarin red stains can aid in diagnosis

Differential Diagnosis

- Vasculitis (small or medium vessel): calciphylaxis is usually localized to high fat areas, intensely tender, and presents gradually over time. By the time of diagnosis thick eschars are common, whereas vasculitis tends to be more acute. Biopsy can help differentiate.
- Vasculopathy:
  - Cryoglobulinemia: usually present with less dramatic cutaneous lesions, with findings smaller and more distal; serologies and histopathology can differentiate
  - Anti-phospholipid antibody syndrome: many patients with calciphylaxis will have APLAs, and if present treatment should cover both entities
- Panniculitis: Calciphylaxis often causes secondary damage and inflammation in the fat and can present similarly; the clinical setting (ESRD) and biopsy can be helpful in distinguishing
- Medication induced (Warfarin necrosis): the history and timing is essential in differentiating these entities

Essential Work-Up

- Deep and large skin biopsy are necessary to evaluate pathology; if infection is being considered, tissue culture
- Comprehensive metabolic panel (BUN/Cr, Ca, Ph)
- Serum parathyroid hormone (PTH) level; ESRD patients commonly have associated hyperparathyroidism (secondary or tertiary)
- Hypercoaguable work-up (Prothrombin time, activated partial thromboplastin time, anti-phospholipid antibody panel [lupus anticoagulant/DRVV, anti-cardiolipin, B2-glycopreotin1 Abs])
- Vitamin K testing may be important
- Newer studies suggest that some imaging modalities can help detect and follow the extent of calcification
- In some settings, consider further workup:
  - If high clinical suspicion for hypercoaguable state an appropriate work-up should be ordered including antithrombin III, factor V Leiden level, prothrombin mutations (GP2021A), homocysteine level, Protein C/S
    Protein C level, protein S level may be abnormal in acutely ill hospitalized patients
- If clinically indicated, consider cryoglobulin testing and/or vasculitis work-up (ANA, ANCA)

Treatment

- Pain management is essential and treatment requires a multi-disciplinary approach including nephrology consultation

- Treatment should focus on the prevention of additional calcium-phosphate deposition and vascular damage via:
  - Normalization of the calcium-phosphate product by low calcium dialysis
  - Minimize calcium or phosphate containing medications and calcium sparing diuretics
  - Use of phosphate binders (combination of calcium acetate and magnesium carbonate more beneficial than calcium carbonate binders)
- Normalization of parathyroid hormone via medications or surgical intervention
- Consider bisphosphonate therapy
- Consider vitamin K testing and supplementation
- Consider pentoxifylline
- Removing additional potential triggers:
  - Convert patients from warfarin to alternate means of anticoagulation when clinically appropriate
  - Avoid prednisone if possible
- Consider IV sodium thiosulfate (in select cases, consider IL sodium thiosulfate); this may assist with the removal of circulating calcium in addition to the break-down of existing vessel calcification
- There is mixed evidence regarding thrombolytic agents, which carry high risk of bleeding complications; use remains controversial
- Wound care is needed to aid in healing and help prevent secondary bacterial infection:
  - Enzymatic debridement (collagenase), frequent dressing changes with a moist wound bed
  - Surgical evaluation and gentle debridement of devitalized tissue
  - Hyperbaric oxygen may be helpful in some patients but data does not demonstrate clear benefit
  - Monitor for signs of superinfection with a low threshold to add topical antimicrobial agents
  - Metronidazole cream or gel if malodorous
  - Mupirocin if honey-to-serous colored drainage
  - Consideration of other topical antimicrobials including acetic acid soaks also can be used
- Patients are at high risk of overt infection and bacteremia; physicians should have a low threshold to initiate antibiotics if systemically ill

Suggested Readings

1. Weenig RH, Sewell LD, Davis MDP, et al. Calciphylaxis: natural history, risk factor analysis and outcome. J Am Acad Dermatol. 2007;56:569–79.
2. Vedvyas C, Winterfield LS, Vleugels RA. Calciphylaxis: a systematic review of existing and emerging therapies. J Am Acad Dermatol. 2012;67(6):253–60.

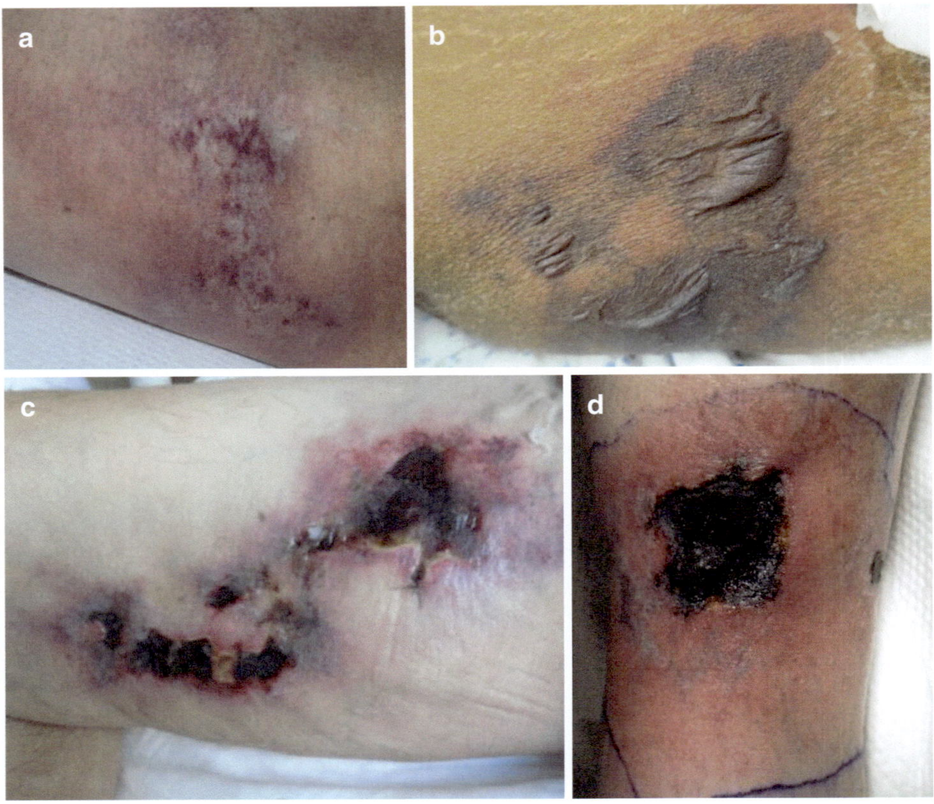

Fig. 57.1 Calciphylaxis: (**a**) Early lesions present with painful subcutaneous plaques often with overlying purpuric to red-brown vaguely angulated plaques; here there is blanching of the skin due to tissue ischemia and impending necrosis. (**b**) This lesion of early calciphylaxis demonstrates typical angulated purpura, but with bullae formation due to hypoperfusion of the epidermis. These blistered areas will erode, ulcerate, and form eschars. (**c**) Here there is more extensive angulated ischemic purpura with eschar formation in the ulcerated areas. (**d**) More developed lesions show similar ischemic changes in the intact skin, but areas of ulceration will develop and rapidly form thick black eschars.

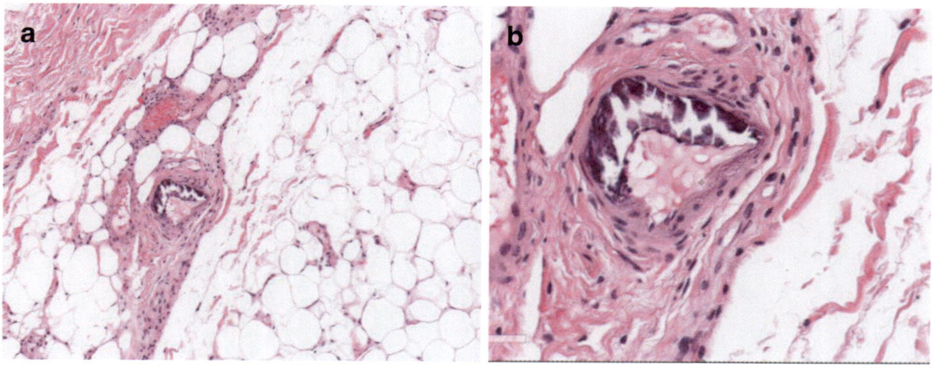

Fig. 57.2 Calciphylaxis (*2×,10×*; *H&E)*: A larger incisional biopsy is often necessary to sample the subcutaneous tissue. (**a**) Overlying epidermal ulceration with associated epidermal and dermal necrosis can be observed. (**b**) Within the small to medium vessels in the deep dermis or within the subcutaneous tissue, there is fibrosis, intravascular thrombi and calcification within the vessels, particularly in the tunica media of the arteriole wall. Calcification within the collagen bundles and adipocytes also can be seen.

Levamisole-Associated Vasculopathy and Vasculitis

58

Grant Ghahramani

Overview

- Levamisole, a veterinary anti-helminthic, is a commonly used adulterant for illegal drugs (cocaine, heroin)
- Its use is associated with agranulocytosis (neutropenia), mixed vasculitis/vasculopathy leading to skin lesions, and autoantibody development that can mimic idiopathic autoimmune diseases
- Retiform purpura tends to develop on the trunk and extremities with predilection for ear helices, nasal tip, and cheeks with scattered areas of necrosis
- Since levamisole-associated disease is essentially only seen in the setting of recreational drug use, a delicate clinical approach is necessary; clinicians should utilize this opportunity to refer patients for substance abuse counseling/treatment when clinically indicated

Clinical Presentation

- Patients develop characteristic large irregular areas of dusky retiform purpura, sometimes with areas of necrosis, with involvement of the "tips" (ears, nose, digits). The ear involvement is a very common feature, and somewhat specific (may occur in cryoglobulinemia as well). There may be hemorrhagic bullous or vesiculopustular lesions with arciform configuration (Fig. 58.1)
- In patients less forthcoming about substance abuse, clinical clues may help confirm clinical suspicion and narrow the differential diagnosis; additionally, this information may be gently used to further discussions concerning the patient's drug use:
  - Perforated septum with intranasal cocaine use
  - Inhaled crack-cocaine may result in burned lips and finger tips, inhalational injury including angioedema and oropharyngeal burns, worsening asthma/bronchospasms, shortness of breath and or pleuritic pain
  - Cocaine causes vasospasm and associated thrombotic risk; history of TIA/stroke, MI, PE may be clue to prior use
  - Peripheral vein scarring ("track marks") and irregular oval shaped hypo-or-hyperpigmented scars related to skin popping are consistent with IVDU

G. Ghahramani, MD
Cotton O'Neil Dermatology, Topeka, KS, USA

M. Rosenbach et al. (eds.), *Inpatient Dermatology*,
https://doi.org/10.1007/978-3-319-18449-4_58

Histopathology

- Features of small vessel vasculitis and/or vasculopathy can be seen:
  - Findings may include leukocytoclastic vasculitis, microvascular thrombosis, and overlying epidermal necrosis (Fig. 58.2)

Differential Diagnosis

- Warfarin-induced skin necrosis: usually affects areas high in adipose tissue, shortly after warfarin initiation
- Septic vasculitis/infectious endocarditis: patients with substance abuse may have both diagnoses, and blood cultures +/− echocardiography should be considered
- Cutaneous small vessel vasculitis: cocaine may cause vasculitis, and thus these diagnoses may coexist; if present, it is important to rule out additional organ involvement and other causes of vasculitis
- Cryoglobulinemia: skin findings also favor the ears and other distal "tips" and this can be hard to clinically distinguish from levamisole abuse; laboratory testing and history are essential
- Anti-phospholipid antibody syndrome: the fixed livedo and jagged retiform purpura clinically overlap with lesions seen in the setting of levamisole; laboratory testing is required

Work-Up

- A thorough history should focus on recreational drug use (cocaine and heroin), additionally, the physical and review of symptoms should assess for associated systemic disease as vasculitis may involve other organs
- CBC: agranulocytosis, specifically neutropenia, can be present
- Urine drug screen
- Levaminsole-specific confirmatory testing is very time-sensitive (half-life <6 h) and not widely available, but if considered early in the disease course may confirm the diagnosis ANA, ANCA antibodies (+MPO, elastase, and PR3), and/or antiphospholipid antibody can be positive
  - Cocaine and levamisole-tainted cocaine abuse can lead to dual-positivity of both c- and p-ANCA antibodies, which is rare in native idiopathic disease and can be helpful sign

Treatment

- Discontinue levamisole containing drugs
- Consider a psychiatry consultation to assist with substance abuse management
- Watch for signs of withdrawal
- Substance abuse therapy; consult psychiatry and social work as needed
- Lesions demonstrate self-resolution; topical wound care can be used to help with healing

Suggested Readings

1. Waller JM, Feramisco JD, Alberta-Wszolek L, McCalmont TH, Fox LP. Cocaine-associated retiform purpura and neutropenia: is levamisole the culprit? J Am Acad Dermatol. 2010;63(3):530–5.
2. Rongioletti F, Ghio L, Ginevri F, Bleidl D, Rinaldi S, Edefonti A, Gambini C, Rizzoni G, Rebora A. Purpura of the ears: a distinctive vasculopathy with circulating autoantibodies complicating long-term treatment with levamisole in children. Br J Dermatol. 1999;140(5):948–51.
3. Chung C, Tumeh PC, Birnbaum R, Tan BH, Sharp L, McCoy E, Mercurio MG, Craft N. Characteristic purpura of the ears, vasculitis, and neutropenia—a potential public health epidemic associated with levamisole-adulterated cocaine. J Am Acad Dermatol. 2011;65(4):722–5.

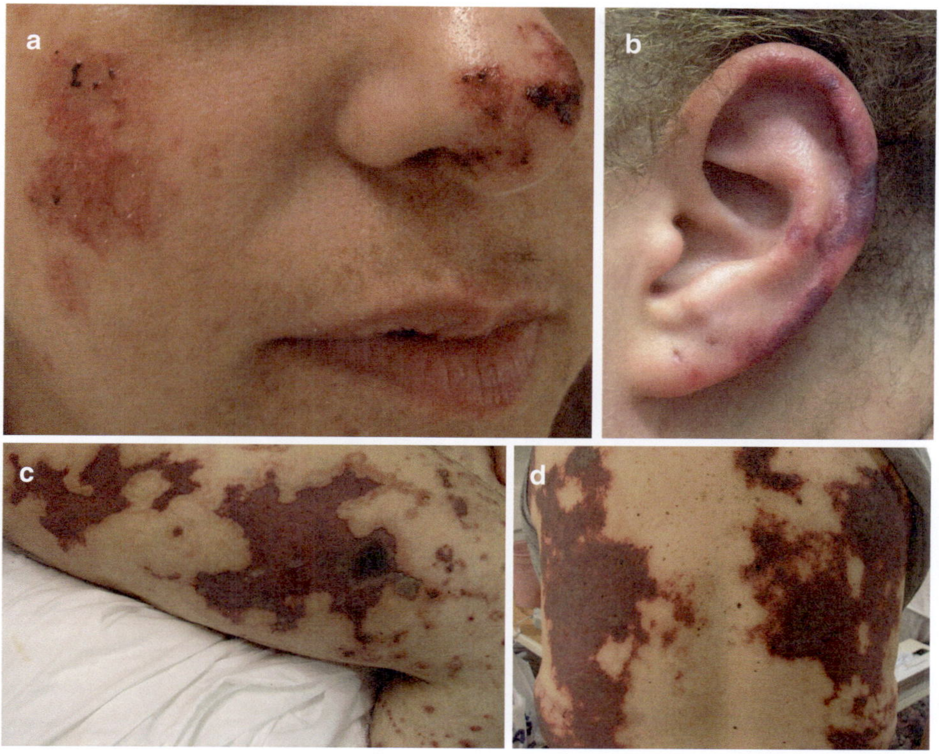

Fig. 58.1 Levamisole-related purpura: (**a**) Characteristic retiform purpura and eschar of the nose and cheeks. (**b**) Angulated stellate retiform purpura of the ears is also common. (**c, d**) There is extensive involvement of the upper thigh (**c**) and back (**d**) in a patient with levamisole-induced vasculitis/vasculopathy.

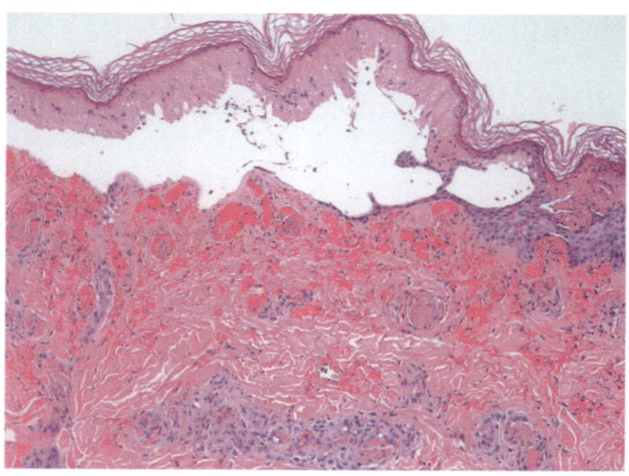

Fig. 58.2 Levamisole-related purpura *(10×; H&E):* Histopathology demonstrates overlying epidermal necrosis with a basket weave stratum corneum. Within the superficial and deep vessels, there can be both microvascular thrombi and/or leukocytoclastic vasculitis. Surrounding red blood cell extravasation also is common.

Part IX

Erythroderma

Erythroderma is generalized redness (often with scaling) covering the majority of the body usually 80–90% or more of the body surface area. It represents the end stage of numerous disorders, with the most common etiologies in the inpatient setting being psoriasis, acute GVHD, medication reaction, malignancy (CTCL or paraneoplastic phenomenon), pityriasis rubra pilaris, superinfected and/or flaring eczematous dermatitis, blistering disorders, and idiopathic.

Diagnosing the cause of erythroderma can be difficult. History, detailed physical exam, biopsy, and supplementary laboratory testing is often required. If erythroderma occurs as an exacerbation of pre-existing condition, the history is essential. However, when erythroderma occurs de novo, diagnosis can be challenging. Skin biopsies, while helpful, are frequently non-diagnostic (though even a non-diagnostic biopsy can help exclude certain entities on the differential). Physicians should maintain a low threshold for re-biopsy, as some etiologies evolve over time, and multiple biopsies may be necessary to arrive at a specific diagnosis. Further work-up may include testing for infections (HIV, HTLV, and more), reviewing medications for drug culprits, evaluating patients for underlying occult malignancy, or using advanced diagnostic techniques such as T-cell receptor gene rearrangement, flow cytometry, and high throughput sequencing.

Regardless of the underlying etiology, there are some general common rules to keep in mind when managing erythroderma. Patients may experience rapid skin turnover, with high nutritional demands, loss of temperature homeostasis, fluid and electrolyte imbalances, and a risk for high output heart failure due to the extensive dilated cutaneous vasculature, in addition to the potential for secondary infection through inflamed, damaged skin.

Treatment is aimed at identifying and managing the underlying cause of erythroderma, while providing supportive care for the secondary complications. Skin directed therapy with low to mid potency steroids (such as triamcinolone 0.1% ointment dosed in a one pound jar) in a "soak and smear" fashion—where it is applied after bathing or under wet dressings in addition to liberal use of a thick emollient is important. Sauna suits or wet wraps may be available which can help retain moisture. Oral antihistamines can sometimes help with pruritus. Pain control is important, particularly if there is severe skin inflammation and epidermal breakdown. Crusted, eroded skin should be evaluated for secondary infection, especially with staph or herpes. Blood cultures should be considered in acutely flaring patients or patients with fever or signs of sepsis, but may be falsely positive when collected through damaged (frequently colonized) erythrodermic skin.

Systemic therapy should be administered only after thorough evaluation, and the particular agent often requires an experienced inpatient dermatologist consultant. While infliximab can lead to rapid resolution in erythrodermic psoriasis, it can exacerbate CTCL, for instance. Appropriate systemic treatment depends on identifying the specific underlying cause; if there is doubt, it is best to select agents which are not contraindicated in the management of any of the entities that remain on the differential diagnosis.

Medication-Induced Erythroderma

59

Molly Moye

Overview

- Erythroderma refers to a diffuse, often exfoliative, dermatitis involving 80–90% of the skin.
  - Erythroderma most commonly results from generalization of an existing chronic dermatosis (atopic dermatitis, psoriasis, other), followed by drug-induced, malignancy associated (CTCL, Hodgkin lymphoma, paraneoplastic) or idiopathic causes (etiology may be unknown in up to 25% of cases)
- Drug-induced erythroderma refers to the development of erythroderma within days to weeks of initiation of a new medication and typically has a more acute onset and resolution than other forms of erythroderma
  - The most common classes of medications implicated are antiepileptics, antihypertensives, and antibiotics, but all medications should be considered as potential causes of erythroderma
  - In addition to the scheduled medication, hospitalized patients may have exposures to additional potential culprits including radiocontrast dye, dialysate exposure during renal replacement therapy, and perioperative medications during procedures
- Incidence rates are variable but notable increased in the setting of HIV (causing approximately 40% of erythroderma case) with ethambutol a common offender; heightened rates also seen in the pediatric population following anti-seizure or antibiotic use

Clinical Presentation

- Diffuse erythema of 90% or more of the body surface area with or without associated scale (variably exfoliative) with associated pruritus (Fig. 59.1)
- Clinical clues of a drug-induced etiology include:
  - Abrupt onset, previous morbilliform eruption, multiple, varied cutaneous morphologic lesions present together
- Extensive erythema is followed in 2–6 days by exfoliative scaling
  - Pruritus can be severe, leading to scratching and lichenification in more chronic processes
  - Due to the abrupt onset of drug-related erythroderma, signs of chronicity are typically absent (patients lack palmoplantar keratoderma, alopecia, lichenification, dyspigmentation)
- May be accompanied by fever, chills, malaise, and reactive peripheral lymphadenopathy
- Skin colonization and superinfection, particularly with *Staphylococcus aureus,* is common

M. Moye, MD
Forefront Dermatology, Louisville, KY, USA
e-mail: mollymoye@me.com

M. Rosenbach et al. (eds.), *Inpatient Dermatology*,
https://doi.org/10.1007/978-3-319-18449-4_59

- Other complications of erythroderma include:
  - Peripheral edema
  - Thermoregulatory disturbances
  - Hypoproteinemia
  - Hypovolemia and reflexive tachycardia
  - Electrolyte abnormalities, e.g. hypernatremia, hypocalcemia
  - Anemia, folate deficiency
  - High-output congestive heart failure

Histopathology

- Biopsies of erythroderma are usually nonspecific, showing hyperkeratosis, mild acanthosis, and focal parakeratosis (Fig. 59.2)
  - No findings definitively suggest a drug-induced etiology but eosinophils may be suggestive

Differential Diagnosis

- Other causes of erythroderma include:
  - Psoriasis: patients may have more classic plaques, and history of prior psoriasis
  - Cutaneous T-cell lymphoma: patients may have lymphadenopathy, ectropion, thick plaques or tumors, but ultimately flow cytometry may be necessary to exclude CTCL
  - Pityriasis rubra pilaris: may have an orange hue, islands of sparing, follicular prominence, palmoplantar keratoderma, and often suggestive histopathology
  - Paraneoplastic erythroderma: all cases of erythroderma without a clear trigger warrant thorough systemic evaluation
  - Graft-versus-host disease: erythroderma post-transplant is highly suspicious; diarrhea and liver function abnormalities may also suggest GvH

Work-Up

- Perform a detailed history and physical to identify clues to the underlying cause of erythroderma
  - A drug-chart depicting timings of medication exposure relative to the onset of cutaneous symptoms can be helpful in identifying potential culprits
- Skin biopsy can be helpful to rule out other causes of erythroderma (inflammatory dermatoses, cutaneous T cell lymphoma)
  - Additional tests as warranted to exclude other underlying causes of erythroderma, e.g. flow cytometry, lymph node biopsy
- Baseline labs including complete blood count, chemistry panel, and liver function tests
- Monitor for cardiac failure, sepsis, temperature instability, and electrolyte imbalances

Treatment

- Discontinue all drugs that could potentially be the culprit drug and simplify drug regimen as much as possible, eliminating all unnecessary medications
  - Patients with suspected drug-induced erythroderma should undergo close clinical evaluation for signs of other serious drug reactions with appropriate work-up and treatment as clinically indicated:
    - Epidermal duskiness/detachment (concerning for SJS/TEN)
    - Small pustules (suggestive of AGEP)
    - Facial involvement and edema (concerning for DRESS)
- Acute management of fluid and electrolyte imbalances, temperature instability, nutrition, and secondary infections (Fig. 59.2)

- Supportive care including emollients and maintenance of fluid homeostasis with IV fluids, if needed, while erythrodermic
  - Topical steroids can enhance patient comfort (particularly ointment-based vehicles, ideally applied after the skin is moistened by bathing or wet-wraps), and systemic steroids can be used at the discretion of the clinician
- Adjunctive therapies:
  - Antihistamines for pruritus
  - Antibiotics for secondary bacterial infections, particularly *Staphylococcus aureus*

Suggested Readings

1. Khaled A, Sellami A, Fazaa B, et al. Acquired erythroderma in adults: a clinical and prognostic study. J Eur Acad Dermatol Venereol. 2010;24:781–8.
2. Li J, Zheng HY. Erythroderma: a clinical and prognostic study. Dermatology. 2012;225:154–62.
3. Wilson DC, Jester JD, King LE. Erythroderma and exfoliative dermatitis. Clin Dermatol. 1993;11:67072.

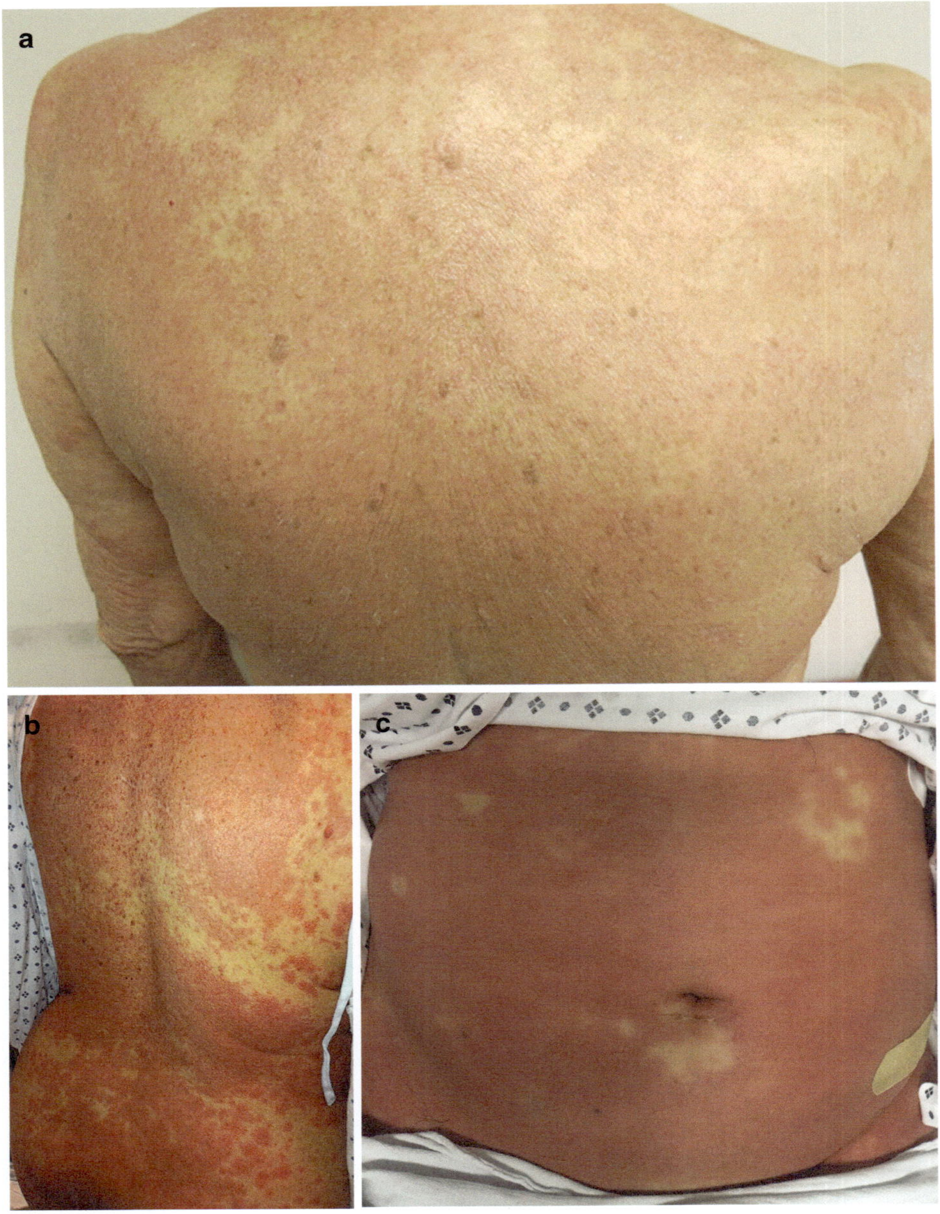

Fig. 59.1 Erythroderma due to a medication: (**a**) Widespread nearly confluent erythematous macules over more than 80% of the body due to combination antibiotic therapy. Erythrodermatous drug eruptions will usually not lead to ectropion of the eyelids (differentiating it from CTCL). If there is facial involvement with edema, DRESS should be suspected. (**b**) Near-confluent blanchable erythematous macules extending to patches. (**c**) Diffuse confluent erythema.

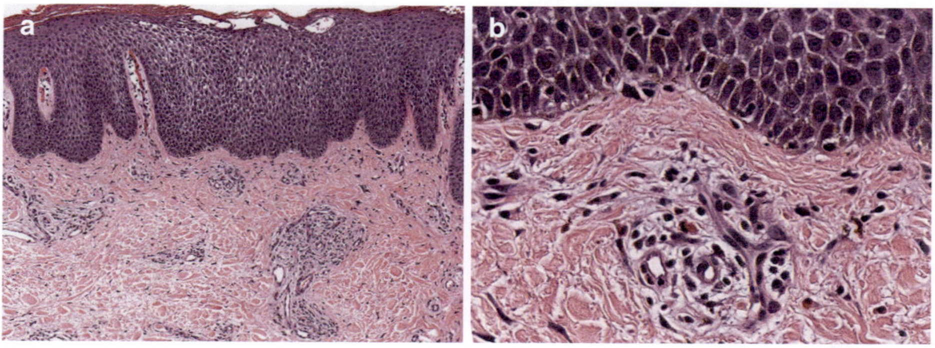

Fig. 59.2 Medication-induced erythroderma *(5×, 40×; H&E)*: (**a**) The epidermis can have variable features including acanthosis, spongiosis, and some may exhibits psoriasiform features. (**b**) There are eosinophils present in the perivascular and interstitial inflammatory infiltrate. These findings are nonspecific and CTCL cannot be excluded based on histologic assessment alone. If there is clinical suspicion for CTCL then ancillary studies (such as flow cytometry or T-cell reception gene rearrangement) should be considered.

Atopic Dermatitis and Erythroderma

60

Joy Wan

Overview

- Erythroderma refers to a diffuse often exfoliative dermatitis involving >90% of the skin for which an underlying etiology is not determined in a significant subset of cases
  - In cases with an established etiology, erythroderma most commonly results from generalization of an existing chronic dermatosis, followed by drug-induced, malignancy associated (CTCL, Hodgkin lymphoma, paraneoplastic) or idiopathic causes
- Acute flare and generalization of moderate to severe atopic dermatitis (AD) is a common cause of secondary erythroderma
  - Underlying triggers may include discontinuation of immunosuppressive therapy/steroids, new medications, systemic illness, or skin superinfection
- Clinical clues to underlying atopic dermatitis may include:
  - Pre-existing personal history of atopy or atopic dermatitis
  - Pre-existing eczematous patches and plaques especially in flexural areas
  - Severe pruritus and lichenification
  - Prurigo nodularis: pruritic nodules on the extremities
  - Elevated serum immunoglobulin E levels and eosinophilia

Clinical Presentation

- Diffuse erythema of 90% or more of the body surface area with or without associated scale (variably exfoliative) with associated pruritus (Fig. 60.1)
- Extensive erythema followed in 2–6 days by exfoliative scaling
  - Weeping and serous crusting is more common in erythroderma due to atopic dermatitis than other causes
  - Palmoplantar keratoderma, non-scarring alopecia, and ectropion can occur in long-standing severe erythroderma but are uncommon in atopic dermatitis (and may suggest CTCL)
  - Pruritus can be severe, leading to scratching and lichenification (focused in flexures, neck, face—including eyelids, and dorsal aspects of hands and feet)
- May be accompanied by fever, chills, malaise, and reactive peripheral lymphadenopathy Skin colonization and superinfection, particularly with *Staphylococcus aureus,* is common

J. Wan, MD
Children's Hospital of Philadelphia, University of Pennsylvania, Philadelphia, PA, USA
e-mail: joy.wan@uphs.upenn.edu

M. Rosenbach et al. (eds.), *Inpatient Dermatology*,
https://doi.org/10.1007/978-3-319-18449-4_60

- Additional complications of erythroderma include:
  - Peripheral edema
  - Thermoregulatory disturbances
  - Hypoproteinemia
  - Hypovolemia and reflexive tachycardia
  - Electrolyte abnormalities, e.g. hypernatremia, hypocalcemia
  - Anemia, folate deficiency
  - High-output congestive heart failure

Histopathology

- Biopsies of erythroderma are usually nonspecific, showing hyperkeratosis, mild acanthosis, and focal parakeratosis, and can mask features of the underlying disease
- Histologic clues to underlying atopic dermatitis may include mild to moderate spongiosis, acanthosis, dermal eosinophils, dermal edema, and parakeratosis

Differential Diagnosis

- Other causes of erythroderma include:
  - Psoriasis: patients may have more classic plaques, and history of prior psoriasis
  - Cutaneous T-cell lymphoma: patients may have lymphadenopathy, ectropion, thick plaques or tumors, but ultimately flow cytometry may be necessary to exclude CTCL
  - Pityriasis rubra pilaris: may have an orange hue, islands of sparing, follicular prominence, palmoplantar keratoderma, and often suggestive histopathology
  - Paraneoplastic erythroderma: all cases of erythroderma without a clear trigger warrant thorough systemic evaluation
  - Graft-versus-host disease: erythroderma post-transplant is highly suspicious; diarrhea and liver function abnormalities may also suggest GvH

Work-Up

- Perform a detailed history and physical to identify clues to the underlying cause of erythroderma including personal or family history of early development of asthma and allergic rhinitis
- Baseline labs including complete blood count (may demonstrate eosinophilia), IgE (often elevated), chemistry panel, and liver function tests
- Consider bacterial culture of acutely inflamed, raw, weepy skin or areas of honey-colored crusting (for *Staph*)
- Consider viral culture if prior history of herpetic superinfection or presence of vesicles, punched-out circular erosions, or linear painful fissures
- Skin biopsy can be helpful to rule out other causes of erythroderma
- Additional tests as warranted to exclude other underlying causes of erythroderma e.g. flow cytometry, lymph node biopsy
- Monitor for cardiac failure, sepsis, temperature instability, and electrolyte imbalances

Treatment

- Acute management of fluid and electrolyte imbalances, temperature instability, nutrition, and secondary infections

- Acute treatment of the underlying atopic dermatitis
  - Wet wrap or sauna suit therapy for 7–14 days leads to rapid improvement
    - Skin is gently bathed in lukewarm water (or wet towel wraps) for 5–10 min followed by gentle pat dry. Topical corticosteroid ointment, typically mid-potency (e.g. desonide to face, triamcinolone to body), is applied to the skin, followed by wet wrap or sauna suit
    - Wet wraps consist of two layers of bandages to cover trunk, extremities, and face: a moist first layer soaked in lukewarm water, followed by a dry second layer
    - Alternatively, sauna suit can be used to occlude the skin
    - Leave in place at least 2 h and repeat every 12 h
  - Systemic corticosteroids can be effective for severe acute flares of AD but are usually avoided due to risk of rebound upon discontinuation
- Adjunctive therapies:
  - Antihistamines for pruritus
  - Antibiotics for secondary bacterial infections, particularly *Staphylococcus aureus*
- After acute phase, long-term maintenance therapy for moderate to severe atopic dermatitis should be initiated with close outpatient follow-up with an experienced dermatologist

Suggested Readings

1. Cathcart SD, Theos A. Inpatient management of atopic dermatitis. Dermatol Ther. 2011;24(2):249–55.
2. Rothe MJ, Bialy TL, Grant-Kels JM. Erythroderma. Dermatol Clin. 2000;18(3):405–15.
3. Simon D, Bieber T. Systemic therapy for atopic dermatitis. Allergy. 2014;69(1):46–55.

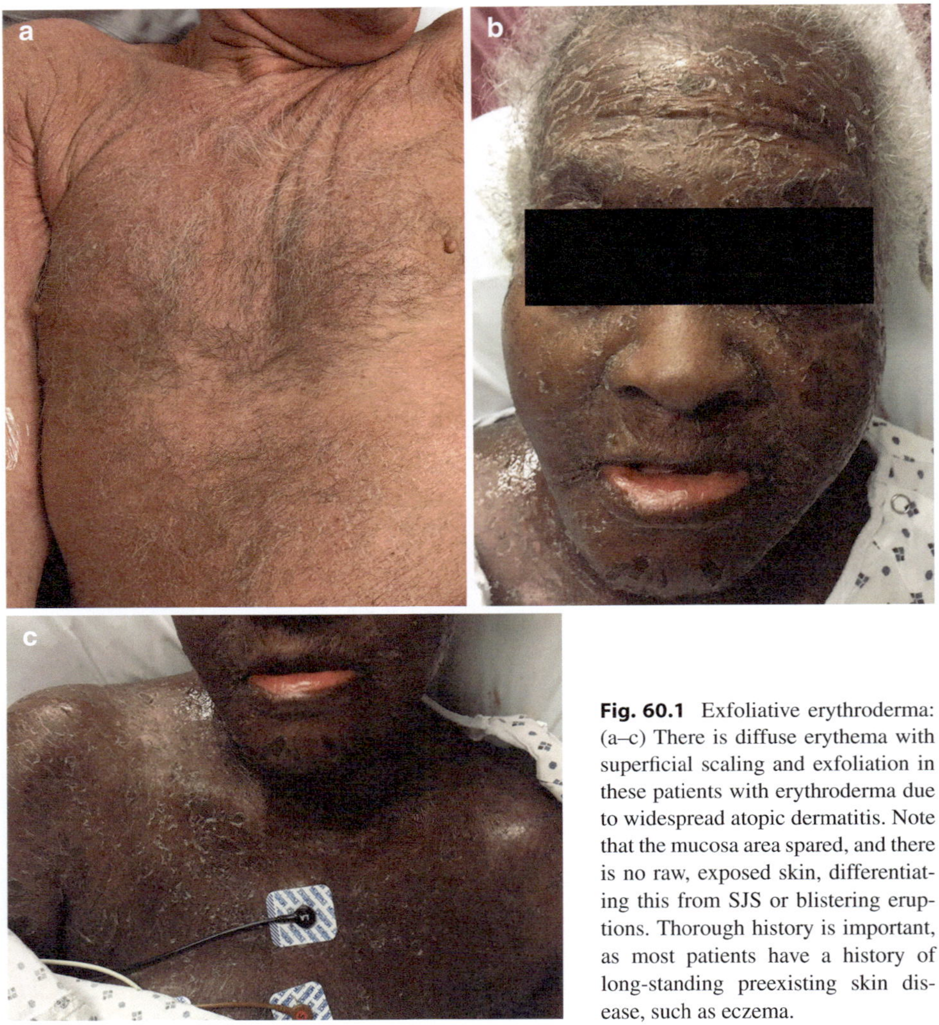

Fig. 60.1 Exfoliative erythroderma: (a–c) There is diffuse erythema with superficial scaling and exfoliation in these patients with erythroderma due to widespread atopic dermatitis. Note that the mucosa area spared, and there is no raw, exposed skin, differentiating this from SJS or blistering eruptions. Thorough history is important, as most patients have a history of long-standing preexisting skin disease, such as eczema.

Psoriasis

61

Krishna A. Mutgi

Overview

- Psoriasis is a chronic papulosquamous inflammatory skin disease with characteristic dry erythematous plaques and adherent silvery scales; lesions are initially well circumscribed but may extend laterally and coalesce leading to move extensive involvement
- There are many clinical forms of psoriasis, chronic plaque psoriasis is the most common overall but patients with pustular psoriasis or erythrodermic psoriasis are more likely to necessitate inpatient treatment as a direct consequence of their disease
  - Chronic plaque psoriasis: symmetrical lesions commonly involve the scalp, back, and extensor surfaces and at sites of previous skin trauma (Koebner phenomenon)
  - Inverse psoriasis: Primarily involves the intertriginous areas and typically lacks scale making misdiagnoses of intertrigo and/or infections common
  - Guttate psoriasis: Abrupt eruption of numerous small (typically <1 cm) psoriasiform lesions which often occur following a streptococcal infection in younger patients without a history of psoriasis
- Erythrodermic psoriasis: Patients with pre-existing psoriasis can develop diffuse exfoliative erythematous dermatitis involving >80–90% of body surface area
- Pustular psoriasis is a severe, often acute, form of psoriasis characterized by the development of sterile neutrophilic pustules on an erythematous base and will be the focus of this chapter
  - Associated with pregnancy, medications (oral contraceptives, lithium, and withdrawal of oral or extensive super potent topical corticosteroids), and infections
  - Various rare clinical subtypes described: Von-Zumbusch type, impetigo herpetiformis, annular type, exanthematic type, localized type

Clinical Presentation

- Patients with pustular psoriasis can present with manifestations ranging from localized disease, commonly on the thighs and/or proximal arms, to widespread erythroderma; with generalized disease patients often have associated fever and malaise (Fig. 61.1)

K. A. Mutgi, MD
Mercy Health Dermatology, Toledo, OH, USA

M. Rosenbach et al. (eds.), *Inpatient Dermatology*,
https://doi.org/10.1007/978-3-319-18449-4_61

- Pustular psoriasis consists of sterile pustules on an erythematous background, some variants include:
  - Von-Zumbusch type—acute (over hours) development and generalization of sterile neutrophilic pustules which can coalesce into broad lakes of pus on an erythematous base progressing to erythroderma and accompanied by fever and malaise
  - Impetigo Herpetiformis—occurs in pregnancy and characterized by symmetrical erythematous patches with sterile pustules starting on the flexures and intertriginous areas and expanding centrifugally in the third trimester, associated with increased fetal mortality
  - Annular type—subacute development of sterile pustules that advance centrifugally with leading edge pustulation and central resolution
  - Exanthematic type—acute development of small pustules occurring within a few days after a triggering medication such as lithium and resolving quickly upon discontinuation; clinical and histological overlap with acute exanthematous pustulosis
  - Localized type—development of pustules within preexisting psoriatic plaques, development of pustules limited to the palms and soles (palmoplantar pustulosis) or development of pustules limited to the distal fingers, nail folds and nail beds (Acrodermatitis continua of Hallopeau)

Histopathology

- Spongiform neutrophilic intraepidermal pustules tend to be large and are often associated with parakeratosis with overlying neutrophils (Figs. 61.2 and 61.3)
- Variable acanthosis with elongated rete ridges (psoriasiform hyperplasia) is present and more evident in older lesions

Differential Diagnosis

- Acute Generalized Exanthematous Pustulosis: often the critical differential, AGEP and pustular psoriasis can be indistinguishable; biopsies may show eosinophils in AGEP, or a history of psoriasis can suggest a pustular flare, but distinguishing the two requires history and clin-path correlation
- Disseminated Candidiasis: can mimic pustular psoriasis clinically and pathologically, but special stains should distinguish candida
- Folliculitis: in folliculitis pustules are based on hair follicles, and larger than the non-follicular pustules of psoriasis
- Dermatomyositis: plaque psoriasis and dermato can both have similar pink scaly patches, but histology should distinguish
- Erythroderma: differentiating between erythrodermic psoriasis and other causes of erythroderma can be a challenge and often comes down to a prior history of plaque psoriasis

Work-Up

- History and physical examination with an emphasis on eliciting personal, medication, or family history of psoriasis and potential triggers (medications, infections including strep or HIV, recent steroid taper and withdrawal)
  - Medications should be considered in cases of new-onset psoriasis (long and growing list including beta blockers, ACE inhibitors, lithium, TNF-inhibitors, hydroxychloroquine, and more)
- Punch biopsy, especially if preexisting diagnosis of psoriasis cannot be identified on history or physical examination
- Complete blood count with left shift, elevated ESR and CRP are all consistent with the diagnosis but nonspecific
- Hypocalcemia and folate deficiency can be seen in cases of rapid skin turnover (erythrodermic/pustular psoriasis)
- Electrolytes, especially in erythrodermic patients, should be monitored and abnormalities corrected

- Blood cultures should be considered for erythrodermic patients or if fevers, chills, or other signs of systemic infection are observed, as bacteremia can both precipitate and complicate psoriasis flares
- Culture or scraping of a pustule may be helpful to rule out infection

Treatment

- Aggressive topical therapy can be helpful in patients while awaiting evaluation for infection/comorbidities or with contraindications to systemic suppression
  - "Soak and Smear" with wet towel wraps or bathing, followed by thick application and use of a full 1 pound jar of triamcinolone ointment, with a 'sauna suit' over the layer of ointment can rapidly clear patients even with extensive disease
- For hospitalized patients with severe erythrodermic or pustular psoriasis, systemic therapy is often required. Patients should be evaluated for concomitant superinfection with appropriate antimicrobial therapy prior to systemic immunosuppression.
  - First line agents:
    - Cyclosporine—rapid onset with improvement in 1–2 weeks;
    - Infliximab—rapid onset with improvement in 1–2 weeks;
    - Methotrexate—slower onset of action
    - Acitretin—slower onset, useful for chronic maintenance in patients with pustular disease (teratogenic and can reside in fat with prolonged effects, avoid use in women of childbearing potential)
  - Second line agents:
    - Etanercept, Adalimumab, PUVA (often not used in acutely inflamed skin as can burn patients and induce worsening of disease through koebnerization)
- Topical steroids, vitamin D analogs and calcineurin inhibitors can be helpful adjuncts or used as monotherapy in patients with more limited disease

Suggested Readings

1. Robinson A, Van Voorhees AS, Hsu S, et al. Treatment of pustular psoriasis: from the Medical Board of the National Psoriasis Foundation. J Am Acad Dermatol. 2012;67(2):279–88.
2. Mengesha YM, Bennett ML. Pustular skin disorders: diagnosis and treatment. Am J Clin Dermatol. 2002;3(6):389–400.

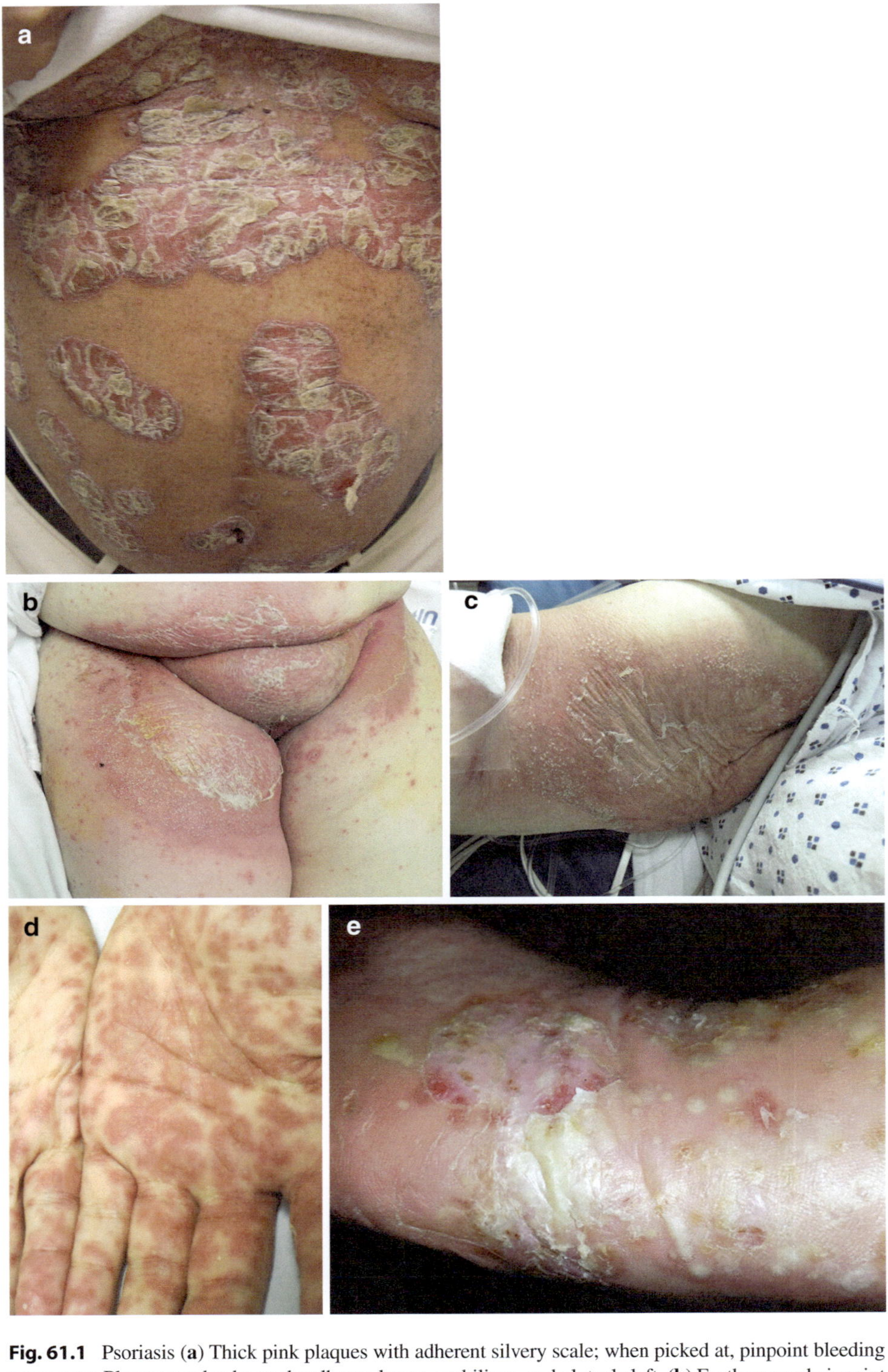

Fig. 61.1 Psoriasis (**a**) Thick pink plaques with adherent silvery scale; when picked at, pinpoint bleeding may occur. Plaques tend to be on the elbows, knees, umbilicus, and gluteal cleft. (**b**) Erythema and pinpoint pustules favor body fold areas in pustular psoriasis. (**c**) The erythema may have a concentrated wall of pustules, as shown here extending from the axilla. (**d**) Deep-seated pustules involving the palms. (**e**) Extensive pustules on the soles in palmoplantar pustular psoriasis, in this case due to a TNF-inhibitor.

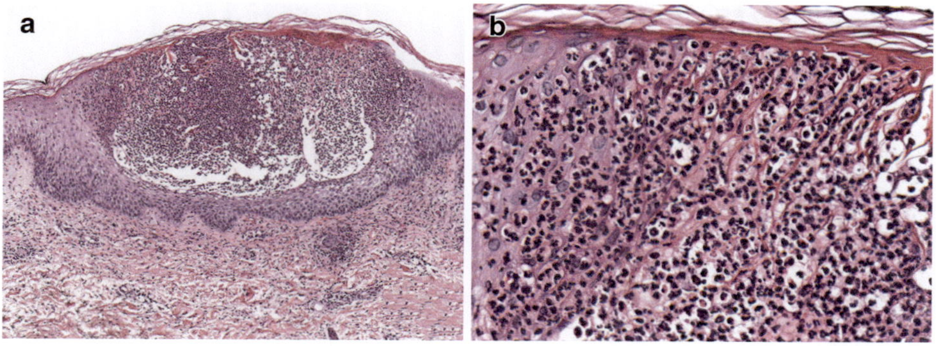

Fig. 61.2 Pustular psoriasis (*5×, 40×; H&E*): (**a**) The epidermis exhibits psoriasiform change with club-shaped elongated rete ridges and overlying parakeratosis. The epidermis is spongiotic with intraepidermal neutrophilic macropustules. (**b**) The abundant neutrophils are concentrated within the pustules and also intercalate between surrounding keratinocytes. These macro-pustules, typical of pustular psoriasis, are a larger-scale version of the pustules of Kogoj seen in psoriasis.

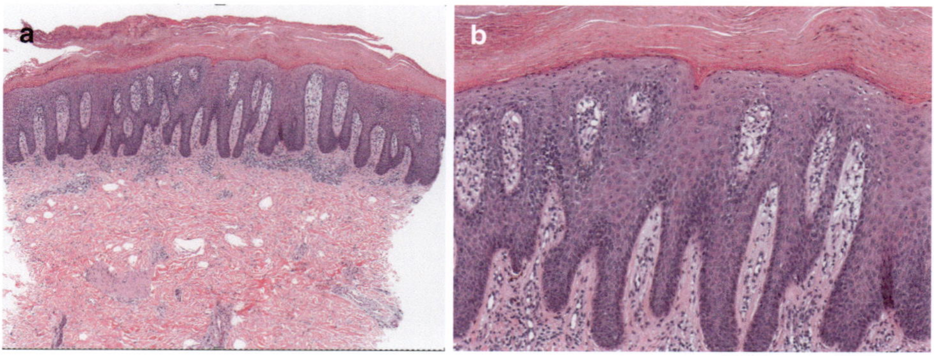

Fig. 61.3 Psoriasis (*2.5×, 10×; H&E*): (**a**) There is parakeratosis which in the current case is confluent but may exist in mounds (not shown), there is psoriasiform hyperplasia with regular elongation of the thickened rete ridges. Collections of neutrophils can commonly be seen in the s. corneum (munro abscesses). (**b**) High power demonstrates dilated vessels in the papillary dermis with mixed perivascular inflammation; extravasated RBCs maybe seen.

62 Cutaneous T-Cell Lymphoma

Nahid Y. Vidal

Overview

- Cutaneous lymphomas are mainly T-cell in origin (CTCL), and although the majority of these cases are mycosis fungoides (MF), CTCL should not be used synonymously with MF
  - Other primary CTCL subtypes include variants of MF, Sézary syndrome (SS), anaplastic large T-cell cutaneous lymphoma, lymphomatoid papulosis, and subcutaneous panniculitis-like T-cell lymphoma
  - Additionally, any systemic T-cell lymphoma can theoretically take residence in the skin as a secondary form of CTCL
- MF is usually an indolent disease affecting elderly patients with favorable prognosis in early stages
- SS is the leukemic variant of MF characterized by erythroderma, peripheral blood involvement (proven circulating clonal atypical T cells referred to as Sézary cells) and lymphadenopathy
- Cutaneous manifestations are variable in MF and staging is based on both the type of cutaneous eruption (patch, plaque, tumor, erythrodermic) and its distribution
  - MF/SS staging is complex and also dependent on nodal, visceral, blood involvement and molecular assessment of clonality
- Staging and outcomes:
  - Patients with T1 disease: <10% skin involvement (stage 1A):
    No difference in survival with age matched controls; low risk of progression
  - Patients with T2 disease ± nodal involvement: ≥10% skin involvement (stage 1B-2):
    Overall favorable prognosis, although nodal disease is considered a negative prognostic factor
    Approximately 25% progress to more advanced disease with a subset dying as a result of MF
  - Patients with tumors (T3) (stage 2B):
    On average patients survive 4–8 years; mortality typically MF related
  - Patients with erythroderma ± SS, diffuse nodal and visceral involvement (Stage 3, 4):
    Median survival 2–4 years with MF related mortality
  - Presence of nodal, visceral, and/or blood involvement will result in higher staging (see to the EORTC guidelines for details)

N. Y. Vidal, MD
Section of Dermatology, Department of Surgery, Dartmouth-Hitchcock Medical Center, Lebanon, NH, USA

Geisel School of Medicine, Hanover, NH, USA
e-mail: nahid.y.vidal@hitchcock.org

M. Rosenbach et al. (eds.), *Inpatient Dermatology*,
https://doi.org/10.1007/978-3-319-18449-4_62

- In MF/SS the most common cause of death is opportunistic infection
- Patients with MF/SS are at increased risk for developing a secondary malignancy, typically lymphoma

Clinical Presentation

- The development of distinct skin lesions and definitive MF diagnosis is often proceeded by months to years of nonspecific, often scaling dermatoses with associated nondiagnostic histology
- Cutaneous eruptions may be generalized, as is seen in erythroderma, or may present as localized lesions which may evolve and spread; commonly associated with pruritus (Fig. 62.1)
  - Non-sun exposed areas are typically involved initially, commonly including the buttocks, upper thighs, lower abdomen, and breasts ("bathing suit region")
- Early lesions may be very subtle with mild erythema and minimal associated scale; increased infiltration results in more prominent patches which can evolve into plaques and tumors
  - Scaly patches and plaques may be dry or weeping
  - Plaques are variable with regard to size (although often >5 cm), shape, color, and distribution
    Plaques can become extensive and coalescence results in generalized involvement; may have intervening areas of normal appearing skin
  - In more advanced lesions, plaques may expand into tumors (exophytic solid lesions with a diameter measuring at least 1 cm)
- Erythroderma refers to erythema over ≥90% total body surface area, which may be exfoliative (with scale); associated with palmoplantar hyperkeratosis, alopecia, dystrophic nails and ectropion of the eyelids
  - Erythroderma may be a presenting sign or a symptom of disease evolution
  - Patients may have associated fevers and chills
  - Lymphadenopathy is frequently present in advanced stage disease
- Atypical presentations include folliculotropic, hypopigmented, pigmented-purpuric dermatosis-like, poikiloderma, and panniculitic CTCL. Peripheral edema and cutaneous vasodilation are common, leading to insensible losses

Histopathology

- MF: Can be difficult to diagnose depending on the stage at time of biopsy and prior treatments; frequently multiple biopsies, and additional extended diagnostic testing, are required (Fig. 62.2)
  - Lesions may have a variably-dense lichenoid infiltrate and epidermotropism with atypical enlarged angulated hyperchromatic lymphocytes infiltrating or "tagging" the basal layer of the epidermis
  - Pautrier's microabscesses (collections of atypical lymphocytes) may form within the epidermis with relatively little associated spongiosis
  - Papillary fibrosis with irregularly arranged collagen fibers and deeper infiltrates are seen in plaque stage
  - Epidermitropism may be less evident in thick plaques/tumors
    Instead, confluent sheets of atypical lymphocytes are present in the dermis and subcutaneous fat
  - Lymphocytic folliculotrophism, syringotropism may be evident; intrafollicular mucin (follicular mucinosis) may be seen and is suggestive of MF
- SS: (Fig. 62.3)
  - Can vary from indistinct pathology to specimens showing features indistinguishable from late stage MF
  - Bland biopsies in SS may be misleading; flow cytometry is an important component of the workup
- Common immunohistochemical pattern: elevated CD4:CD8 ratio, with many cells staining CD3+, CD4+, CD7−, CD8−, CD26−. CD30+ staining of large cells can be a sign of large cell transformation

Differential Diagnosis

- Psoriasis: patients may have more classic plaques, and history of prior psoriasis
- Pityriasis rubra pilaris: may have an orange hue, islands of sparing, follicular prominence, palmoplantar keratoderma, and often suggestive histopathology
- Paraneoplastic erythroderma: all cases of erythroderma without a clear trigger warrant thorough systemic evaluation
- Graft-versus-host disease: erythroderma post-transplant is highly suspicious; diarrhea and liver function abnormalities may also suggest GvH
- Rarely, erythrodermic presentations of: seborrheic dermatitis, dermatomyositis, sarcoidosis, leukemia cutis, pemphigus, lichen planus

Work-Up

- CBC with differential and pathology review of the buffy coat smear for Sézary cells
  - Sèzary cells are atypical T-lymphocytes which classically have cerebriform nuclei
- Skin biopsy should be performed, ideally of an untreated area as topical steroids may minimize epidermotropism
- Assess for lymphadenopathy and arrange LN biopsy if clinically suspicious
- T-cell receptor gamma rearrangement studies to assess for clonality shoulds be performed; this is typically a PCR molecular assay
  - Testing can be performed on peripheral blood and fresh or paraffin embedded tissue
  - A positive result, signifying the detection of a clone, is not synonymous with neoplasia; clonality can be present in reactive processes
  - Matching clones in different skin and peripheral blood specimens is most convincing of a neoplastic process
- Flow cytometry on peripheral blood can also be used to immunophenotype lymphocytes allowing for the assessment of CD4/CD8 ratio (elevated in MF), loss of T-cell antigens, and clonality; classically MF cells are CD4+, CD7−, CD26−
- Assess for visceral involvement:
  - Hepatic function panel (to look for hepatic involvement)
  - Uric acid and lactate dehydrogenase (LDH) levels—which may be markers of bulky/aggressive disease
  - Metabolic profile to evaluate renal status, acid-base balance, electrolyte abnormalities
  - Case by case basis: CXR, CT Chest/abdomen/pelvis, MRI of the brain, PET imaging
- HIV testing and other tests that may help exclude other diagnoses in differential (HTLV-1 testing may be indicated depending on the patient's background and travel history)

Treatment

- Goals of treatment include controlling extent of skin disease and sequelae, improve quality of life, and halt progression of disease; complete remission is very rare for erythrodermic MF or SS

For All Patients

- Skin directed therapy to control symptoms and calm inflammation
  - Wet towel wraps followed by thick layer of ointment based mid-potency topical steroids (triamcinolone 0.1% ointment) or using "soak and smear method"
- Symptomatic treatment of pruritus and pain
- Monitoring and management of secondary complications due to cutaneous vasodilation such as high output heart failure, peripheral edema, insensible losses, nutritional deficiencies (due to high skin turnover), renal/electrolyte imbalances

- Evaluating for infection with low threshold for empiric antibiotic therapy
  - Gram positive bacteremia is a frequent complication through impaired skin barrier

Systemic, Additional Treatments

- Early stage MF treatments include skin directed therapy with topical steroids, topical nitrogen mustard, or phototherapy
- More advanced patch, plaque, tumor stage, erythrodermic MF or SS systemic therapies to be used include:
  - Extracorporeal photopheresis (ECP), low-dose MTX, oral bexarotene, gemcitabine, doxorubicin, HDAC-inhibitors (SAHA, romidepsin), Denileukin diftitox, PUVA (combined with INF-alpha, bexarotene), Interferons, retinoids, multi-agent systemic chemotherapy, total skin electron beam therapy. Multimodality therapy is frequently used.
- Allogenic stem cell transplantation may be considered in advanced stages of CTCL or transformed mycosis fungoides

Suggested Readings

1. Yamashita T, Abbade LT, Marques ME, et al. Mycosis fungoides and Sézary syndrome: clinical, histopathological and immunohistochemical review and update. An Bras Dermatol. 2012;87(6):817–28.
2. Dugas-Breit S, Schulze HJ, et al. New and established treatment options for mycosis fungoides and Sézary syndrome-an update. J Dtsch Dermatol Ges. 2014;12(7):561–9. https://doi.org/10.1111/ddg.12376.
3. Moriarty B, Whittaker S. Diagnosis, prognosis, and management of erythrodermic cutaneous T-cell lymphoma. Expert Rev Hematol. 2014;12:1–13.
4. Olsen E, Vonderheid E, Pimpinelli N, et al. Revisions to the staging and classification of mycosis fungoides and sèzary syndrome: a proposal of the Internationaal Society for Cutaneous Lymphoma (ISCL) and the cutaneous lymphoma task force of the European Organization of Research and Treatment of Cancer (EORTC). Blood. 2007;110:1713–22.

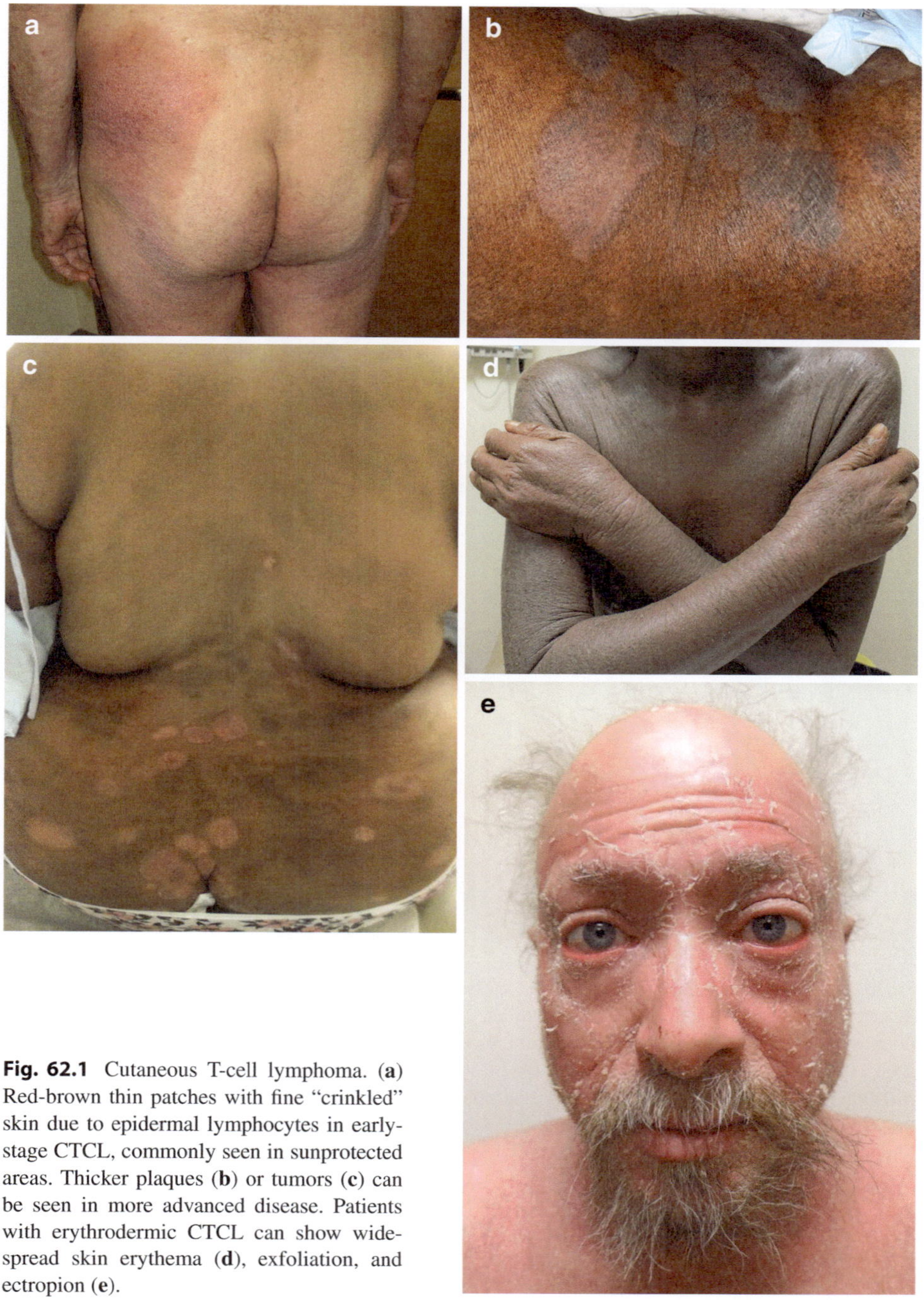

Fig. 62.1 Cutaneous T-cell lymphoma. (**a**) Red-brown thin patches with fine "crinkled" skin due to epidermal lymphocytes in early-stage CTCL, commonly seen in sunprotected areas. Thicker plaques (**b**) or tumors (**c**) can be seen in more advanced disease. Patients with erythrodermic CTCL can show widespread skin erythema (**d**), exfoliation, and ectropion (**e**).

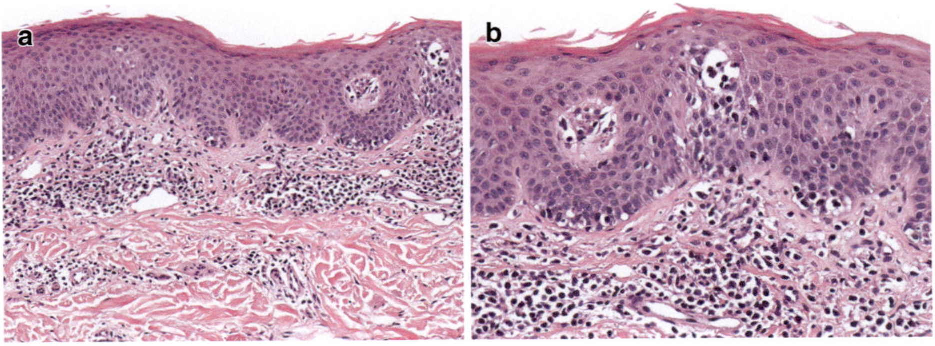

Fig. 62.2 Cutaneous T-cell lymphoma *(10×, 20×; H&E):* Histopathology varies depending on the stage of the disease. (**a**) Atypical lymphocytes often line up and tag the dermal epidermal junction with epidermotropism (atypical lymphocytes within the epidermis with an overall paucity of spongiosis). There is a superficial lichenoid inflammation infiltrate composed of atypical lymphocytes with hyperchromatic nuclei. (**b**) Pautrier microabscesses are characteristic features and characterized by intraepidermal collections of atypical cells.

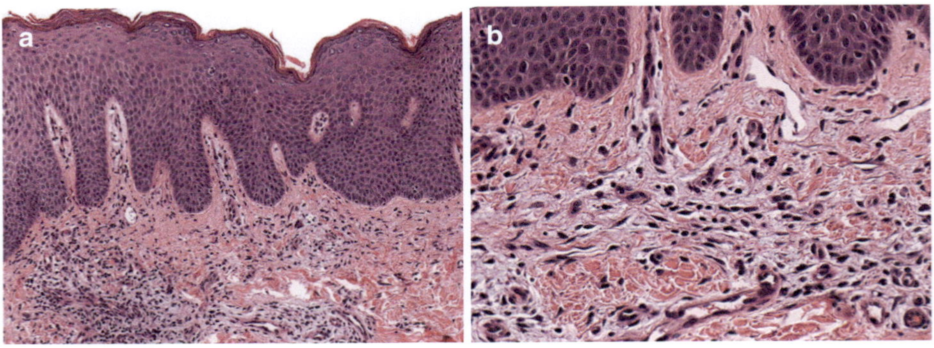

Fig. 62.3 Sèzary Syndrome *(10×, 20×; H&E):* The patient has cutaneous T-cell lymphoma (CTCL) and Sèzary syndrome (SS) with a high blood burden of disease. The histopathology in patients with SS is often nonspecific. If there is clinical suspicion in the absense of clear histology, then additional workup such as TCR-gene rearrangement and/or flow cytometry is warranted. (**a**) There can be variable epidermal changes including acanthosis, epidermal atrophy, and variable spongiosis. In this case, there is acanthosis with a superficial lymphocytic infiltrate. (**b**) Within the dermis, there is an infiltrate of atypical lymphocytes. Significant epidermotropism often is lacking as in this case.

Pityriasis Rubra Pilaris

63

Pooja Chitgopeker

Overview

- Pityriasis rubra pilaris (PRP) is a rare inflammatory dermatosis of unknown etiology characterized by distinctive clinical lesions including red-orange plaques ("salmon colored") with fine scale, hyperkeratotic fissuring lesions of the palmoplantar surfaces, and follicular hyperketatotic papules ("nutmeg grater")
- An uncommon cause of erythroderma
- Classified into six subtypes based on age of onset, clinical course, morphology and prognosis. Main distinctions are adult, juvenile, or HIV-associated

Clinical Presentation

- Clinically there are red-orange ("salmon colored") perifollicular "nutmeg-grater" papules which extend into confluent plaques, often with intervening areas of normal appearing skin, with a cephalocaudal spread (Fig. 63.1)
  - Palms and soles frequently develop an orange hue, become waxy and hyperkeratotic with the potential to fissure which can be quite painful
  - Scaling on the face and scalp is pityriasiform and coarser on the lower half of the body
  - Nail findings include thick nail plates with a rough surface, yellow-brown discoloration and subungual debris
  - Ectropion may sometimes occur along with keratitis and corneal perforation
- Oral mucosa may be affected with white spots and lines, pale blue lines and erythematous lesions over buccal mucosa, gingivae and tongue
- Reactive lymphadenopathy may occur if large surface area is affected

P. Chitgopeker, MD
University of Iowa, Iowa City, IA, USA
e-mail: pooja-chitgopeker@uiowa.edu

M. Rosenbach et al. (eds.), *Inpatient Dermatology*,
https://doi.org/10.1007/978-3-319-18449-4_63

Histopathology

- Psoriasiform epidermal hyperplasia with hypergranulosis with overlying alternating parakeratosis and orthokeratosis in both vertical and horizontal directions ("checkerboard pattern")
- Follicular plugs with "shoulder parakeratosis", in which parakeratosis is present adjacent to the keratin-plugged follicle (Fig. 63.2)

Differential Diagnosis

- Psoriasis: erythrodermic psoriasis may be hard to distinguish, but will often have more scale, fewer "skip areas," and less palmoplantar keratoderma; biopsy can be helpful
- Cutaneous T cell lymphoma, Sezary syndrome: may be impossible to distinguish and should have low threshold to perform T-cell receptor gene rearrangement and flow cytometry
- Generalized drug-induced hypersensitivity reaction: may lack the follicular accentuation, islands of sparing, and palmoplantar thickening
- Acute graft vs. host disease (aGVHD): timing and history are critical, as there can be extensive overlap; classic features of PRP are rarely seen even in erythrodermic aGVH

Work-Up

- Thorough history and physical exam focusing on clinical course, age of onset, history of other pre-existing skin disorders and family history
- Skin biopsy to help establish histopathological findings and exclude other entities
- HIV test
- Age appropriate investigation for internal malignancy as PRP may be paraneoplastic
- It is essential to rule out CTCL/Sezary and TCR-gene rearrangement and flow are often indicated

Treatment

- Often resistant to both topical and systemic therapies
- First line topical therapy include: emollients, keratolytics, topical tretinoin, topical corticosteroids in soak and smear method with wet towel wraps and thick ointment-based medium potency topical steroids
- Systemic treatment first line include retinoids, phototherapy, or methotrexate
- Second line systemic treatments include: cyclosporine, PUVA, acitretin + phototherapy, TNF alpha inhibitors; immunosuppressants should be used with caution and cutaneous T-cell lymphoma should be excluded prior to initiation

Suggested Readings

1. Klein A, Lantdhaler M, Karrer S. Pityriasis rubra pilaris. A review of diagnosis and treatment. Am J Clin Dermatol. 2010;11(3):157–70.
2. Bell SL, Patel AN, Leach IH, Cohen SN. Consider triggers for pityriasis rubra pilaris. Clin Exp Dermatol. 2014;39(3):403–5.

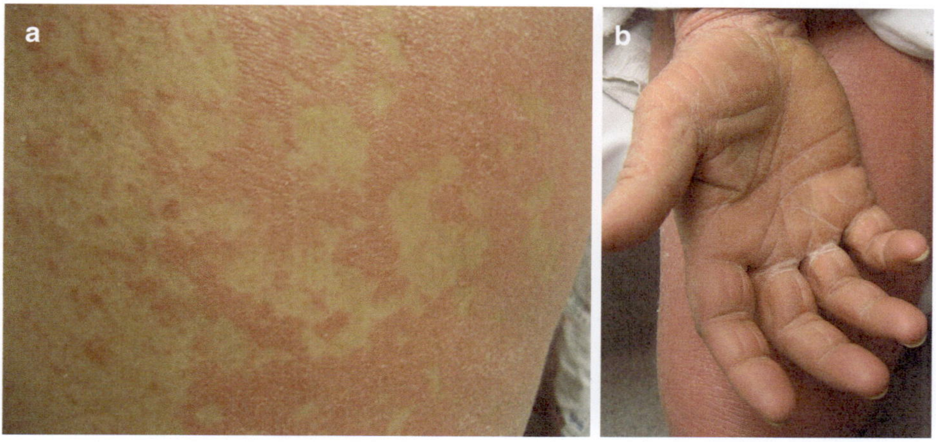

Fig. 63.1 Pityriasis rubra pilaris: (**a**) Orange-pink dermatitis with islands of sparing and some follicular prominence (resembling a "nutmeg grater"). (**b**) Waxy keratoderma typical of pityriasis rubra pilaris.

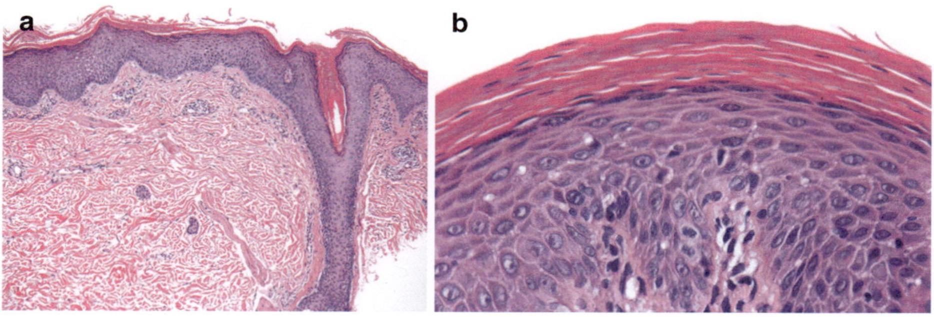

Fig. 63.2 Pityriasis rubra pilaris (*10X, 40X; H&E*): (**a**) Histopathology can demonstrate psoriasiform hyperplasia with follicular plugging, shoulder parakeratosis (adjacent to hair follicles), and varying parakeratosis. The underlying superficial dermis often contains a surprisingly mild inflammatory infiltrate (compared to striking clinical appearance). (**b**) Checkerboard parakeratosis is characteristic with parakeratosis alternating with hyperkeratosis in both horizontal and vertical direction. There is a mild superficial lymphocytic infiltrate.

Part X

Inflammatory and Autoimmune Conditions

Autoimmune diseases can cause a wide array of multisystem manifestations, including a broad spectrum of skin findings. This chapter covers both classic rheumatologic-dermatologic entities such as the connective tissue/collagen vascular diseases (lupus, dermatomyositis, systemic sclerosis) and autoimmune blistering diseases (bullous pemphigoid, pemphigus vulgaris, and pemphigus foliaceous), as well as other inflammatory dermatoses such as pyoderma gangrenosum and erythema nodosum. These entities are often as challenging to manage as they are to diagnose; this section is focused primarily on aiding the consulting clinician in recognizing and accurately diagnosing each of these entities, rather than addressing the long-term evaluation and chronic management of these complex medical/dermatologic diseases.

Autoimmune blistering diseases are often a source of confusion for non-dermatologists. When blisters are present, a skin biopsy can offer an incredible amount of information which can help determine at what level of the skin the blister is occurring, and what inflammatory cells are present, helping narrow down the differential diagnosis. Important additional workup includes a biopsy of peri-lesional, uninvolved skin for immunofluorescence studies, and confirmatory serologic antibody testing, to help hone in on a specific diagnosis. Patients may present to the hospital with new onset autoimmune blistering disease, flares of pre-existing diseases (which should always be carefully evaluated for signs or symptoms of superinfection—a widespread HSV infection in a patient with pemphigus can closely mimic a flare of the blistering disease), or can develop blisters while in-house, in which case drug-induced blistering diseases should be considered. This is a particular concern in the case of linear IgA bullous dermatosis, which may occur after antibiotic use (particularly with vancomycin).

Similarly, rheumatologic dermatologic entities may be seen as part of the initial disease onset, where patients can present with a diverse range of cutaneous findings, or as part of a flare of a pre-existing autoimmune disease. Beyond the cutaneous findings, pathologic evaluation of these eruptions can often be helpful in confirming the presence of a connective tissue disease, but many of these entities share similar histopathologic findings. Making an accurate diagnosis often involves supplementation with lab findings, serologic testing, radiographic imaging, and may require consultation with other specialists, particularly rheumatologists. An inpatient dermatologist should keep in mind that when asked to evaluate patients with these multisystem processes, consulting teams may request a skin biopsy. While pathology can be overlapping in many of the entities on the differential, it is important for a consulting dermatologist to remember to treat not just the patient, but the consulting team as well. When there is a hospitalized patient with a constellation of multiple organ system findings and evidence of widespread inflammation, performing a skin biopsy to demonstrate interface dermatitis may not yield a specific diagnosis, but can be a helpful clue in the puzzle to piecing together the diagnosis.

Pyoderma Gangrenosum

64

Inbal Sander

Overview

- Pyoderma gangrenosum (PG) is a painful ulcerating neutrophilic dermatosis which primarily involves the skin, commonly the lower legs or sites of prior trauma (pathergy); approximately half of cases develop in patients with an underlying systemic disease, most commonly inflammatory bowel disease
  - Less common associated diseases include inflammatory arthritis, hematologic malignancies, and monoclonal gammopathy (most often IgA)
- PG is a diagnosis of exclusion—other causes of cutaneous ulceration must be ruled out

Clinical Presentation

- Lesions typically present as a tender nodule or sterile pustule and then quickly enlarge and erode into painful, exudative, rapidly expanding ulcers with gray-purple/violaceous, overhanging borders. May heal with criss-crossed cribiform scaring (Fig. 64.1)
- 25–40% of cases may display pathergy, induction of lesions or worsening of lesions after trauma, including at IV sites or after biopsy
- Five recognized subtypes:
  - Classic: purple-gray edematous border with exudative central ulcer
  - Bullous: intense edema that then ulcerates; significant overlap with Sweet syndrome
  - Pustular: single or studded pustules can be the first sign of PG but often expand into classic morphology
  - Vegetative: more exophytic with interconnected superficial tracts and small cysts, often resembling a deep/endemic fungal infection
  - Peristomal: usually displays more classic morphology but located around ostomy sites in patients with IBD/Crohn disease
- May have accompanying fever, malaise, myalgias and arthralgias
- Can rarely involve lungs, heart, central nervous system, gastrointestinal tract, eye, liver, spleen and lymph nodes; the lung is the mostly commonly involved extracutaneous organ
- There can be discordance between PG activity and the associated systemic disease activity

I. Sander, MD
Johns Hopkins School of Medicine, Baltimore, MD, USA

M. Rosenbach et al. (eds.), *Inpatient Dermatology*,
https://doi.org/10.1007/978-3-319-18449-4_64

Histopathology

- Diffuse dermal neutrophilic inflammation, extending beyond area of ulceration; may have accompanying vasculitis but should not be vasculocentric (Fig. 64.2)
- Stains for organisms negative; accompanying tissue cultures should be negative

Differential Diagnosis

- Infection (bacterial, fungal, viral, mycobacterial, protozoal): It is important to correlate neutrophilic dermatoses with negative special stains and cultures to exclude infection
- Ulcers due to vascular insufficiency: typically more ragged, irregular, less violaceous/edematous rim, and less exudative
- Systemic vasculitides: GPA can present with "malignant pyoderma" closely resembling PG, and the two can also coexist—ANCA serologies are important in ruling out GPA
- Exogenous tissue injury: accidental intra-articular injection of crystalline material can lead to "Nicolau syndrome" which can resemble PG, but usually has less edematous borders and less exudate
- Sweet's syndrome (acute febrile neutrophilic dermatosis): Sweets and PG share similar pathophysiology and can be impossible to distinguish; neutrophilic dermatoses may be diagnosed as Sweets in the setting of myelodysplasia and the same presentation called PG in the setting of IBD
- Cutaneous Crohn's disease: usually occurs closer to the perianal region and biopsy may have more granulomas, but can be challenging to distinguish
- Lymphoma: may cause ulcerative lesions and is one of the main differential diagnoses requiring biopsy to completely exclude prior to labeling a patient with PG

Work-Up

- A thorough history and physical to evaluate for an associated systemic disease is warranted
- Biopsy and tissue culture are critical in the new diagnosis of PG to exclude exclude infectious, vasculitic or malignant etiologies (despite risk of pathergy)
  - Biopsy should be taken from the edge of the ulcer, approximately 80–90% normal skin with a small sliver of ulcer border ideally
- Other diagnostic tests may include anti-nuclear antibody (ANA), rheumatoid factor, anti-neutrophil cytosplasmic antibody (ANCA) to exclude other etiologies of ulcers
  - Further studies, including bone marrow biopsy, serum protein electrophoresis with immunofixation, urine protein electrophoresis, fecal occult blood testing, imaging, or colonoscopy/endoscopy or capsule endoscopy may be indicated

Treatment

- The main principles are: identifying and controlling any associated systemic disease, using anti-inflammatory/suppressive agents to stop the neutrophilic inflammation, and careful wound care to facilitate healing
- Anti-inflammatories regimens depend on extent of disease
  - Topical medications are important as primary treatment or more commonly as adjuncts to systemic therapy: Topical corticosteroids, tacrolimus, and cyclosporine (ophthalmic preparations) are used most commonly
  - Intralesional steroids to the ulcer edge may be helpful, particularly in peristomal disease
  - First line agents include systemic corticosteroids, TNF inhibitors (particularly infliximab), or cyclosporine.
  - Oral antineutrophilic agents (i.e. colchicine and dapsone), minocycline, and other nonsteroidal immunosupressives (mycophenolate mofetil, azathioprine, methotrexate) have shown benefit
- Local wound care:
  - Relies on absorptive dressing (hydrocolloids, foams and aliginates) for exudative lesions and moisture-retentive occlusive dressing (like films and hydrogels) for healing, dry lesions.
  - Avoid "Wet-to-dry" dressings and surgical debridement because of pathergy risk
- Pain control if often essential as active PG may be exquisitely painful

Suggested Readings

1. Ahronowitz I, Harp J, Shinkai K. Etiology and management of pyoderma gangrenosum: a comprehensive review. Am J Clin Dermatol. 2012;13(3):191–211.
2. Callen JP. Pyoderma gangrenosum. Lancet. 1998;351:581–5.
3. Binus AM, Qureshi AA, Li VW, Winterfield LS. Pyoderma gangrenosum: a retrospective review of patient characteristics, comorbidities and therapy in 103 patients. Br J Dermatol. 2011;165(6):1244–50.

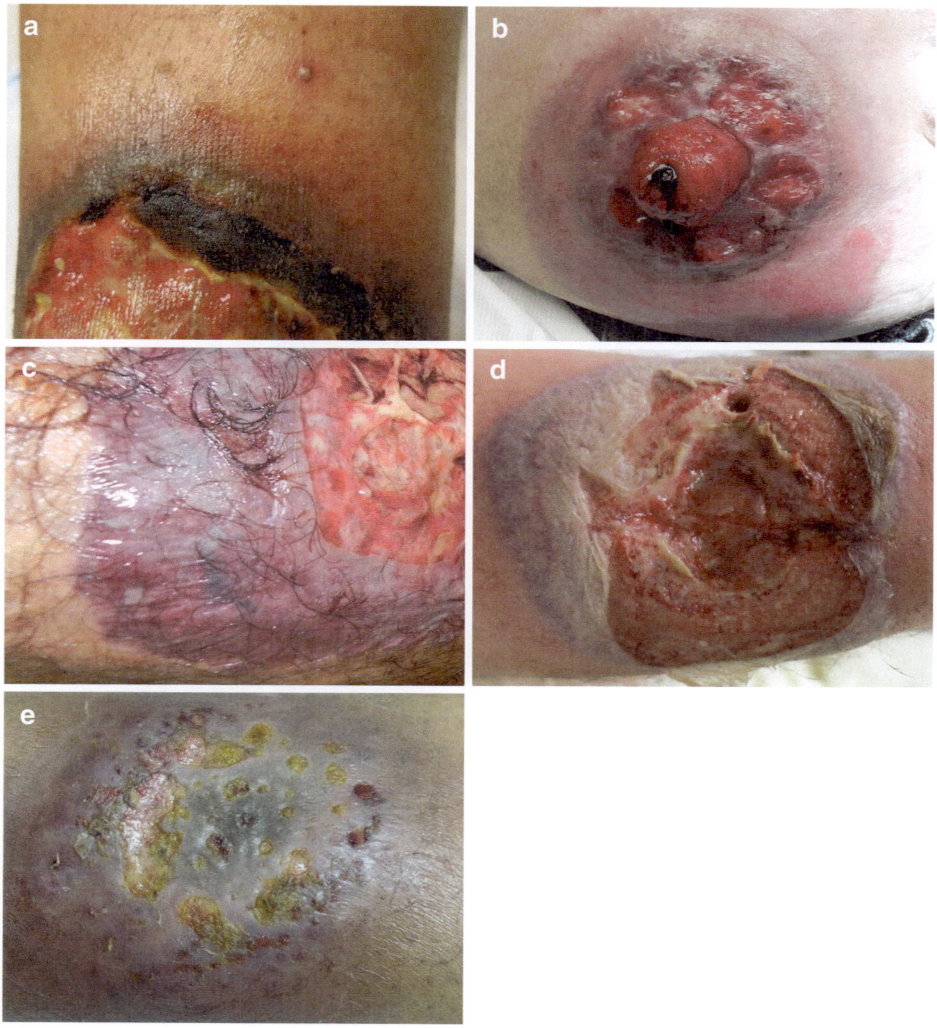

Fig. 64.1 Pyoderma gangrenosum: (**a**) Large leg ulcer demonstrating a violaceous or "gun-metal" gray inflammatory border and adjacent violaceous pustule typical of active and incipient pyoderma gangrenosum, respectively. (**b**) Peristomal pyoderma gangrenosum with friable, necrotic, and violaceous tissue breaking apart in a manner resembling cheesecloth. (**c**) Large, swollen plaque of pyoderma gangrenosum on the calf exhibiting typical purple-gray "undermined" border as the dermal neutrophilic inflammation extends outward, leaving behind a superficial layer of epidermis. (**d**) Deep, limb-threatening pyoderma gangrenosum of the left arm with violaceous, necrotic border. (**e**) Vegetative type of pyoderma gangrenosum with epidermal thickening and numerous areas of ulceration.

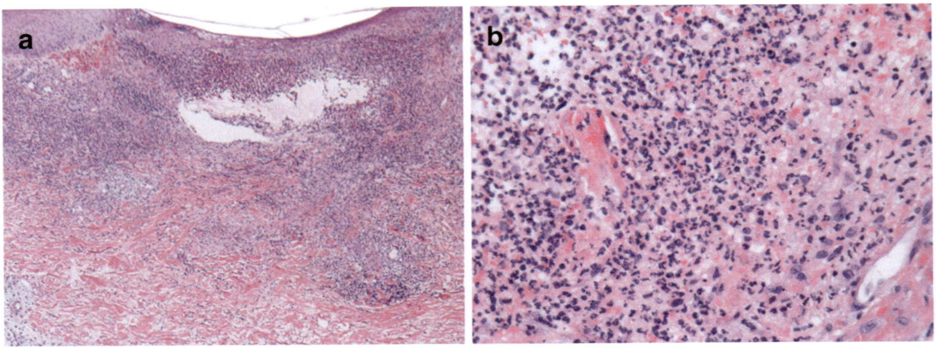

Fig. 64.2 Pyoderma gangrenosum *(5×, 40×; H&E)*: (**a**) Low power demonstrates epidermal necrosis or an overlying ulceration with diffuse neutrophilic infiltrate within the dermis. (**b**) On high power, there are numerous neutrophils. Infection needs to be excluded with infectious stains and negative tissue cultures.

Panniculitis/Erythema Nodosum

65

Misha Rosenbach

Overview

- Panniculitis is inflammation of the fat and is divided into two main forms based on the location of the inflammation, septal or lobular
  - This distinction is problematic since panniculitis typically does not exclusively involve one component of the subcutis; however, predominant involvement of the septa can be a helpful diagnostic clue
- Complicated clinical category as panniculitis can result from an extensive list of associated diseases, medications, or infections but often has similar presentation
  - Distribution, histology, and history are helpful in elucidating etiology
- The most common form of panniculitis is erythema nodosum (EN), which will be the main focus of this section
  - EN is the prototypic septal panniculitis which typically involves the bilateral lower legs with a symmetrical distribution and can occur as either an acute or chronic process
  - Most common in women in their 20–40s but can affect anyone
  - EN can arise as an idiopathic disease, or as a sign of strep infection, GI bacterial infections, endemic pulmonary fungal infections (coccidioidomycosis), medications (especially female hormones), sarcoidosis, IBD (primarily Crohn's), neutrophilic dermatoses (Behçet's and Sweet syndrome), pregnancy, and other less common associations

Clinical Presentation

- Patients present with red, ill-defined, subcutaneous nodules that are tender to palpation but do not typically ulcerate; established or involuting lesions may appear bruise-like (Fig. 65.1)
  - Lesions tend to persist for weeks and heal without residual scars but recurrences may occur in up to 1/3 of cases
  - More chronic forms do exist such as erythema nodosum migrans
- Generally on the lower legs; EN tends to be bilateral and symmetrical, whereas other forms of panniculitis may favor the posterior calves, thighs, or high fat areas
  - Confluent areas of fat inflammation may have broad erythema which can resemble cellulitis; the bilaterality of EN would be highly atypical in cellulitis

M. Rosenbach, MD
Department of Dermatology, Perelman School of Medicine, University of Pennsylvania, Philadelphia, PA, USA
e-mail: Misha.Rosenbach@uphs.upenn.edu

M. Rosenbach et al. (eds.), *Inpatient Dermatology*,
https://doi.org/10.1007/978-3-319-18449-4_65

- Patients may present with a variety of symptoms related to associated/underlying disease which may include arthritis, respiratory findings (cough, dyspnea, abnormal chest X-ray), and/or diarrhea

Histopathology

- EN may have different features depending on stage of the panniculitis; inflammation is centered on the interlobular septum, with potential spillover into adjacent lobules (Fig. 65.2)
  - Neutrophils are predominant in early lesions with associated histiocytes and rare giant cells; later lesions contain a mixed, possibly granulomatous infiltrate with giant cells
- Lobular panniculitis favors a diagnosis other than EN and may show different features depending on the cause:
  - Vasculitis can indicate erythema induratum (associated with TB)
  - Large atypical cells may indicate panniculitic T-cell lymphoma
  - Hyalinization of adipocytes with overlying features of lupus and
  - Lymphoplasmacytic infiltrate may be a clue to lupus panniculitis
  - Ghost adipocytes, saponification, and calcification can be a clue to pancreatic panniculitis

Differential Diagnosis

- EN should be distinguished from other forms of panniculitis
  - Traumatic panniculitis: antecedent trauma, focal lesion, often at a single site, and with less erythema/red-brown color
  - Lipodermatosclerosis: bilateral bound-down lower legs leading to the characteristic “inverted champagne bottle” look, not discrete nodules
  - Erythema induratum: usually on the posterior calves, and may be more supporative and drain purulent discharge
- Cellulitis: rapid onset and unilaterality should distinguish from EN
- Medium vessel vasculitis: can share clinical overlap and histology and serologic testing may be required
- Abscesses: may display a central pustule and fluctuance, but sometimes an I&D or biopsy and culture are required

Work-Up

- Although classic cases of EN may be diagnosed clinically, without biopsy in the inpatient setting a biopsy if often warranted as critically ill patients often require and expedient diagnosis and EN can be a reaction to numerous systemic diseases and the biopsy may assist with determining etiology
  - Atypical presentations should prompt a biopsy
- A thorough workup to identify associated systemic diseases is indicated in all cases of EN
  - Basic lab work, pregnancy test, Chest X-ray, and evaluation for infection (including strep throat, gastrointestinal illnesses, and endemic pulmonary infections) are warranted
  - Further workup should be based on history and review of systems and may include serologies (ANA, RF), imaging, colonoscopy and more

Treatment

- Identification of any potential underlying disease is essential, with treatment based on the triggering systemic process or removal of the inciting medication
- Mild cases of EN may respond to bed rest, elevation, and/or NSAIDs; more severe cases may require initial prednisone with transition to other agents
  - Second line agents include colchicine, dapsone, hydroxychloroquine, and saturated solution of potassium iodide

Suggested Readings

1. Requena L, Yus ES. Panniculitis. Part I. Mostly septal panniculitis. J Am Acad Dermatol. 2001;45(2):163–83.
2. Requena L, Yus ES. Panniculitis. Part II. Mostly lobular panniculitis. J Am Acad Dermatol. 2001;45(3): 325–61.
3. Blake T, Manahan M, Rodins K. Erythema nodosum—a review of an uncommon panniculitis. Dermatol Online J. 2014;20(4):22376.

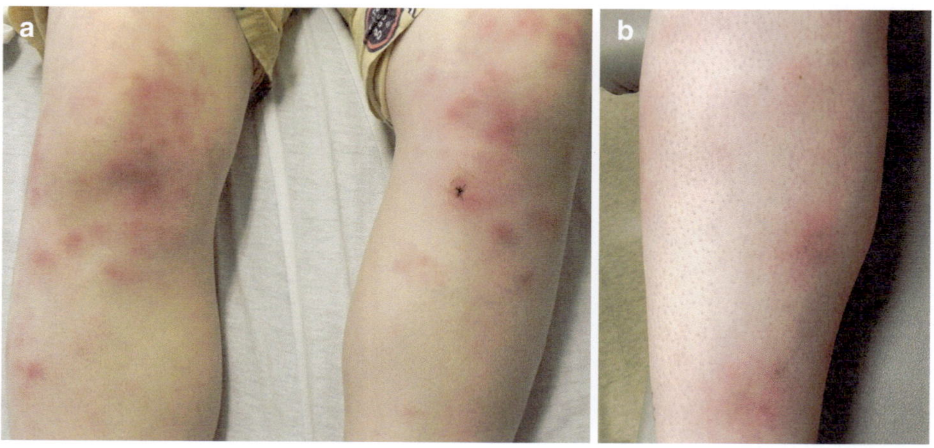

Fig. 65.1 Erythema nodosum (EN): (**a**) Bilateral anterior shin ill-defined tender red nodules characteristic of EN. (**b**) Tender subcutaneous, erythematous nodules on the anterior lower legs.

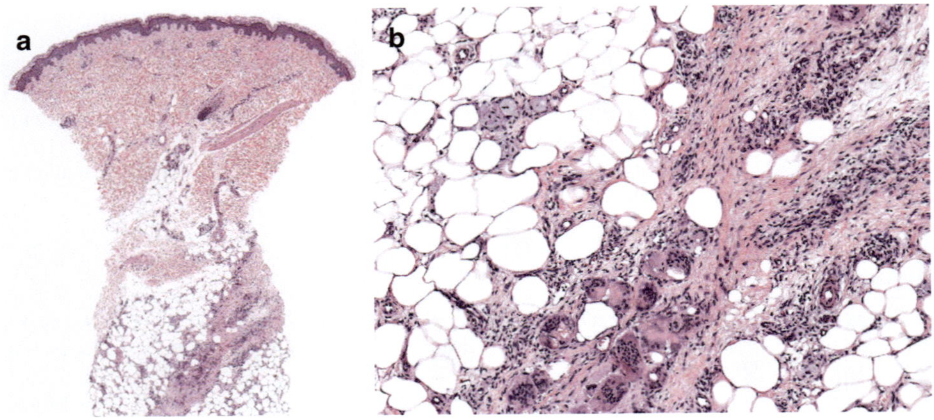

Fig. 65.2 Septal panniculitis (*2.5×*, *20×*; *H&E*): (**a**) Low power demonstrates inflammation within the subcutaneous tissue and widening of the septae. (**b**) Numerous collections of multinucleated giant cells and neutrophils in the thickened septae are characteristic features of erythema nodosum.

Lichen Planus

66

Misha Rosenbach

Overview

- Lichen planus (LP) is an inflammatory mucocutaneous papulosquamous dermatosis characterized by pruritic hyperkeratotic violet papules and plaques
  - Most commonly presents in adults 40–50 years old
- Classified based on distribution (oral, vulvovaginal, nail, classic/skin) and clinical appearance of lesions
  - While most patients with cutaneous disease have oral lesions (75%) the reverse is not true; in many cases patients have isolated oral LP
- Etiology unknown, thought to be potentially autoimmune in nature caused by cytotoxic T-cell driven basal keratinocyte apoptosis (FAS-ligand driven) resulting in chemokine/cytokine release and epidermotropic T-cell migration
- Thought to be mediated by exposure to exogenous antigens such as:
  - Viruses: HCV, possibly HHV-6/7, reports of rare association with HBV vaccine
  - Metal contact allergens are implicated in oral LP (such as gold teeth fillings)
  - Drugs (lichenoid drug reactions): ACE-Is, antimalarials, TNF-alpha inhibitors, diuretics, bisophosphonates
    - Lichenoid drug reactions may be photodistributed, but often are clinically indistinguishable from idiopathic LP
- Koebner phenomenon: lesions may to develop in sites of skin injury such as tracking within surgical scars or at sites of excoriation

Clinical Presentation

- Round to polygonal pruritic violaceous papules often with delicate white reticular striations (Wickham striae) which may coalesce to form extensive plaques favoring flexoral surfaces of the upper extremities, anterior surface of the lower extremities, dorsum of the hands, oral mucosa and genitalia (Fig. 66.1)
  - Wickham striae may be the predominant feature of mucosal lesions; mucosal lesions may be erosive and longstanding erosive mucosal lesions can transform into oral SCC
- There are a multiple variants of LP which are often self-limited; LP more commonly persists in the setting of nail, hypertrophic or mucosal LP

M. Rosenbach, MD
Department of Dermatology, Perelman School of Medicine, University of Pennsylvania, Philadelphia, PA, USA
e-mail: Misha.Rosenbach@uphs.upenn.edu

M. Rosenbach et al. (eds.), *Inpatient Dermatology*,
https://doi.org/10.1007/978-3-319-18449-4_66

  - Variants include: annular LP (often in intertriginous/genital region), bullous LP, hypertrophic LP (increased risk SCC, symmetric and chronic), actinic LP, lichen planopilaris (folliculocentric with potential for scarring alopecia) and atrophic LP (lichen-sclerosis-like lesions), among others

Histopathology

- Interface dermatitis obscures the DEJ with civette body formation representing apoptotic basal keratinocytes and a dense band of lymphocytic (lichenoid) inflammation (Fig. 66.2)
  - Basal keratinocytes appear flattened like the more mature/differentiated cells in the superficial epidermis; this is referred to as basal squamatization
- The epidermis is acanthotic and rete may develop a "sawtooth" appearance; wedge-shaped hypergranulosis and compact overlying orthokeratosis are classic

Differential Diagnosis

- Lichenoid drug reaction: can be challenging to distinguish; anecdotally lichenoid medication reactions may spare the mucosa or have less developed Wickham's striae, and biopsy may have more eosinophils
- Lichenoid GVHD: can be indistinguishable beyond a prior history of allogeneic transplant
- Lichen sclerosis: usually localized to the genitalia and more atrophic; biopsy may be helpful but can be hard to differentiate
- Psoriasis: can develop at sites of trauma (Koebnerize), but more often pink with thick white scaly flakes; there may be substantial overlap but histopathology should distinguish the two
- Lupus (CLE, DLE): Hypertrophic LP can be hard to differentiate from hypertrophic lupus lesions, and other morphologies share some overlap as both are interface reactions—clinical pathologic correlation is required
- SCC: hypertrophic LP lesions can be hard to distinguish from squamous cell carcinoma, and indeed longstanding LP lesions (particularly mucosal erosions) can undergo malignant degeneration
- Scabies: both LP and scabies have a predilection for wrist lesions, and are pruritic, but the pattern and distribution of lesions is often sufficient to distinguish the two

Work-Up

- All patients should undergo a thorough history for potential triggers
- Testing for hepatitis C is recommended, with additional viral testing when there is a suggestive antecedent trigger
- Potential inciting medications should be stopped or adjusted
- Skin biopsy may be helpful but is not always required
- All patients should have a thorough evaluation of mucosa (genitalia and oral, potentially with an oral medicine consultation)
  - Patients with oral involvement should be followed with periodic examinations

Treatment

- Lichen planus is often self-limited (2–3 year duration), but given the pruritus usually requires treatment
- Topical steroids (mid- to high-potency) may be used as initial treatment
- Severe or extensive cases may require systemic corticosteroids for rapid relief
- Phototherapy can be helpful (NBUVB or PUVA) and patients may be started on light therapy de novo or as a steroid sparing agent
- Patients have been treated with systemic, immunomodulatory, and immunosuppressive agents such as retinoids, antimalarials, mycophenolate mofetil, and methotrexate and more in widespread, recalcitrant, or intensely symptomatic cases

Suggested Readings

1. Atzmony L, Reiter O, Hodak E, Gdalevich M, Mimouni D. Treatments for cutaneous lichen planus: a systematic review and meta-analysis. Am J Clin Dermatol. 2016;17(1):11–22.
2. Gorouhi F, Davari P, Fazel N. Cutaneous and mucosal lichen planus: a comprehensive review of clinical subtypes, risk factors, diagnosis, and prognosis. Sci World J. 2014;2014:742826.
3. Pickert A. Concise review of lichen planus and lichenoid dermatoses. Cutis. 2012;90(3):E1–3.

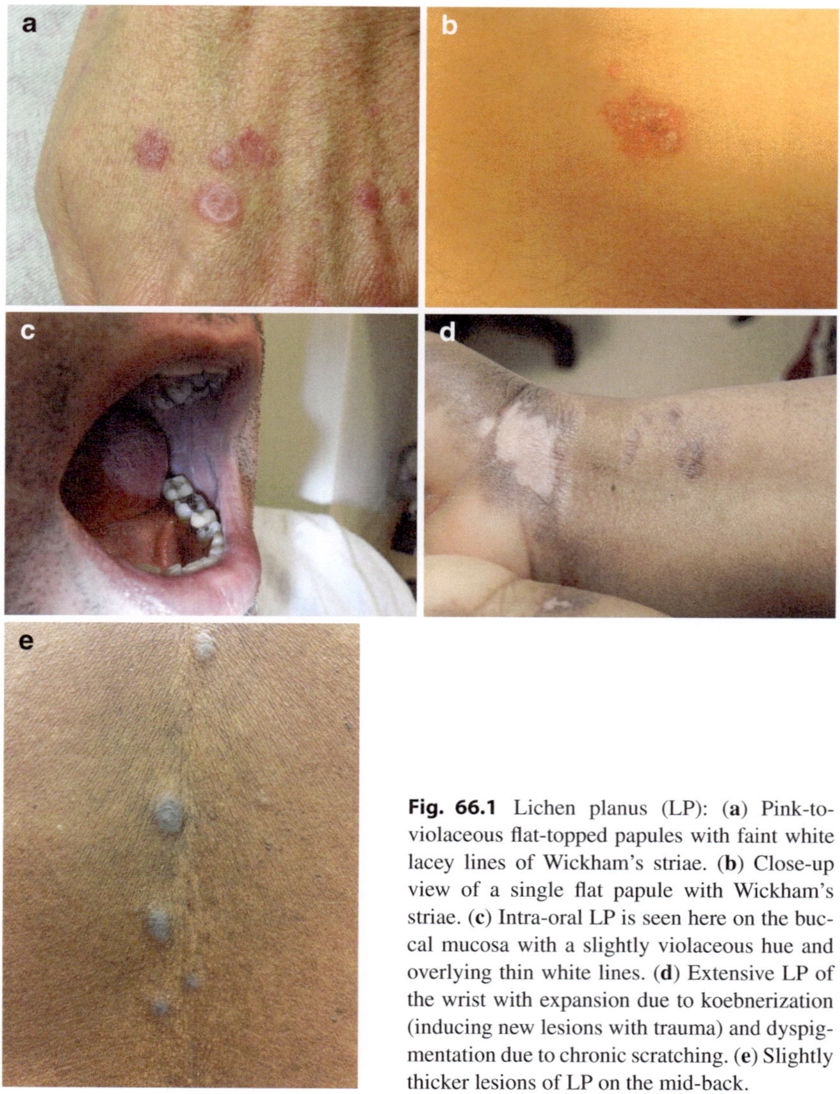

Fig. 66.1 Lichen planus (LP): (**a**) Pink-to-violaceous flat-topped papules with faint white lacey lines of Wickham's striae. (**b**) Close-up view of a single flat papule with Wickham's striae. (**c**) Intra-oral LP is seen here on the buccal mucosa with a slightly violaceous hue and overlying thin white lines. (**d**) Extensive LP of the wrist with expansion due to koebnerization (inducing new lesions with trauma) and dyspigmentation due to chronic scratching. (**e**) Slightly thicker lesions of LP on the mid-back.

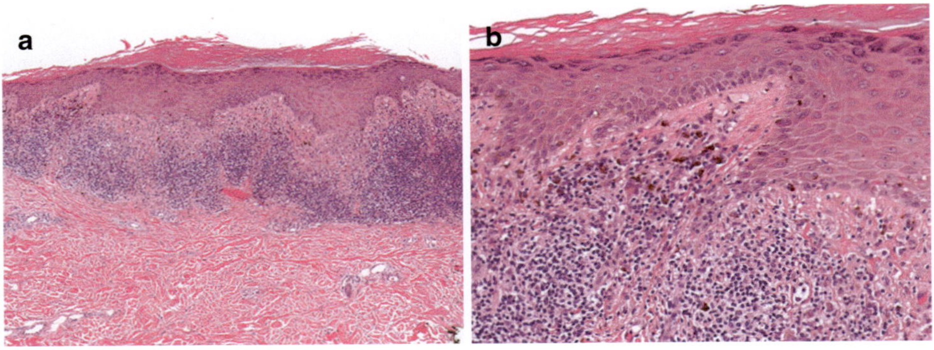

Fig. 66.2 Lichen planus (*2.5*×, *10*×): There is overlying compact hyperkeratosis, the epidermis is acanthotic with a prominent granular layer and a "saw tooth" pattern to the irregular rete ridges with a pronounced interface and lichenoid predominantly lymphocytic infiltrate with necrotic basal keratinocytes forming pink colloid bodies.

67 Dermatomyositis

Pooja Chitgopeker

Overview

- Dermatomyositis (DM) is an idiopathic autoimmune inflammatory disease which can present with variable skin signs, muscle inflammation, and systemic symptoms
  - Classic DM: a photodistributed violaceous poikiloderma favoring the chest and back (Shawl sign), eyelids (helitrope sign), and extensor surfaces (Gottron's papules and sign) with associated inflammatory myositis typically presenting as proximal muscle weakness
  - Amyopathic DM: Skin-limited disease without myositis; these patients still are at risk for systemic manifestations. Notably DM patients can present with isolated skin findings with delayed development of myositis
  - Hypomyopathic DM: Patients lack clinically evident muscle weakness but have myositis based on imaging and laboratory testing
- Systemic associations include: increased risk for internal malignancy (25% of patients with dermatomyositis), interstitial lung disease, cardiac involvement and arthritis

Clinical Presentation

- Photodistributed pruritic violaceous erythema and poikiloderma commonly prominent over areas of taught, stretched, tight skin (Fig. 67.1)
  - Poikiloderma refers to skin with epidermal atrophy, mixed hyper/hypopigmentation, and telangiectasias.
- Violaceous/lilac erythema around the eyes (heliotrope sign), on the anterior chest (V-neck), and upper back/shoulders (Shawl) is common
  - Heliotrope sign may be accompanied by periorbital edema and facial erythema which may vary in intensity throughout the disease course
- Violaceous lesions are usually prevalent on extensor surfaces:
  - Gottron's papules: flat-topped papules develop from lichenification of established lesions over the finger and hand joints
  - Gottron's sign: erythema knuckles, elbows and/or knees
  - Holster sign: lateral hips
  - "Inverse Gottron's": erythema of the creases on the palmar aspect of the fingers, often with ulceration, associated with a phenotype with severe interstitial lung disease

P. Chitgopeker, MD
University of Iowa, Iowa City, IA, USA
e-mail: pooja-chitgopeker@uiowa.edu

M. Rosenbach et al. (eds.), *Inpatient Dermatology*,
https://doi.org/10.1007/978-3-319-18449-4_67

- Violeacous erythema of the proximal nail fold with atrophy, nail fold telangiectasias, and cuticular dystrophy and nail fold telangiectasias are characteristic
- Broad areas of dermatomyositis erythema often display some fine white scale
- Flagellate erythema and cutaneous calcinosis are rare findings; atypical variants of dermatomyositis can include follicular prominence and pityriasis-rubra-pilaris-like changes
- The myositis typically presents with proximal muscle weakness, often of the muscles of the neck and extremities
  - Patients may have trouble combing hair, or rising from seated positions to standing
  - Muscle weakness of internal musculature (swallowing/dysphagia) or bulbar muscles is uncommon
- Systemic symptoms of fatigue and malaise; in patients with interstitial lung disease dyspnea may be a common symptom

Histopathology

- Epidermal atrophy with basement membrane degeneration and interface vacuolar dermatitis with interstitial mucin deposition in the dermis and a sparse perivascular lymphocytic infiltrate (Fig. 67.2)
  - When Grotton's papules are biopsied the epidermis is acanthotic not atrophic but the underlying changes will be the same
- Colloidal iron stain may help to identify the presence of mucin

Differential Diagnosis

- Systemic lupus erythematous: the malar rash of lupus typically sharply spares the nasolabial creases, unlike DM, and when on the hands lupus affects the spaces between the knuckles, whereas DM is localized to the PIP/DIP/MCP joints, but there can be substantial overlap and indeed patients can have true overlap syndromes/mixed connective tissue disease.
- Psoriasis: plaques with fine scale may develop on extensor surfaces in DM and can be clinically confused with psoriasis, and biopsy may be required
- Airborne or allergic contact dermatitis: DM often has a photodistributed component, and will spare the sub-mental chin, whereas airborne reactions should not, but biopsy can be helpful in differentiating

Work-Up

- All patients should have a thorough physical exam and history to elicit potential signs or symptoms of dermatomyositis and internal involvement, including careful muscular exam and thorough review of systems for atypical muscle involvement such as bulbar disease or esophageal weakness
- Chest X-ray and pulmonary function testing (including DLco) and/or high resolution CT chest to evaluate for interstitial lung disease
- EKG to assess for cardiac involvement of myositis
- General labs: Complete blood count with differential, comprehensive metabolic panel
- Serum creatinine kinase, serum aldolase
  - If CK/aldolase are normal but muscle involvement is still suspected, MRI of affected muscles to identify inflammation and subsequent muscle biopsy may be indicated; electromyography (EMG) may identify subclinical disease
- Age appropriate malignancy screening is indicated in all patients, plus additional imaging for gynecologic/ovarian malignancies in women; Consider full body CT chest/abdomen/pelvis or a PET scan.
- Emerging data is coming to light regarding dermatomyositis subphenotypes with specific antibodies which may portend a higher risk of malignancy (such as anti-TIF1-gamma or NXP2 in some populations), more mild disease (Mi2), or severe lung disease (anti-MDA5 antibodies) for instance
  - If available, consider specific myositis antibody panel testing

Management

- Patients should be regularly seen to monitor treatment and screened for potential underlying malignancy or delayed muscle or lung involvement
- Skin directed therapy with strict photoprotection and topical corticosteroids
- Hydroxychloroquine may help some patients, however, 25% of patients with dermatomyositis may develop an antimalarial-associated morbilliform rash
- Oral prednisone when there is muscle involvement or extensive skin involvement to control symptoms quickly
- Steroid sparing agents such as methotrexate, azathioprine, mycophenolate mofetil (which may be helpful in some cases both for cutaneous involvement and interstitial lung disease)
- Intravenous Immunoglobulin (IVIG) may be effective for recalcitrant skin disease, whereas rituximab may help treat some cases of recalcitrant lung disease

Suggested Readings

1. Femia A, Vleugels R, Callen J. Cutaneous dermatomyositis: an updated review of treatment options and internal associations. Am J Clin Dermatol. 2013;14:291–343.
2. Braunstein I, Werth V. Treatment of dermatologic connective tissue disease and autoimmune blistering disorders in pregnancy. Dermatol Ther. 2013;26(4):354–63.

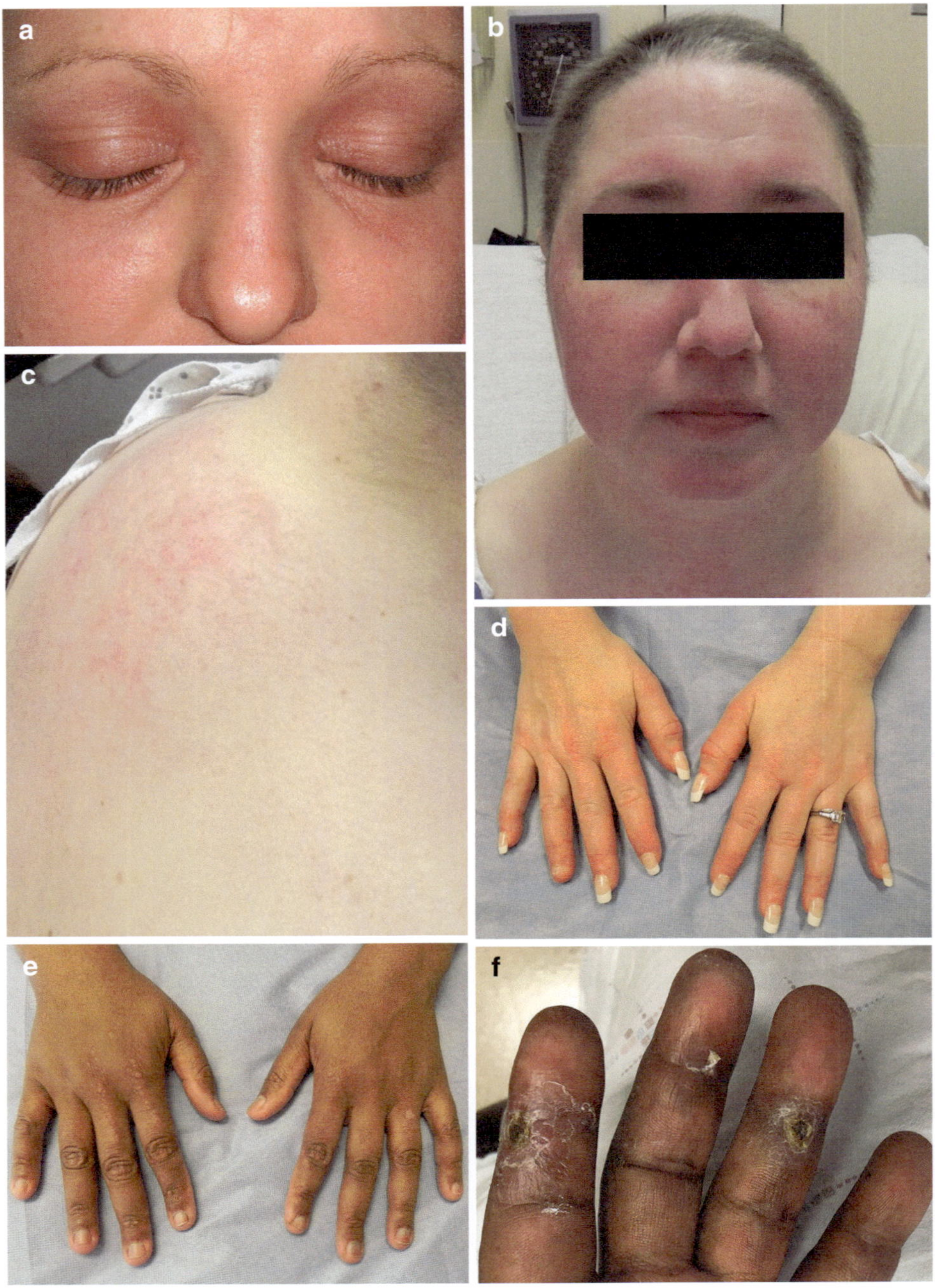

Fig. 67.1 Dermatomyositis: (**a**) Violaceous erythema of the eyelids (heliotrope sign). (**b**) Violaceous erythema extending across the face and V-neck area of the upper chest. (**c**) Erythema across the upper back (shawl sign). (**d**) Erythema over the MCPs, DIPs, and PIPs (Gottron sign) with prominent erythema of the proximal nail fold. (**e**) Papules over the MCP, DIP, and/or PIP joints (Gottron's papules). (**f**) Ulcerations of the folds on the palmar aspects of the fingers, "inverse Gottron's sign," can be seen in patients with anti-MDA dermatomyositis, which is frequently amyopathic but can severely affect the lungs.

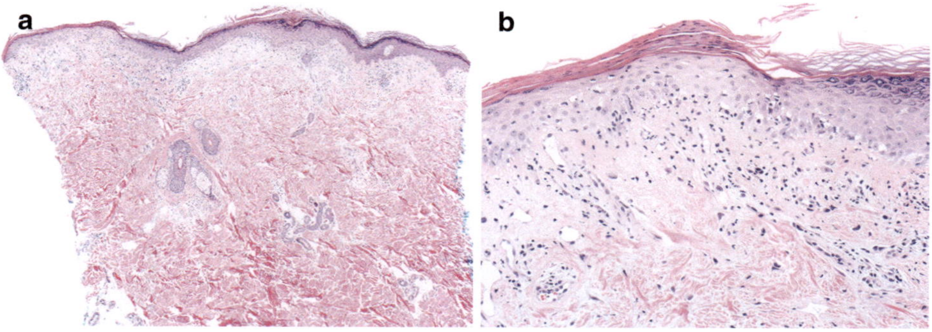

Fig. 67.2 Dermatomyositis (*4X, 20X; H&E*): (**a**) Histopathology demonstrates changes at the dermal-epidermal junction and within the superficial dermis. (**b**) There is a subtle interface dermatitis with associated baso-vacuolar change. Features are overall subtle and slight increase in dermal mucin also can be seen.

Lupus

68

Pooja Chitgopeker

Overview

- Lupus represents a heterogeneous group of diseases which range from skin-only autoimmune processes to widespread systemic disease
- The classic form is systemic lupus erythematous (SLE), an autoimmune systemic disease with protean clinical manifestations related to potentially extensive, varied multiorgan involvement
  - Associated symptoms are most commonly related to manifestations in the skin/mucous membranes (highly variable including malar rash, alopecia, discoid lesions and oral/nasal ulcers), joints (arthritis and arthrlagias), vasculature (Raynaud's phenomenon, vasculopathies including APLAs and vasculitis) and kidneys (commonly glomerulonephritis), with rare pulmonary, cardiac, or central nervous involvement
  - Diagnosis based on ACR classification system requires at least four of the following criteria:
    - Malar rash, photosensitivity, discoid rash, oral ulcers, arthritis, serositis, renal disease, neurologic disease, hematologic abnormalities, ANA, immunologic disorders as evidenced by anti-DNA/anti-SM/evidence APLAs
  - A newer classification system, the systemic lupus international collaborating clinics (SLICC) classification system, uses 17 criteria, requiring four criteria including one clinical and one immunologic criteria
- Cutaneous lupus is broadly divided into three different categories:
  - Acute cutaneous lupus erythematosus (ACLE): the classic malar erythema, typically associated with systemic disease; skin inflammation tends to be superficially restricted (epidermis/superficial dermis)
  - Subacute cutaneous lupus erythematosus (SCLE): two main types—psoriasiform and annular, both are photodistributed, with characteristic anti-Ro/ssA antibodies, and frequently drug-induced; minority of patients will have systemic involvement though may meet ACR criteria for SLE; superficially restricted disease (epidermis/superficial dermis)
  - Chronic cutaneous lupus erythematosus (CCLE) that is further subdivided to encompass:
    - Discoid lupus (DLE): 5–25% with systemic involvement, classic dyspigmented, atrophic/scarring, scaling photodistributed lesions; superficial and deep involvement and variable adnexal involvement with a propensity to scar
    - Lupus profoundus: rare deep plaques/nodules with possible overlying discoid lesions; subcutaneous involvement causing a potentially disfiguring panniculitis

P. Chitgopeker, MD
University of Iowa, Iowa City, IA, USA
e-mail: pooja-chitgopeker@uiowa.edu

M. Rosenbach et al. (eds.), *Inpatient Dermatology*,
https://doi.org/10.1007/978-3-319-18449-4_68

Chilblain lupus: painful red to purple papules/plaques often on fingers and toes associated with coldness; dermal involvement

Lupus tumidus: Indurated urticarial-like plaques; dermal involvement typically with epidermal and adnexal sparing

  - Bullous lupus: rare vesiculobullous eruption which results from autoantibodies to type VII collagen primarily in young women of African descent in their 20–40s; patients usually have overt systemic lupus and also discoid lesions

- Patients with connective tissue diseases may have overlap syndromes with other diseases, and often have elevated rates of other autoimmune diseases in general

Clinical Presentation

- ACLE is frequently associated with active systemic disease (Fig. 68.1a, b)
  - Classic lupus malar erythema (butterfly rash): typically a transient, sun-exacerbated, non-scarring rash, tends to strikingly spare the nasolabial creases
  - Most patients will exhibit some degree of photosensitivity
- SCLE is strikingly photodistributed and localized to sun exposed skin including upper trunk, the upper V of the back, and extensor aspects of the upper extremities (Fig. 68.1c)
  - Annular variant: annular scaly erythematous plaques with slightly raised red borders and central clearing that produce a polycyclic array
  - Papulosquamous variant is also seen, and can look psoriasiform
  - Lesions often do not scar
  - Drug induced SCLE is quite common and can be seen secondary to hydrochlorothiazide, proton pump inhibitors, terbinafine, tumor necrosis factor alpha inhibitors, and a long and growing list of agents
- CCLE: DLE is the most common skin manifestation of lupus (Fig. 68.1d, e)
  - Lesions are found either localized to the face, scalp, and ears or generalized occurring above and below the neck involving extensor forearms and hands

    Patients with localized, limited disease on the head are less likely to have systemic involvement

    Generalized DLE is rare but can be challenging to treat and often patients have systemic internal organ involvement in these casese
  - Well demarcated, scaly, erythematous macules or papules which develop into indurated discoid plaques that extend into the hair follicle resulting in scarring alopecia and follicular plugging
  - Lesions eventually become atrophic and scarred with variable dyspigmentation
- CCLE: Lupus profundus is a form of lupus affecting the fat, causing a panniculitis which presents as painful firm subcutaneous nodules (often with with overlying DLE) in areas with increased fat deposition such as upper arms, legs, face and breasts; these can also appear as atrophic "dells" (Fig. 68.1g)
- CCLE: Chilblains lupus presents as painful violaceous papules, plaques, and nodules in cold exposed areas such toes and fingers, but also occasionally on the nose, elbows, knees and lower legs; can resemble frostbite
- CCLE: Tumid lupus presents with erythematous, indurated, "juicy" urticarial-like plaques without scale or follicular plugging; lesions resolve without scarring (Fig. 68.1f)
- Bullous lupus presents acutely with tense subepidermal vesicles and bullae with clear or hemorrhagic contents that occur over normal skin or inflamed skin (often occurring on sites of involvement of cutaneous lupus, such as discoid lupus lesions) (Fig. 68.3)
- Non-specific cutaneous findings can be present that occur in other autoimmune connective tissue diseases: Raynaud's phenomenon, nailfold telangectasias and erythema, vasculitis, diffuse non-scarring alopecia, livedoid vasculopathy, palmar erythema

Histopathology

- Biopsy of new lesions are most helpful
- Histological findings depend on the subtype but there is overlap in histology in ACLE, SCLE and DLE including interface dermatitis with vacuolar degeneration, lymphohistiocytic inflammatory infiltrate (both superficial and deep), frequently with mucin deposition (Fig. 68.2)
- ACLE: Dermal changes can be subtle but vacuolar degeneration can be pronounced

- SCLE: Interface dermatitis with vacuolar change and variable keratinocyte apoptosis and associated epidermal atrophy with dermal edema and mucin
- DLE: Superficial and deep inflammatory infiltrate with periadnexal inflammation, superficial interface dermatitis with vacuolar change with scattered apoptotic keratinocytes, there is prominent hyperkeratosis, follicular plugging and scarring with a thickened basement membrane and an atrophic basal layer in established lesions
- Lupus profundus: often with deep inflammation in the fat with rims of lymphocytes around some of the adipocytes and hyalinization of the fat lobules
- Tumid lupus: Prominent mucin deposition with a variable inflammatory infiltrate typically with epidermal sparing
- Bullous lupus: Subepidermal blistering with dermal edema and perivascular inflammation in the superficial and mid dermis with a predominance of neutrophils in the upper dermis with microabscesses within dermal papillae and large deposits of mucin are commonly found in the reticular dermis consistent with underlying SLE (Fig. 68.4)
  - Direct immunofluorescence demonstrates IgG ± IgM, IgA, and complement (c3) in a linear or granular pattern at the basement membrane zone
  - Salt split skin shows immune reactant deposition along the dermal side where type VII collagen is found

Differential Diagnosis

Differential diagnosis varies with the subtype of CLE. As most are photodistributed, it is important to rule out a sun burn, photo-toxic drug reaction (by medication history and timing), UV-recall reaction (in the setting of chemotherapy), and chronic photodermatitis (such as patients with HIV or certain forms of chronic contact dermatitis).

- ACLE: the striking nasolabial sparing is often a helpful clue
  - Rosacea: telangiectasias, papules, and pustules may be a clue
  - Seborrheic dermatitis: greasy scale of the eyebrows, nasolabial creases, and scalp
  - Erysipelas: acute, painful, red, hot, and accompanied by fever
  - Dermatomyositis: often involves the nasolabial creases, but it is important to look for other skin signs of dermato and serologic/systemic involvement in lupus
- SCLE:
  - Psoriasis: can have substantial overlap, but SCLE is photoexposed and psoriasis is often helped by sun
  - Granuloma annulare: not usually as scaly or widespread, but biopsy may help
  - Tinea corporis: can be very similar, but KOH prep should demonstrate hyphae, or biopsy may distinguish
- DLE:
  - Lichen planus: can share similar clinical appearance; LP has less tendency to scar, and may show Wickham's striae, but can be challenging clinically and histologically
  - Lichen planopilaris: if the characteristic scarring alopecia with erythema and scale around adjacent follicles is present, it is helpful, but the two entities may have substantial clinical and histological overlap (fortunately, treatments overlap too)
  - Sarcoidosis: can have substantial clinical overlap as sarcoid can even involve the conchal bowl of the ear; biopsy should distinguish the two
  - Squamous cell carcinoma: some chronic forms of DLE, especially hypertrophic variants, are nearly impossible to distinguish from SCC, and SCC can develop at sites of longstanding DLE—biopsies should be performed to help differentiate
- Lupus profundus:
  - Subcutaneous panniculitic-like T-cell lymphoma: this is primarily a histological differential but it is important to try to exclude SPTCL when making a diagnosis of lupus profundus
- Bullous lupus (BLE):
  - Bullous pemphigoid: BP tends to be on the thighs with urticarial lesions, versus photodistributed with discoid lesions in BLE, but biopsy can differentiate (Figs. 68.3 and 68.4)
  - Epidermolysis Bullosa Acquisita: may be substantial overlap and similar antigenic target, and can be challenging to distinguish requiring clinical, pathological, and serological correlation

  - Linear IgA bullous dermatosis/Dermatitis herpetiformis: histologically all three of these show neutrophils at the dermal/epidermal junction, but the clinical presentation should be different enough to distinguish

Work-Up

- Skin biopsy can help establish diagnosis of cutaneous lupus
- Direct immunofluorescence (DIF) can be helpful in cases were histopathology is equivocal and in cases of bullous lupus
  - Immunoglobulins and complement are typically found at the dermal-epidermal junction and around hair follicles
  - Deposits are usually granular and contain IgG and IgM
  - Biopsies for DIF should be performed from sun protected, uninvolved skin ("lupus band test")—though this is rarely needed to confirm a diagnosis of lupus anymore
- CBC to evaluate for anemia, thrombocytopenia, leukopenia, and BMP to screen for renal disease
- Antibody testing:
  - ANA screen—typically positive in most patients. SLE with negative results can be seen in patients with CLE with or without systemic involvement; the very rare "ANA-negative" lupus is less common in the modern age of more advanced testing; if lupus is suspected and ANA is negative, often Ro or La antibodies are present
  - Other antibodies specific for SLE: anti dsDNA, anti Smith, ribosomal P
  - Antiphospholipid antibodies if there is a history of clotting or pregnancy loss,
  - Other serologies are often sent to diagnose or exclude overlap syndromes, inflammatory arthritis, or mixed connective tissue disease; these are often performed and interpreted in conjunction with a rheumatologist
- Complement levels (C3, C4) are important and may be low during lupus flares
- A thorough medication history is essential, particularly in cases of SCLE

Treatment

- Strict sun protection with broad-spectrum sunscreen, hats, sun protective clothing, and sun avoidance is essential in all cases of lupus
- Patients with systemic lupus should be managed in conjunction with a rheumatologist
- Skin involvement can be managed in a variety of ways:
  - Topical or intralesional corticosteroids are the mainstay of treatment for limited lesions; topical calcineurin inhibitors also can be utilized
  - Antimalarials are considered first line systemic treatment for skin lupus, and may reduce or delay progression from skin lupus to systemic involvement in some cases
  - Second line treatments include methotrexate, thalidomide, dapsone and mycophenolate mofetil
  - If cutaneous bullous lupus predominates, it responds well to dapsone (Check G6PD levels prior to dosing dapsone), though sometimes rituximab may be necessary

Suggested Readings

1. Okon L, Werth V. Cutaneous lupus erythematosus: diagnosis and treatment. Best Pract Res Clin Rheumatol. 2013;27(3):391–404.
2. Parodi A, Cozzani E. Cutaneous manifestations of lupus erythematosus. G Ital Dermatol Venereol. 2014;149(5):549–54. Epub 2014 Jul 31.
3. Contestable J, Edhegard K, Meyerle J. Bullous systemic lupus erythematous: a review and update to diagnosis and treatment. Am J Clin Dermatol. 2014;15(6):517–24.
4. Grover C, Khurana A, Singal A. Bullous systemic lupus erythematous. Indian J Dermatol. 2013;58(6):492.
5. Petri M, Orbai AM, Alarcon GS, et al. Derivation and validation of systemic lupus international collaborating clinics classification criteria for systemic lupus erythematosus. Arthritis Rheum. 2012;64:2677–86.

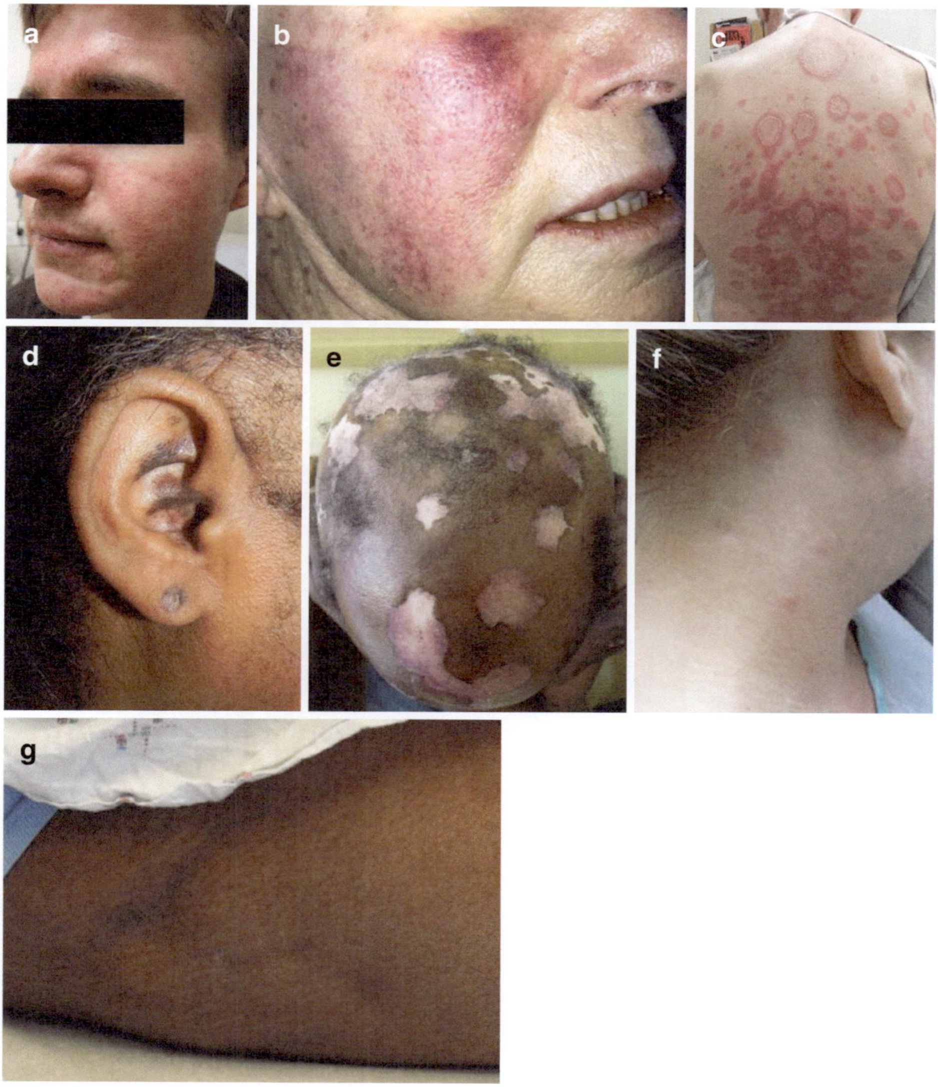

Fig. 68.1 Lupus: (**a**, **b**) Malar rash with sparing of the melolabial folds a male patient (**a**) and female (**b**) with acute cutaneous lupus. Patient b was profoundly thrombocytopenic and may have bled into her rash, leading to the brighter red/purple color. (**c**) Erythematous annular and polycyclic scaling plaques on the upper body in a patient with subacute cutaneous lupus (SCLE). (**d**) Atrophic and hyperpigmented scarring of the ear and conchal bowl typical of discoid lupus erythematosus (DLE). (**e**) Extensive pink-purple active inflammation in areas of atrophic scarring and dyspigmentation in a patient with extensive scalp chronic cutaneous lupus (DLE). (**f**) Indurated pink papules due to deep inflammation and extensive mucin deposition in a patient with tumid lupus. (**g**) Delling of the skin in high fat areas can result from lupus panniculits; sometimes discoid lupus lesions are present overlying the panniculitis.

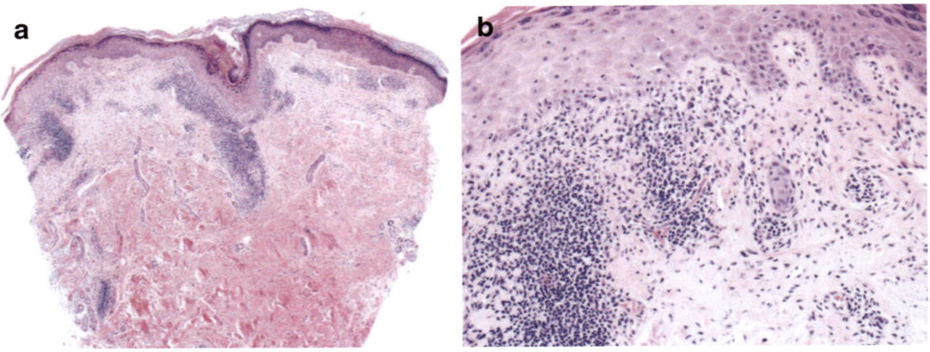

Fig. 68.2 SLE (*2X, 20X, H&E*): (**a**) On low power, there is a superficial interface dermatitis with a superficial and deep perifollicular and pereccrine lymphoplasmacytic infiltrate with follicular plugging. (**b**) The lymphoplasmacytic infiltrate predominates along the dermal-epidermal junction resulting in basovacuolar change at with dyskeratotic cells. Increased dermal mucin also is seen as blue discoloration in the dermis. Basement membrane thickening also can be observed (not shown here).

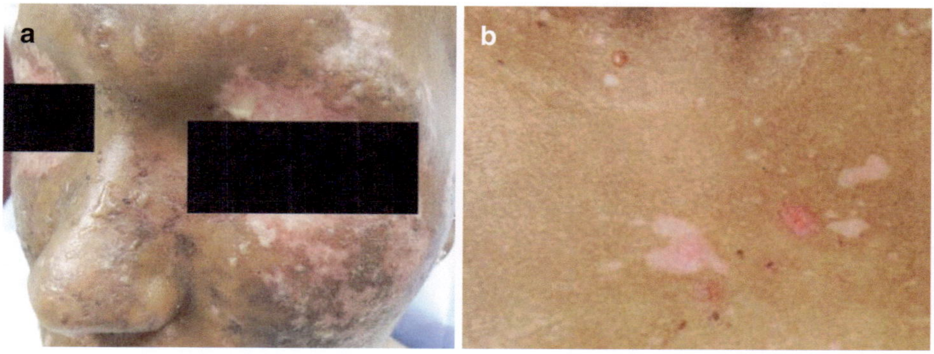

Fig. 68.3 (**a**) Bulla may develop overlying areas of discoid lupus lesions, or de novo on otherwise uninvolved skin. Tense bullae on sun-exposed areas of the face in a patient who also has atrophic and dyspigmented scarring from coexisting discoid lupus erythematosus. (**b**) The chest of a patient with more mild bullous lupus, demonstrating dyspigmentation and scarring of discoid lupus and scattered small bullae from the bullous component.

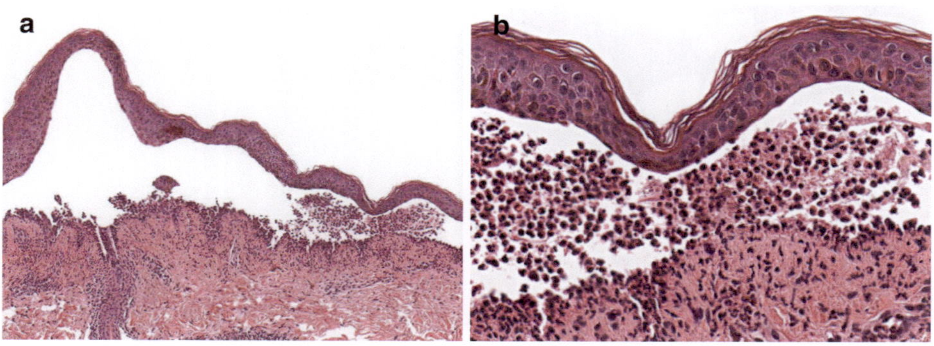

Fig. 68.4 Bullous lupus erythematous (*5X, 20X; H&E*): (**a**) There is a subepidermal bullae with associated papillary dermal edema and abundant neutrophils. (**b**) Neutrophils are located in perivascular, interstitial and intravesicular regions. Although difficult to appreciate in this biopsy, one should assess for interstitial mucin. DIF will demonstrate IgG and complement with variable IgM and IgA in a linear or granular bandlike pattern at the dermal-epidermal junction (not shown).

Bullous Pemphigoid

69

Aileen Y. Chang

Overview

- Bullous pemphigoid (BP) is a chronic autoimmune blistering disease more commonly seen in the elderly.
- Due to autoantibodies targeting components of hemidesmosomes which assist in epidermal-stromal adhesion at the basement membrane zone, resulting in sub-epidermal separation of the entire epidermia and tense bullae clinically
  - Target antigens include:
    BP180, an anchoring filament which associates the hemidesmosome with the lamina densa
    BP230, an intracellular protein that connects the intermediate filaments with the hemidesmosome
- Drug-induced BP occurs rarely, either presenting as an acute, self-limited illness that resolves with removal of the drug or as a chronic illness that behaves as the spontaneous form of the disease
  - Offending agents include furosemide, penicillamine, penicillin, sulfasalzine, captopril, and PD-1 inhibitors

Clinical Presentation

- Presents as a widespread pruritic urticarial plaques with tense, intact blisters commonly involving the thighs and flexural areas, with oral involvement present in up to one-third of cases (Fig. 69.1)
  - Patients may have a non-bullous prodromal phase with nonspecific pruritic eczema and urticarial-like plaques prior to the development of blistering disease
- Ruptured bullae result in areas of denudation which typically remain fixed in size and resolve without scarring
  - Cicatricial pemphigoid (benign mucosal pemphigoid): Lesions tend to be limited to the mucosa, most commonly the oral and conjunctiva, with vesicles which quickly rupture resulting in erosions, ulcers and scarring; approximately one quarter of patients will have associated skin findings
    Notably some patients with cicatricial pemphigoid have antibodies against laminin 3-3-2/epiligrin, which may be a marker for increased risk of internal malignancy
  - Pemphigoid gestationis: Pregnant women, often later in pregnancy or even after delivery, develop bullous lesions typically of the trunk and extremities. The fetus is generally not affected by the disorder, which usually spontaneously resolves but may need treatment, and may recur especially with subsequent pregnancies or OCP use

A. Y. Chang, MD
Department of Dermatology, University of California, San Francisco, CA, USA
e-mail: aileen.chang@ucsf.edu

M. Rosenbach et al. (eds.), *Inpatient Dermatology*,
https://doi.org/10.1007/978-3-319-18449-4_69

Histopathology

- Eosinophil-rich subepidermal blister with an underlying superficial inflammatory infiltrate containing lymphocytes, histiocytes, and eosinophils (Fig. 69.2)
- Direct immunofluorescence will reveal linear IgG and/or C3 at the basement membrane zone; salt split skin may allow for more specific visualization of fluorescence on the epidermal side or "roof" of the blister

Differential Diagnosis

- Epidermolysis bullosa acquisita (EBA): also presents with tense bullae, but may have more scarring or milia formation; salt split skin and ELISA testing can help distinguish
- Linear IgA bullous dermatosis: the tense bullae of LABD are often grouped in clusters, with neutrophils on histology, and a distinct immunofluorescence pattern
- Pemphigus vulgaris: the bullae are more flaccid, and the mucosa are generally more severely affected; histology and immunofluorescence are distinct
- Dermatitis herpetiformis: severe pruritis resultant erosions mean bullae are rarely seen, and the lesions tend to be clustered on the knees/elbows/buttocks; histology can distinguish

Important Work-Up

- Patients' medication history should be carefully reviewed for potential triggering agents, which should be stopped if suspected
- Usually two biopsies are performed: one is for routine staining and is taken on the edge of an intact bulla or simply shaving off an entire small blister, the other is for direct immunofluorescence (DIF) and is taken from normal skin near the involved area and placed in Michel's fixative
- Salt split skin studies can help differentiate BP from EBA, and will show IgG and/or C3 bound to the epidermal side of the split/blister's roof in BP and the dermal side/blisters base in EBA
- Enzyme-linked immunosorbent assay (ELISA) for BP180 and BP230 to assess for circulating antibodies in the patient's serum
- Patients should get routine blood work; CBC may display a peripheral eosinophilia, but labs are more important to monitor for medication-related adverse events or comorbidities

Treatment

- Topical clobetasol is effective for moderate to severe BP; topical application may be difficult for the elderly without assistance.
- Most hospitalized patients have severe disease and usually receive oral or IV therapy.
- Prednisone is utilized as a first-line agent to achieve rapid disease control, with transition to steroid-sparing agents for long-term therapy
  - Goal is to achieve lowest maintenance dose to prevent new blister formation
- Steroid-sparing agents include:
  - Azathioprine, mycophenolate, methotrexate, and cyclophosphamide; rituximab or IVIG may be helpful in some cases, and there is emerging data for the use of omalizumab in select patients; plasmapheresis is rarely used
  - Monotherapy with these agents can occasionally control disease
  - Tetracycline antiobiotics with or without niacinamide, dapsone, and topical steroids can control some patients; the BLISTER trial demonstrated that doxycyline is an effective monotherapy

Suggested Readings

1. Joly P, Roujeau JC, Benichou J, et al. A comparison of oral and topical corticosteroids in patients with bullous pemphigoid. N Engl J Med. 2002;346(5):321.
2. Stavropoulos PG, Soura E, Antoniou C. Drug-induced pemphigoid: a review of the literature. J Eur Acad Dermatol Venereol. 2014;28(9):1133–40.
3. Ruocco E, Wolf R, Caccavale S, Brancaccio G, Ruocco V, Lo Schiavo A. Bullous pemphigoid: associations and management guidelines: facts and controversies. Clin Dermatol. 2013;31(4):400–12.
4. Lo Schiavo A, Ruocco E, Brancaccio G, Caccavale S, Ruocco V, Wolf R. Bullous pemphigoid: etiology, pathogensis, and inducing factors: facts and controversie. Clin Dermatol. 2013;31(4):391–9.

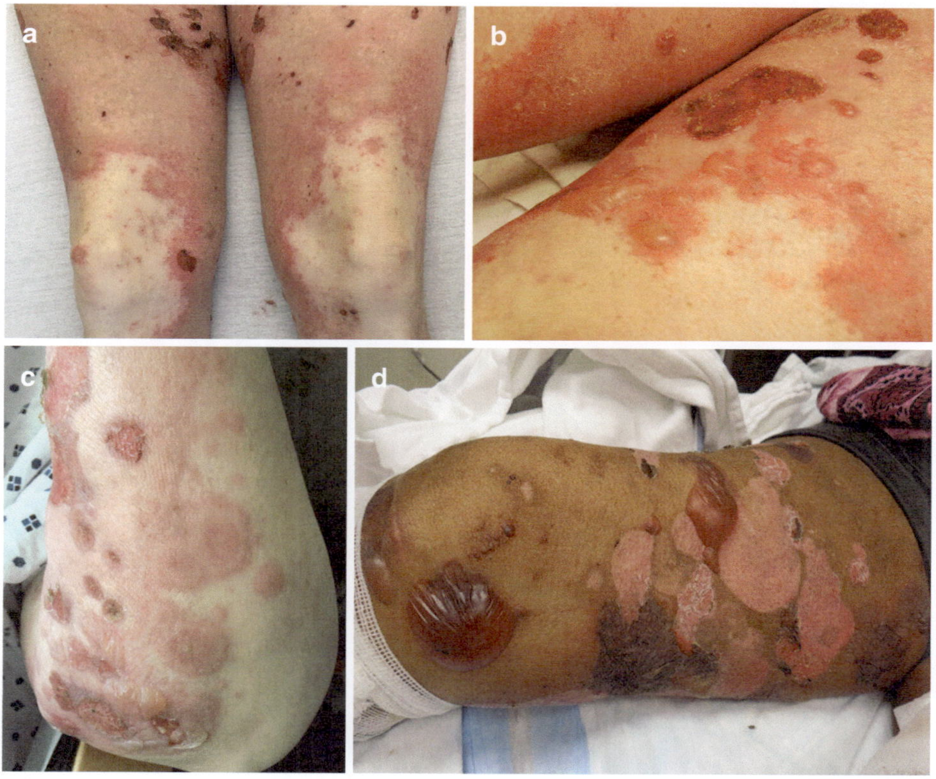

Fig. 69.1 Bullous pemphigoid: (**a**) Urticarial plaques (seen at the distal edge of the eruption here) with tense intact bullae are often seen first on the thighs in older patients. (**b**) This closeup demonstrated the underlying urticarial plaques with superimposed tense bullae. (**c**) In early disease urticarial plaques may predominate, but tense blisters on the urticarial lesions as seen here is characteristic. (**d**) Large bullae may become hemorrhagic, and can rupture leading to areas of denuded skin.

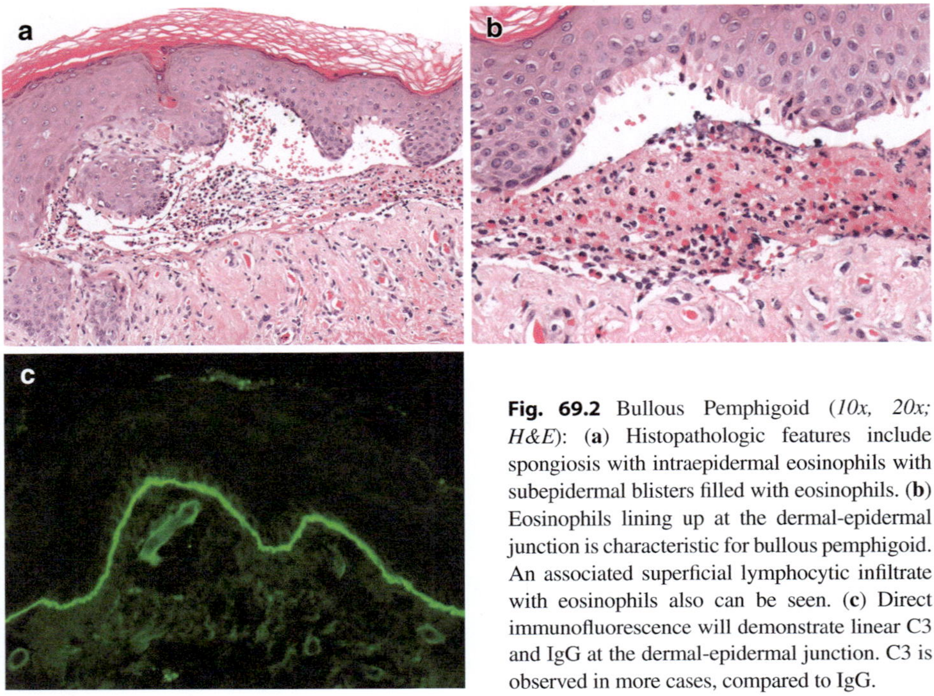

Fig. 69.2 Bullous Pemphigoid (*10x, 20x; H&E*): (**a**) Histopathologic features include spongiosis with intraepidermal eosinophils with subepidermal blisters filled with eosinophils. (**b**) Eosinophils lining up at the dermal-epidermal junction is characteristic for bullous pemphigoid. An associated superficial lymphocytic infiltrate with eosinophils also can be seen. (**c**) Direct immunofluorescence will demonstrate linear C3 and IgG at the dermal-epidermal junction. C3 is observed in more cases, compared to IgG.

Pemphigus Foliaceus

70

Aileen Y. Chang

Overview

- Pemphigus foliaceus (PF) is a rare, autoimmune blistering disease with autoantibodies (IgG) to desmoglein1 (Dsg1), a component of desmosomes involved in keratinocyte adhesion
  - Dsg1 is concentrated in the superficial component of the epidermis, causing patients to develop flaccid skin bullae with superficial intraepidermal splitting.
    - Dsg1 is the same target as seen in bullous impetigo/staphylococcal scalded skin
    - Dsg3 predominates in deeper layers of the epidermis and throughout the mucosa; anti-Dsg3 autoantibodes are associated with pemphigus vulgaris (PV: anti-Dsg3: mucosal lesions; anti-Dsg1 and 3: mucocutaneous disease). In PF, there is sufficient Dsg3 throughout the mucosal surfaces to compensate for the loss of Dsg1 adhesion from the pathogenic autoantibodies, thus PF does not affect the mucosa.
  - Drug induced pemphigus and paraneoplastic pemphigus also involve Dsg1/3; paraneoplastic pemphigus tends to have multiple and variable additional targets (including plakins), while IgA pemphigus may also target desmocollins
    - Drug induced pemphigus is most commonly caused by penicillamine or other thiol (SH) compounds, including captopril. Medications rarely induce pemphigus, but drug-induced PF is more common than drug-induced PV.
    - Paraneoplastic pemphigus is most commonly associated with non-Hodgkin's lymphoma and chronic lymphocytic leukemia and is characterized by an severe erosive-ulcerative stomasitis often with oropharynx and lip involvement in addition to palm/sole erythema multiforme-like involvement

A. Y. Chang, MD
Department of Dermatology, University of California, San Francisco, CA, USA
e-mail: aileen.chang@ucsf.edu

M. Rosenbach et al. (eds.), *Inpatient Dermatology*,
https://doi.org/10.1007/978-3-319-18449-4_70

Clinical Presentation

- PF results in small, superficial blisters which are not usually seen at presentation as they are transient and easily ruptured; instead, scaly erythematous eroded lesions with adherent crusts predominate, favoring the face, scalp, chest, and back are typical (Fig. 70.1)
  - Nikolsky sign (horizontal, tangential pressure to the mucosa and/or skin leads to skin separation) may be positive and lesions may be associated with pain or burning
  - Erosions are more shallow than the deep denudation seen in PV
  - Characteristically, mucosal involvement is absent

Histopathology

- Superficial erosions are most commonly seen, with splitting in the superficial component of the epidermis, often at the granular layer (Fig. 70.2)
- Histologically indistinguishable from staphylococcal scalded skin syndrome and bullous impetigo (may see gram positive cocci in the latter but this is not definitive as PF is also prone to secondary skin infection)

Differential Diagnosis

- Bullous impetigo/staphylococcal scalded skin syndrome: clinically and histologically nearly identical; cultures, DIF, and ELISA testing can distinguish
- Pemphigus vulgaris: involves the mucosa, which is spared in PF; pathology, DIF and ELISA can further distinguish
- Linear IgA bullous dermatosis: ringed clusters of tense bullae are seen, with distinctive pathology/immunofluoresence
- Seborrheic dermatitis: PF may favor the face/chest, but is generally more raw and eroded than typical seborrheic dermatitis; biopsies can be diagnostics

Important Work-Up

- Biopsy is required and usually two biopsies are done:
  - One is taken from an early, small vesicle or from the edge of a new erosion for routine processing
  - The other is for direct immunofluorescence (DIF) and is taken from perilesional uninvolved skin and placed in Michel's fixative or saline (not formalin)
- Enzyme-linked immunosorbent assay (ELISA): Patients with pemphigus foliaceus will have antibodies against Dsg1

Treatment

- Treatment is generally less aggressive than in PV, as overall morbidity and mortality are lower in PF
- Topical steroids may be adequate in mild cases, in more severe cases oral prednisone is used
- Steroid-sparing agents, such as dapsone, azathioprine or mycophenolate may be beneficial
- If drug-induced, the offending medication should be identified and removed immediately
- Patients may have superinfection with concurrent *Staphylococcus aureus* or herpes simplex virus, which should be identified and eradicated if present

Suggested Readings

1. Martin LK, Werth VP, Villaneuva EV, et al. A systematic review of randomized controlled trials for pemphigus vulgaris and pemphigus foliaceus. J Am Acad Dermatol. 2011;64(5):903.
2. Stern RS, Shear NH. Cutaneous reactions to drugs and biological modifiers. In: Arndt KA, LeBoit PE, Robinson JK, Wintroub BU, editors. Cutaneous medicine and surgery, vol. 1. Philadelphia: W.B. Saunders; 1996. p. 412.

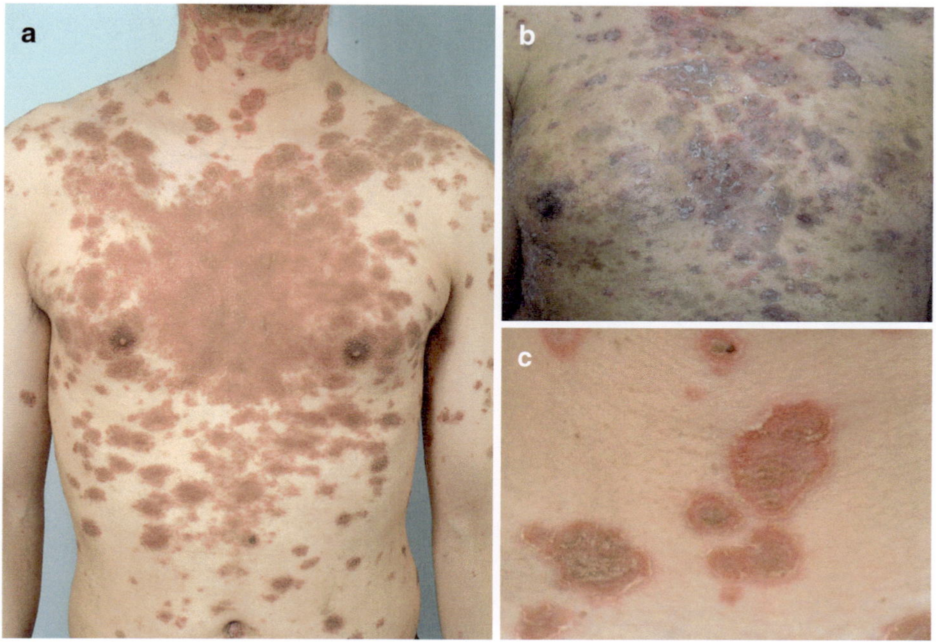

Fig. 70.1 Pemphigus foliaceous: (**a**) There are widespread very superficial erosions with incredibly fragile bullae which often rupture spontaneously, leaving an adherent patch of denuded epidermis which can resemble "cornflakes," or brawny scale. (**b**) Pemphigus is common in patients of Indian/Asian ancestry, and may look "dusky" on a background of darker skin. (**c**) Close up of PF with superficial blistering leaving raw erosions, which can be mistaken for pemphigus vulgaris.

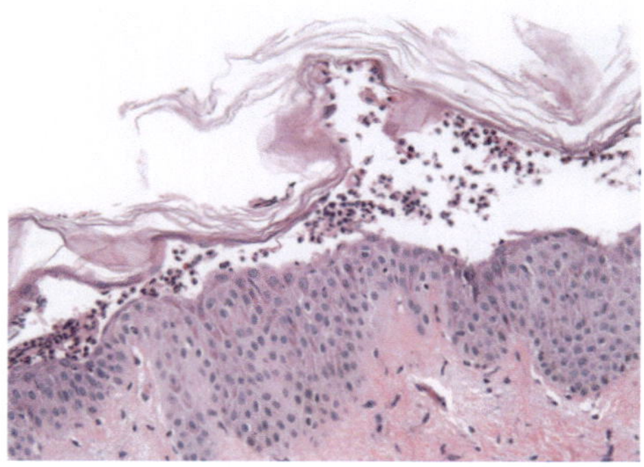

Fig. 70.2 Pemphigus foliaceous (*10x; H&E*): Histopathology demonstrates spongiosis with intraepidermal acantholysis and separation superficially within the granular layer. Neutrophils and eosinophils often are observed within the epidermis. Within the dermis, there is a superficial lymphocytic infiltrate with scattered eosinophils. DIF demonstrates intercellular IgG and C3 within the superficial layers of the epidermis.

Pemphigus Vulgaris

71

Aileen Y. Chang

Overview

- Pemphigus Vulgaris (PV) is a rare, autoimmune blistering disease with autoantibodies to desmoglein 3 (Dsg3) and variably to desmoglein 1 (Dsg1), which are components of desmosomes involved in cell-cell adhesion of keratinocytes in the epidermis
  - Dsg1 is more expressed in the superficial component of the epidermis, whereas Dsg3 is expressed throughout the epidermis, though with more expression towards the base
  - Antibodies against Dsg1 cause a superficial split, as Dsg3 compensates for the loss of Dsg1-related adhesion towards the base of the epidermis (as seen in pemphigus foliaceous). Antibodies against Dsg3 cause a blister at the supra-basal layer, just above the basal keratinocytes, which remain bound to the dermis by the hemidesmosomes, as there is no Dsg1 towards the base to compensate (as seen in pemphigus vulgaris)
  - Dsg3 predominates in the mucosa, so patients with isolated anti-Dsg3 autoantibodes develop mucosal PV; it is thought that the retention of unaffected Dsg1 in the non-mucosal skin helps compensate for the loss of Dsg3 and prevents skin involvement
  - Many patients with PV have antibodies against both Dsg1 and Dsg3 and get severe mucosal as well as variable cutaneous bullae and erosions
  - Drug induced pemphigus and paraneoplastic pemphigus also involve Dsg1/3; paraneoplastic pemphigus tends to have variable additional targets (including plakins) while IgA pemphigus may also target desmocollins
    - Drug induced pemphigus is most commonly associated with penicillamine or other thiol (SH) compounds, including captopril, and may induce PF more commonly than PV
    - Paraneoplastic pemphigus is most commonly associated with non-Hodgkin's lymphoma and chronic lymphocytic leukemia and is characterized by a severe erosive-ulcerative stomasitis often with oropharynx and lip involvement in addition to palm/sole erythema multiforme-like lesions

A. Y. Chang, MD
Department of Dermatology, University of California,
San Francisco, CA, USA
e-mail: aileen.chang@ucsf.edu

M. Rosenbach et al. (eds.), *Inpatient Dermatology*,
https://doi.org/10.1007/978-3-319-18449-4_71

Clinical Presentation

- Flaccid bullae which rupture readily and leave broad painful erosions, with raw, red eroded mucosal surfaces (Fig. 71.1)
- Often presents initially in the oropharynx, with a tendency to become more generalized and heal with post-inflammatory pigment alteration but not scarring
- The distribution of lesions will vary depending on whether the patient has mucosal (anti-Dsg3) or mucocutaneous (anti Dsg1 and 3) disease
- Mucosal lesions appear as bright red, raw erosions with a propensity to involve the buccal and palatine mucosa
  - Most patients will develop oral lesions, and conjunctiva is also a common site of involvement; larynx, esophagus, urethral, vulvovaginal and penile involvement can also occur
  - Lesional location will result in variable symptoms, for example, patients may develop dysphonia from larynx involvement and/or dysphagia secondary to esophageal lesions
- Flaccid bullae with clear fluid are more often visualized on cutaneous surfaces but due to their fragility tend to be infrequent and painful erosions predominate which often continue peripheral extension post-eruption
  - Nikolsky sign is positive
  - Eroded areas are prone to infection which a leading cause of morbidity and mortality

Histopathology

- If an intact blister is biopsied suprabasal epidermal acantholysis resulting in an intraepidermal blister with "tombstoning" of basal keratinocytes which remain fixed to the underlying dermis by their intact hemi-desmosomes (Fig. 71.2)
- DIF exhibits intercellular IgG deposition creating a net-like or "chicken wire" pattern

Differential Diagnosis

- Bullous pemphigoid: clinically has tense bullae and urticarial plaques, with less common/less intense mucosal involvement; pathology can distinguish the two
- Bullous lupus erythematosus: usually patients have other signs of lupus (malar rash, discoid lesions) and meet ACR criteria for lupus; histologically with neutrophils at the d/e junction
- Pemphigus foliaceus: should spare the mucosa, and pathology shows the separation higher in the epidermis, but ELISA can definitively distinguish
- Paraneoplastic pemphigus: can share substantial overlap; usually patients have severe hemorrhagic mucosal disease and multiple autoantibody targets, but clinicians should keep this entity in mind
- Stevens-Johnson syndrome: clinical lesions will often have a dusky nonblanching center and deep dark inflammation around areas of bullae, and pathology will show more epidermal necrosis
- Oral lichen planus: can closely mimic oral erosions of PV; if Wickham's striae are present can help clinically, but ELISA testing may be necessary to distinguish

Work-Up

- Biopsy is required and usually two biopsies are done:
  - One is taken from an early, small vesicle or from the edge of a new erosion for routine processing
  - The other is for direct immunofluorescence (DIF) and is taken from perilesional uninvolved skin and placed in Michel's fixative or saline
- Check serum Dsg1 and Dsg3 ELISA:
  - IgG anti-Dsg1: PF
  - IgG anti-Dsg 3: Mucosal restricted PV
  - IgG anti Dsg 1/3: Mucocutaneous PV
- If severe mucosal disease or treatment refractory, consider paraneoplastic pemphigus in association with lymphoproliferative disorders and appropriate associated work-up

Management

- Prednisone reduces antibody production and is the mainstay of initial therapy
- In severe cases or cases of extensive ocular disease, sometimes plasmapheresis and/or rituximab (or cyclophosphamide) should be considered
- Steroid-sparing agents, such as azathioprine or mycophenolate, should be initiated early to enable steroid taper and are indicated long-term; Dapsone has also been used
- Rituximab is increasingly used as first-line initial therapy due to potential for long-term remission and is indicated for refractory disease, with or without intravenous immunoglobulin (IVIG) or plasmapheresis
- Patients may have superinfection with concurrent *Staphylococcus aureus* or herpes simplex virus, which should be identified and eradicated if present
- Patients with ocular disease or genital disease should prompt consultation from the appropriate specialists
- Pain control and appropriate wound care with moist, non-adherent dressings to open erosions are essential

Suggested Readings

1. Martin LK, Werth VP, Villaneuva EV, et al. A systematic review of randomized controlled trials for pemphigus vulgaris and pemphigus foliaceus. J Am Acad Dermatol. 2011;64(5):903.
2. Ahmed AR, Shetty S. A comprehensive analysis of treatment outcomes in patients with pemphigus vulgaris treated with rituximab. Autoimmun Rev. 2015;14(4):323–31.

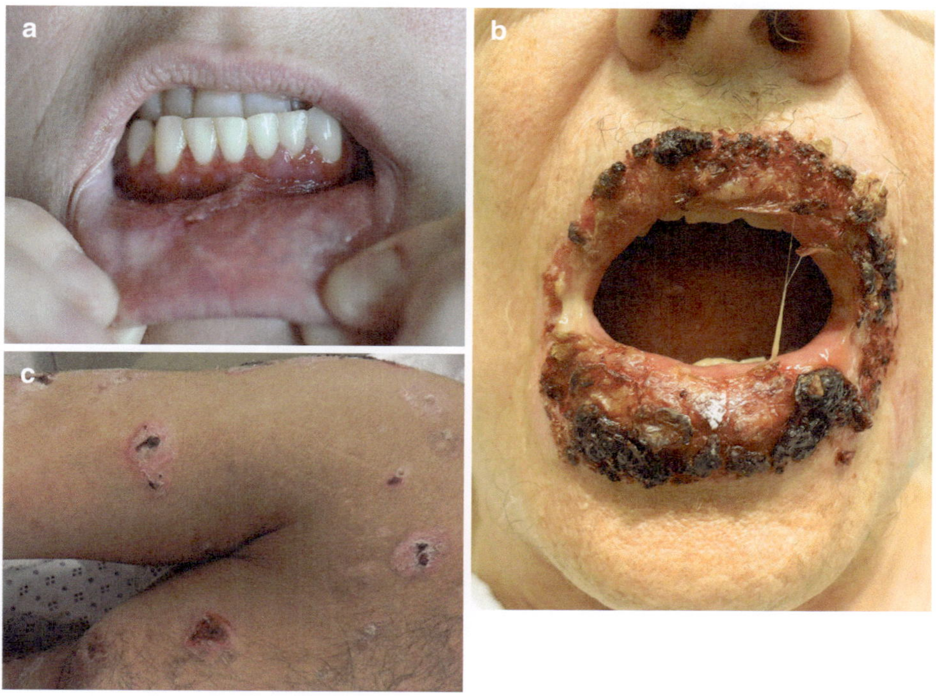

Fig. 71.1 Pemphigus vulgaris: (**a**) Painful gingival erosions. (**b**) Hemorrhagic crusted lips of pemphigus vulgaris. (**c**) Patients may also have cutaneous involvement, resulting in fragile bullae and erosions.

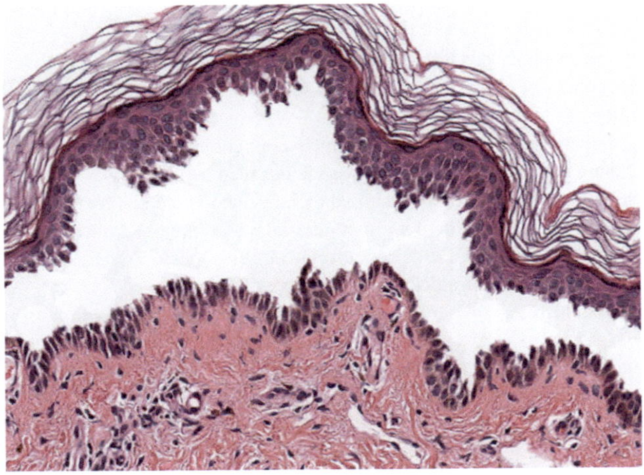

Fig. 71.2 Pemphigus vulgaris (*10×*; *H&E*): There is suprabasal acanthyolysis with intraepidermal bulla formation leaving a row of basal keratinocytes. Associated spongiosis and intraepidermal spongiosis with a superficial perivascular infiltrate composed of lymphocytes and eosinophils also can be seen. Direct immunofluorescence demonstrates a "net-like" pattern due to IgG/complement depoisition between keratinocytes in the deeper portion of the epidermis, where desmogelein 3 predominates.

Linear IgA Bullous Dermatosis 72

Aileen Y. Chang

Overview

- Linear IgA bullous dermatosis (LABD) is an acquired IgA autoimmune blistering disease characterized subepidermal tense bullae in an annular (or less commonly herpetiform or linear) arrangement
- LABD is due to circulating IgA antibodies that target the basement membrane zone, specifically 97 kDa antigen portion of bullous pemphigoid antigen 2 (BP180). An adult and childhood variant exist (chronic bullous disease of childhood-CBDC) of which the etiology is unknown
- Most commonly drug-induced in adults, the vast majority due to vancomycin, followed by penicillins, cephalosporins, other antibiotics, captopril and other ACE inhibitors, NSAIDs; rarely may be paraneoplastic or idiopathic
  - Chronic bullous disease of childhood (CBDC) is typically idiopathic and on average presents at age 5
- There are rare reported associations with gastrointestinal disease (inflammatory bowel diseases, gluten sensitive enteropathy/Celiac disease), autoimmune diseases, malignancies (including chronic lymphocytic leukemia/B-cell lymphomas and carcinomas of various origin) and infections (varicella zoster virus, upper respiratory infections)

Clinical Presentation

- Tense subepidermal bullae and vesicles arise abruptly and may develop in association with urticarial plaques (as can be seen in bullous pemphigoid) or arise on otherwise normal appearing skin; lesions may be pruritic (Fig. 72.1)
  - Patients may develop annular lesions with peripheral vesiculation referred to as having a "crown of jewel" or "string of pearl" configuration
  - Non-bullous morbilliform variant has been rarely described with vancomyocin use (but nearly all cases, including vancomycin-related, are bullous)
- Patients commonly have a distribution of disease with common involvement of the trunk and extremities (extensor surfaces), with perineal and perioral lesions more commonly seen in CBDC
- Mucous membrane involvement is seen in some adult cases with erosions/ulceration of oral and ocular mucosa

A. Y. Chang, MD
Department of Dermatology, University of California,
San Francisco, CA, USA
e-mail: aileen.chang@ucsf.edu

M. Rosenbach et al. (eds.), *Inpatient Dermatology*,
https://doi.org/10.1007/978-3-319-18449-4_72

Histopathology

- Subepidermal split with predominantly neutrophilic infiltrate; papillary microabscesses; may be seen (Fig. 72.2)
- Eosinophils may be present; more common in the drug-induced variant
- Histology is typically indistinguishable from dermatitis herpetiformis necessitating DIF
  - Characteristic direct immunofluorescence (DIF) with linear deposition of IgA along basement membrane zone (BMZ)

Differential Diagnosis

- Bullous pemphigoid: tense bullae and urticarial plaques, less often in the ringed/annular configuration seen in LABD, but histology, immunofluorescence, and ELISA can distinguish
- Bullous lupus erythematosus: usually seen in conjunction with more typical lupus morphologies (discoid, malar), with patients meeting ACR criteria for lupus; immunofluorescence can distinguish the two
- Dermatitis herpetiformis: generally smaller lesions and erosions rather than tense bullae, but immunofluorescence may be necessary to distinguish the two

Important Work-Up

- Detailed medication history to look for potential drug-induced etiology (particularly vancomycin)
- Biopsy of intact blister or blister edge for H&E; biopsy of perilesional uninvolved skin for DIF

Treatment

- If drug induced, the inciting medication must be identified and stopped
- Dapsone is often utilized as first-line therapy; response is usually seen within days
- In severe disease, systemic steroids may be necessary
  - Dapsone and steroid refractory patients: mycophenolate mofetil, azathioprine, IVIG
- Erythrodermic patients with widespread blistering may benefit from management similar to patients with SJS/TEN
- For limited disease: can try high-potency topical steroids and/or tetracycline class antibiotics with or without nicotinamide
- Although uncommon, cases associated with a gluten sensitive enteropathy may benefit from a modified gluten-free diet

Suggested Readings

1. Venning VA. Linear IgA disease: clinical presentation, diagnosis, and pathogenesis. Immunol Allergy Clin N Am. 2012;32(2):245–53.
2. Ng SY, Venning VV. Management of linear IgA disease. Dermatol Clin. 2011;29(4):629–30.

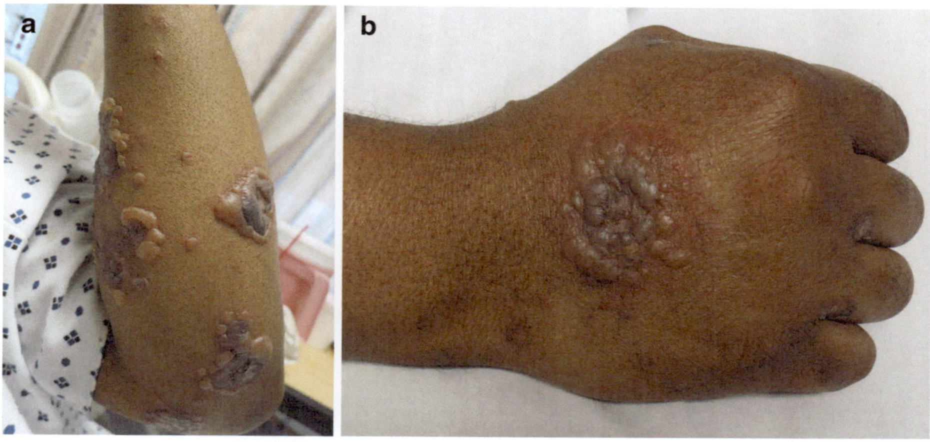

Fig. 72.1 Linear IgA bullous dermatosis: Tense bullae arranged in a typical "crown of jewels," or rosette pattern, on the arm (**a**) and hand (**b**) in a patient after vancomycin exposure.

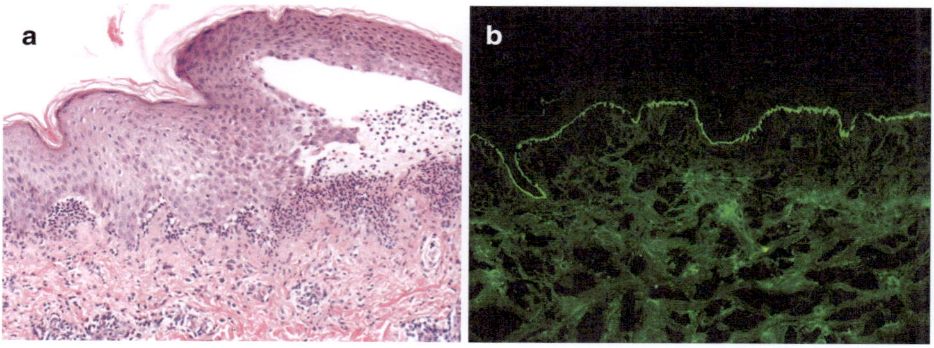

Fig. 72.2 Linear IgA (*10×; H&E, DIF*): (**a**) Histopathology demonstrates a subepidermal bullae with numerous neutrophils lining up along the dermal epidermal junction. (**b**) DIF demonstrates linear IgA along the dermal-epidermal junction.

Dermatitis Herpetiformis

73

Megan H. Noe

Overview

- Cutaneous autoimmune disease in patients with gluten sensitivity secondary to IgA autoantibodies targeting epidermal transglutaminase (TG3); patients classically present with pruritic, grouped papules and vesicles
  - Dermatitis herpetiformis (DH) and celiac disease are associated with HLA-B8, as well as DR3/DQw2
  - TG3 is produced by epidermal keratinocytes and diffuses into the papillary dermis where it locally complexes with circulating IgA anti-TG3; neutrophil chemotaxis and degranulation results in local damage and subepidermal blistering
- More than 90% of patients have evidence of gluten-sensitive enteropathy, however only 20% are symptomatic
  - Patients with DH may also be at higher risk for enteropathy-associated lymphoma
- Associated with autoimmune thyroid disease, specifically Hashimoto's thyroiditis

Clinical Presentation

- Patients present with severe pruritus, often resulting in extensive excoriations in place of primary lesions
- Erosions, excoriated pruritic papules and vesicles typically develop on extensor surfaces (elbows and knees) and buttocks; scalp pruritus also may occur (Fig. 73.1)
- Patients may exhibit symptoms of gluten sensitivity such as indigestion, bloating, increased flatulence and diarrhea related to diet

M. H. Noe, MD, MPH
Department of Dermatology, University of Pennsylvania, Philadelphia, PA, USA
e-mail: Megan.Noe@uphs.upenn.edu

M. Rosenbach et al. (eds.), *Inpatient Dermatology*,
https://doi.org/10.1007/978-3-319-18449-4_73

Histopathology

- Changes in early lesions are focused at the tip of the dermal papillae where edema and neutrophil microabscesses form; in more advanced/classic lesions neutrophils often fill the papillary dermis and are also present within subepidermal vesicles (Fig. 73.2)
- DIF shows granular deposition of IgA at the DEJ with increased concentration in the dermal papillae

Differential Diagnosis

- Other bullous dermatoses (linear IgA bullous dermatosis, bullous pemphigoid, bullous systemic lupus erythematosus): other blistering disorders will often present with visible clinical blisters, which are rare in DH due to the intense pruritus and scratching; histology and immunofluorescence can distinguish. Linear IgA, bullous lupus, and DH all show neutrophils at the dermal/epidermal junction and can be hard to distinguish with pathology alone
- Arthropod bites/bed bugs: may show visible punctum or grouped urticarial papules; biopsies tend to show eosinophils more than neutrophils; immunofluorescence can distinguish
- Scabies: high on the differential as intensely pruritic, but the pruritic lesions of DH are on the elbows/knees/buttocks, not the groin/nipples/axillae/web-spaces; scraping demonstrating mites, or characteristic biopsy can distinguish

Important Work-Up

- Skin biopsy for histopathology of a vesicle or eroded skin lesion
- Direct immunofluorescence of non-lesional normal skin (usually from the elbow)
- Serologic testing for gluten sensitivity including tissue transglutaminase
- GI evaluation with endoscopy for underlying Celiac disease and small bowel lymphoma
- Screening for symptoms of hypothyroidism with TSH, anti-TPO, anti-Tg if indicated

Treatment

- Gluten-free diet is essential even if the cutaneous disease and pruritus resolves with treatment, as patients are at increased risk of GI lymphoma with continued gluten exposure
- Dapsone is first line therapy
  - Baseline CBC, LFT, Cr are recommended
  - G6PD should be tested prior to initiation
  - Agranlocytosis and DRESS are rare but serious side effect that patients should be monitored for
  - Of note, dapsone may result in resolution of skin but not intestinal disease
- Patients intolerant to dapsone can be treated with sulfapyridine

Suggested Readings

1. Boltin D, Petronic-Rosic V. Dermatitis herpetiformis, part 1: epidermiology, pathogenesis and clinical presentation. J Am Acad Dermatol. 2011;64:1017–24.
2. Boltin D, Petronic-Rosic V. Dermatitis herpetiformis, part 2: diagnosis, management, and prognosis. J Am Acad Dermatol. 2011;64:1027–33.
3. Cardones AR, Hall RP III. Management of dermatitis herpetiformis. Dermatol Clin. 2011;29:631–5.

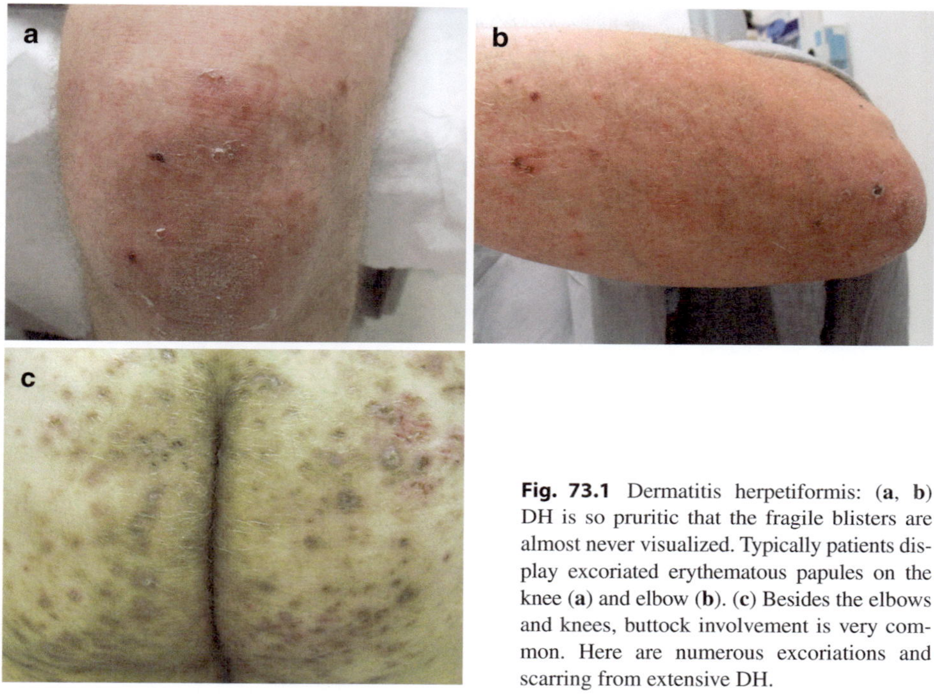

Fig. 73.1 Dermatitis herpetiformis: (**a**, **b**) DH is so pruritic that the fragile blisters are almost never visualized. Typically patients display excoriated erythematous papules on the knee (**a**) and elbow (**b**). (**c**) Besides the elbows and knees, buttock involvement is very common. Here are numerous excoriations and scarring from extensive DH.

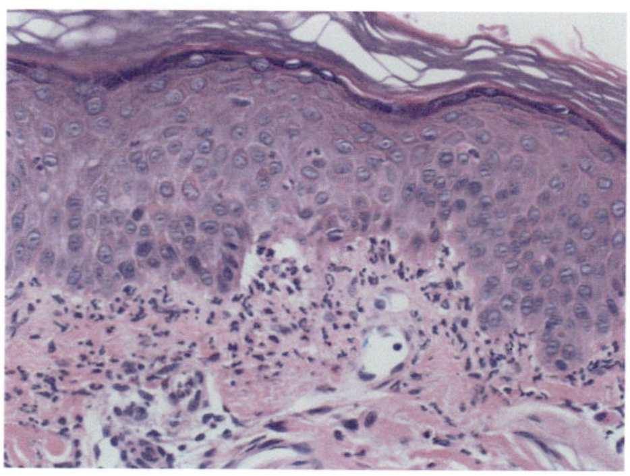

Fig. 73.2 Dermatitis herpetiformis *(40x; H&E; DIF)*. Histopathology demonstrates neutrophilic infiltrate at the dermal-epidermal junction with small separations and potential for larger subepidermal bullae formation. Neutrophilic collections (microabscesses) with within the papillary dermis are characteristic. Eosinophils and acantholysis also can observed. DIF would show granular IgA centered in dermal papillae.

Systemic Sclerosis 74

Lisa Pappas-Taffer

Overview

- Systemic Sclerosis (SSc) is an autoimmune disorder of unknown etiology that causes widespread microvascular damage and excessive collagen deposition
- Classified clinically based on the extent of sclerosis and affected organs; proper classification is important given differences in prognosis
  - Systemic sclerosis (SSc, scleroderma): subdivided into a limited and diffuse form based on extent of skin involvement; earlier and more severe manifestations of internal organ disease are commonly associated with dcSSc. Patients generally display distal symmetric sclerosis, plus sclerodactyly, digital scars, or loss of substance from finger pad "pulp"
    - Limited cutaneous systemic sclerosis (lcSSc): Fibrosis limited to fingers and hands and occasionally face and neck; component of the CREST syndrome: Calcinoisis, Raynaud phenomenon, Esophageal dysmotility, Sclerodactyly, Telangectasias
    - Diffuse cutaneous systemic sclerosis (dcSSc): More extensive fibrosis, including proximal extremities and trunk
- Systemic sclerosis sine scleroderma: internal organ involvement in the absence of cutaneous manifestations
- Extracutaneous involvement may include lung, kidney, heart, and gastrointestinal system
  - Pulmonary hypertension, interstitial lung disease, and renal crisis are the most frequent causes of mortality
  - Survival correlates best with clinical disease subtype (limited vs. diffuse disease, with diffuse disease having increased morbidity and mortality)
- Autoantibody serologies are not diagnostic but are typically positive in 1/3 patients

Clinical Presentation

- Patients have varying amount of firm bound-down skin; a full body skin exam palpating for firmness is required (Fig. 74.1)
  - Early lesions often start with edema, concentrated in the hands. The "puffy hands" stage may be subtle but is often the first sign and amenable to therapeutic intervention
  - Over time, skin becomes indurated stretched and shiny secondary to sclerosis

L. Pappas-Taffer, MD
University of Pennsylvania, Philadelphia, PA, USA
e-mail: lisa.pappas-taffer@uphs.upenn.edu

M. Rosenbach et al. (eds.), *Inpatient Dermatology*,
https://doi.org/10.1007/978-3-319-18449-4_74

- Raynaud phenomenon is present in all patients with systemic sclerosis, and is useful in differentiating from other conditions with sclerodermoid change
- Patients may develop gradual tightening and tapering of the fingers (sclerodactyly)
- Proximal nail fold erythema and/or capillary loop dilation or drop out on exam under magnification
- Additional findings may variably be present, including: healed pitted fingertip ulcerations; flexion contractures of the fingers, calcinosis fingers/extremities; reduced oral aperture; mucocutaneous square shaped ("mat-like") telangectatic macules on the hands, face/oral cavity, chest; hypopigmentation with perifollicular retention of pigment ("salt and pepper")

Histopathology

- A squared-off biopsy due to the sclerosis, demonstrating flattening of rete ridges, dense collagen deposition, fat trapping with loss of peri-adnexal fat and gradual replacement of sebaceous and sweat glands and hair follicles with layered collagen (Fig. 74.2)
- Early, a prominent inflammatory infiltrate at the dermal/subcutaneous junction
- Morphea, sclerodermoid chronic GVHD, and systemic sclerosis can have similar to identical histopathology

Differential Diagnosis

- Sclerodermoid conditions in the absence of Raynaud phenomenon
  - Generalized Morphea: extensive plaques of morphea can closely resemble scleroderma, but patients should not have Raynaud's in morphea
  - Eosinophilic fascitis: can closely mimic scleroderma but patients should not have Raynaud's; biopsy may be helpful if deep enough and with classic findings
  - Scleromyxedema: the range of cutaneous findings can include scleroderma-like changes, but biopsy should show more mucin and patients will often have a paraprotein
  - Scleredema: fixed firm edema usually of the upper back (due to strep, diabetes, paraprotein, or vibration/pressure), biopsy often shows more edema and less tight collagen; importantly the name alone can cause some confusion
  - Nephrogenic systemic fibrosis: shares substantial overlap, though some histological features (CD34+ fibrocytes) and history can help distinguish the two entities
  - Drug/toxin-induced syndromes (toxic oil syndrome from aniline-degraded rapseed oil, eosinophilic myalgia syndrome from contaminated L-tryptophan, polyvinylchloride, bleomycin, or silica exposure): clinically these entities can induce sclerosis and diagnosis is challenging, requiring a careful and thorough history
- Graft-versus-host disease: chronic scleroderma-like GVH is often indistinguishable from de novo scleroderma

Work-Up

- Skin biopsy can be helpful but is not always required
- Autoantibody serologies may be sent for prognosis coupled with limited vs. diffuse clinical classification, but all patients with scleroderma will undergo extensive evaluation for systemic involvement
  - ANA, anti-centromere B, anti-topoisomerase (SCL-70); If negative, may consider anti-RNA-polymerase I and III (anti-RNAP), anti-PM/SCL, and anti-Th/to
    - Discrete: speckled/centromeric ANA pattern relatively specific for lcSCC
    - Nucleolar: ANA pattern: not specific but associated with SSc

Anti-centromere B: more commonly present in lcSCC
SCL-70: more commonly associated with dsSCC and ILD
Anti-RNAP: dsSCC and increased risk of renal crisis

- Screening
  - Pulmonary: high resolution CT scan, pulmonary function testing with DLCO, cardiac echocardiogram
  - GI: consider swallow study or esophagogastroduadenoscopy if symptomatic
  - Renal: daily home blood pressure checks (if diffuse disease)

Treatment

- Consultation with appropriate subspecialties is crucial in these patients with therapy targeted at internal organ involvement; unfortunately, cutaneous treatment is suboptimal
  - Treatment for cutaneous involvement includes: mycophenolate mofetil, methotrexate, UVA-1, PUVA
  - Second-line treatments include: Cyclophosphamide, Imatinib, pulsed dye laser, D-penicillamine, minocycline
- Digital Vasculopathy/Raynaud phenomenon
  - Maintain core body temperature, smoking cessation, avoidance of cold, long-acting calcium channel blockers (nifedipine)
  - If severe, add oral phosphodiesterase-5 inhibitor (sidenafil); or consider IV iloprost 3–5 consecutive days
  - Others: botulinum toxin injections, angiotensin-II receptor blockers (e.g. losartan), prazosin, botulinim toxin, surgical digital sympathectomy

Suggested Readings

1. van den Hoogen F, et al. 2013 classification criteria for systemic sclerosis: an American College of Rheum/European League against Rheumatism collaborative initiative. Arthritis Rheumatol. 2013;65(11):2737–47.
2. Kowal-Bieleck O, Landewe R, Avoouac J, Shwiesko S, Miniati I, et al. EULAR recommendations for the treatment of systemic sclerosis: a report from the EULAR Scleroderma Trials and Research Group (EUSTAR). Ann Rheum Dis. 2009;68:620–8.

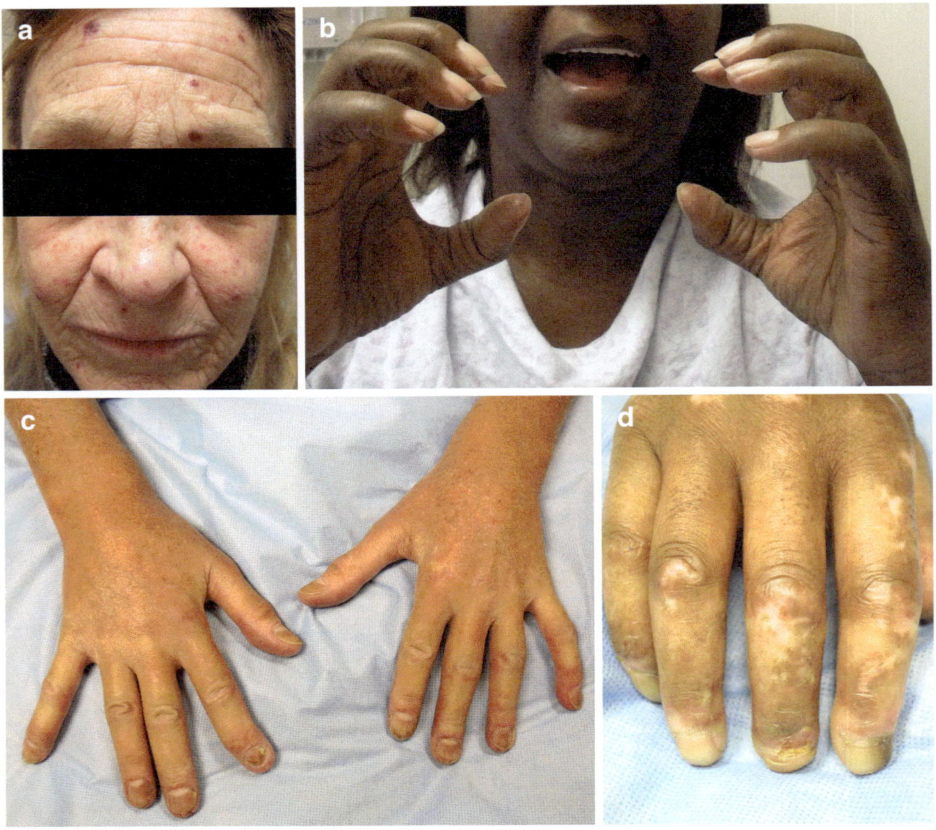

Fig. 74.1 Systemic sclerosis. (**a**) "Mat-like" or squared off telangiectasias on the face in a patient with limited systemic sclerosis (formerly known as CREST syndrome). (**b**) Sclerodactyly and decreased oral aperture in a patient with systemic sclerosis. (**c**) Edema and erythema with loss of skin lines in scleroderma. "Puffy hands" from hand edema can be an early sign of systemic sclerosis. (**d**) Sclerodactyly, resorption/shortening of digits, and digital ulceration in a patient with systemic sclerosis.

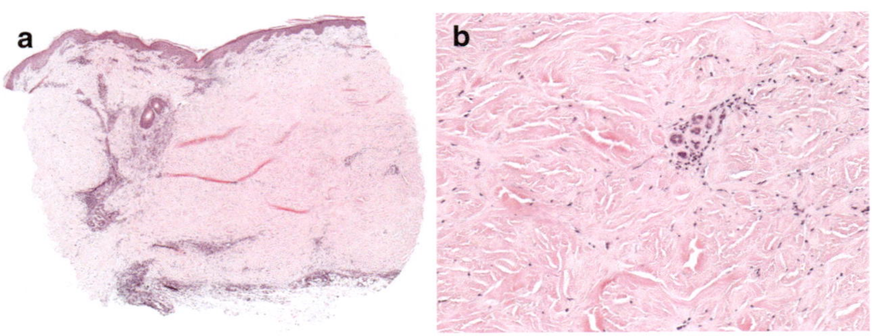

Fig. 74.2 Scleroderma *(4x, 10x; H&E)*: (**a**) Biopsies from scleroderma will appear as a rectangular or "squared off" punch. A lymphoplasmacytic infiltrate concentrated near the dermal-subcutaneous junction often can often be appreciated. (**b**) The dermis is composed of dense, thick, hyalinized and closely packed collagen bundles which "trap" eccine glands and result in loss peri-eccrine gland fat. Differentiating from morphea and scleroderma requires clinical-pathologic correlation.

Systemic Amyloidosis

75

Aileen Y. Chang

Overview

- Amyloidosis is a depositional disease of insoluble protein components which is characterized by the type of material deposited, such as light chains or acute phase reactants, the distribution of disease, systemic versus organ restricted, and associated damage
  - Typically, protein subunits associated with systemic disease circulate in the plasma allowing deposition in the wide range of tissues they come in contact with, while organ restricted amyloidosis is thought to be caused by accumulation of proteins produced by/within the affected organ
- There are over 30 protein subunits which cause amyloidosis and a variety of associated clinical manifestations, some of which are genetic/inherited; this chapter will focus on the ones most commonly encountered in an inpatient setting and those with cutaneous manifestations
  - Primary: AL (amyloid light chain) deposition may be seen in the setting of plasma cells dyscrasias
  - Secondary: AA (acute phase reactant) deposition occurs in patients with chronic inflammation and insufficient clearance
  - Hemodialysis-associated: β_2-microglobulin accumulates in patients with renal failure since it is normally excreted through the kidneys and is not filtered through the dialysis membrane
  - Primary cutaneous (non-familial types): macular amyloidosis, lichen amyloidosis, nodular amyloidosis
    - Macular and lichen amyloidosis are associated with friction/rubbing typically resulting in deposition of amyloid containing keratin derived material and often present in patients with atopic dermatitis and other pruritic conditions such as primary biliary cirrhosis and chronic renal failure
    - Nodular amyloidosis results from AL deposition and is associated with Sjögren syndrome, systemic sclerosis (CREST), and rheumatoid arthritis
- Secondary cutaneous: keratin derived amyloid deposits following PUVA therapy or less commonly conditions like GVHD with keratinocyte apoptosis

A. Y. Chang, MD
Department of Dermatology, University of California,
San Francisco, CA, USA
e-mail: aileen.chang@ucsf.edu

M. Rosenbach et al. (eds.), *Inpatient Dermatology*,
https://doi.org/10.1007/978-3-319-18449-4_75

Clinical Presentation

- Primary amyloidosis is associated with AL deposition in kidneys, liver, heart, gastrointestinal tract, nerves, and skin; patients may have associated plasma cell dyscrasias, primarily multiple myeloma
- Mucocutaneous lesion seen in 30–40% of patients (Fig. 75.1):
  - Waxy papulonodules and plaques near eyes, nose, mouth, mucocutaneous junctions
  - Ecchymoses and pinch purpura, particularly around eyes, oral cavity, or intertriginous areas, seen in 15%
    - Lesions may be induced by minor events, such as emesis leading to facial lesions, lesions in the axilla from patients after repositioning maneuvers in the hospital bed, or purpura after EKG leads or blood pressure measurements
      - Patients are prone to purpuric lesions because amyloid targets blood vessels increasing their fragility and can effect hemostasis
  - Macroglossia is a common manifestation; cutis verticis gyrata, alopecia, and longitudinal nail ridging can also be seen
  - Rarely, bullvous amyloidosis presents with tense, non-inflammatory bullae at areas of trauma and heals with scarring and milia
- Secondary amyloidosis is caused by deposition of AA, an acute phase reactant which is elevated in patients with a chronic inflammatory process such as RA or IBD; it does not specifically involve the skin but vascular deposition may be appreciated on skin biopsy
- Hemodialysis-associated: β_2-microglobulin has a tendency to deposit in synovial membranes leading to carpal tunnel syndrome, bone cysts, destructive spondyloarthropathy; the skin is not a site of involvement
- Primary cutaneous amyloidosis
  - Macular amyloidosis: rippled macular hyperpigmentation on upper back or extensor surface
  - Lichen amyloidosis: pruritic papules on bilateral shins or extensor surfaces; rarely associated with familial syndrome MEN-2A (pheochromocytoma, hyperparathyroidism, medullary thyroid cancer)
  - Nodular amyloidosis: rare, waxy, skin-colored to pink firm plaques and nodules on trunk and extremities composed of AL protein
    - These patients need to be monitored for systemic involvement as AL is produced by clonal plasma cells in skin and progression to primary systemic amyloidosis can occur

Histopathology

- Routine sections will reveal amorphous, eosinophilic fissured masses (Fig. 75.2)
- Congo red stain positive; orange-red color by light microscopy and green birefringence under polarized light
- In macular and lichen amyloidosis the overlying epidermis is often hyperkeratotic and variably acanthotic secondary to persistent rubbing; amyloid expands the dermal papillae and abuts the dermal/epidermal junction
- Nodular amyloidosis may exhibit diffuse deposition of amyloid in the dermis and subcutis often with an associated abundance of plasma cells
- In localized cutaneous amyloidosis there will be an absence of vascular involvement

Differential Diagnosis

- In the inpatient setting, the main form of amyloidosis is systemic, presenting with purpura, which should be distinguished from other causes of bleeding such as thrombocytopenia, anticoagulation, and consumptive processes (such as DIC)
- Other lesions of amyloid carry different differential diagnoses based on the morphologic presentation, and can often be distinguished by biopsy or serologic testing
- For waxy papules of primary systemic amyloidosis, the differential diagnosis may include: papular mucinosis, lipoid proteinosis, adnexal tumors, or scleromyxedema
  - For macular amyloidosis the differential may include notalgia paresthetica, postinflammatory hyperpigmentation, ashy dermatosis
  - For lichen amyloidosis the differential may include lichen simplex chronicus or hypertrophic lichen planus
  - For nodular amyloidosis the differential can include lymphoma cutis, sarcoidosis, or simple lipomas

Important Work-Up

- If there is a specific skin lesion, perform punch biopsy for H&E and Congo red stain; the type of amyloid can be determined at specialized centers by liquid chromatography-mass spectroscopy (Mayo Clinic)
- In absence of specific mucocutaneous lesions, abdominal fat aspiration, fat pad biopsy, or rectal biopsy may detect amyloid deposits around blood vessels
- In systemic and nodular amyloidosis a work-up should be performed to assess for a plasma cell dyscrasia by determining if a light chain restriction is present via SPEP/UPEP with immunofixation electrophoresis and serum free light chains
  - If abnormal light chains are present, proceed to bone marrow aspiration & biopsy

Treatment

- Primary systemic amyloidosis: hematology/oncology should be consulted for systemic treatment such as: melphalan ± prednisone, autologous stem cell transplant, lenalidomide ± dexamethasone with goal of stopping monoclonal light chain production by eliminating clonal plasma cells
- Secondary systemic amyloidosis: treat underlying disease
- Primary cutaneous amyloidosis: topical steroids ± keratolytic agent, UVB or topical PUVA therapy, dermabrasion for macular/lichen amyloidosis; excision, cryotherapy, electrodessication, CO_2 laser for nodular amyloidosis but local recurrence common

Suggested Readings

1. Daoud MS, Lust JA, Kyle RA, Pittelkow MR. Monoclonal gammopathies and associated skin disorders. J Am Acad Dermatol. 1999;40(4):507–35.
2. Groves RW, Black MM. Amyloidosis. In: Bolognia JL, Jorizzo JL, Schaffer JV, editors. Dermatology. St. Louis: Mosby; 2007. p. 702–7.

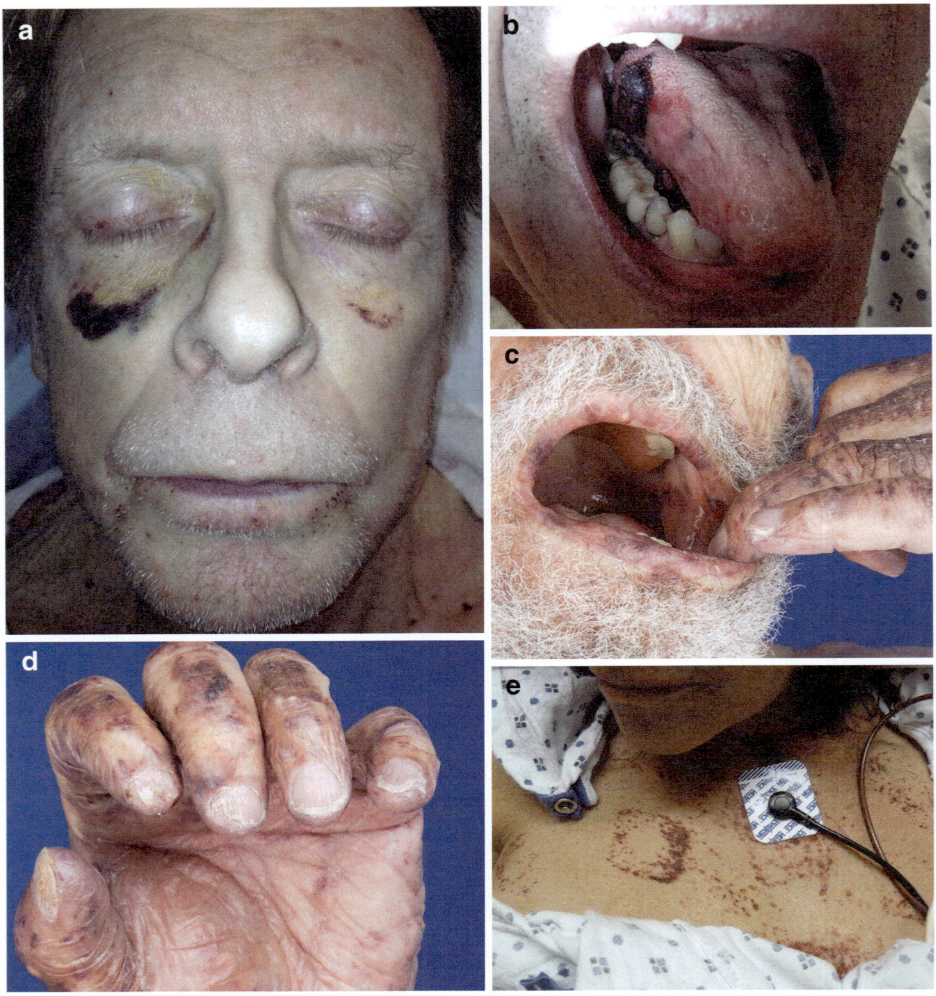

Fig. 75.1 Systemic amyloidosis. (**a**) Pinch purpura of the eyelids in systemic amyloidosis. (**b**) Hemorrhagic plaques on the tongue. (**c**) Purpuric macules and patches on the oral mucosa and fingers. (**d**) Purpura and longitudinal nail ridging and thinning characteristic of systemic amyloidosis. (**e**) Marked skin fragility and purpura due to incidental trauma in a patient with systemic amyloidosis.

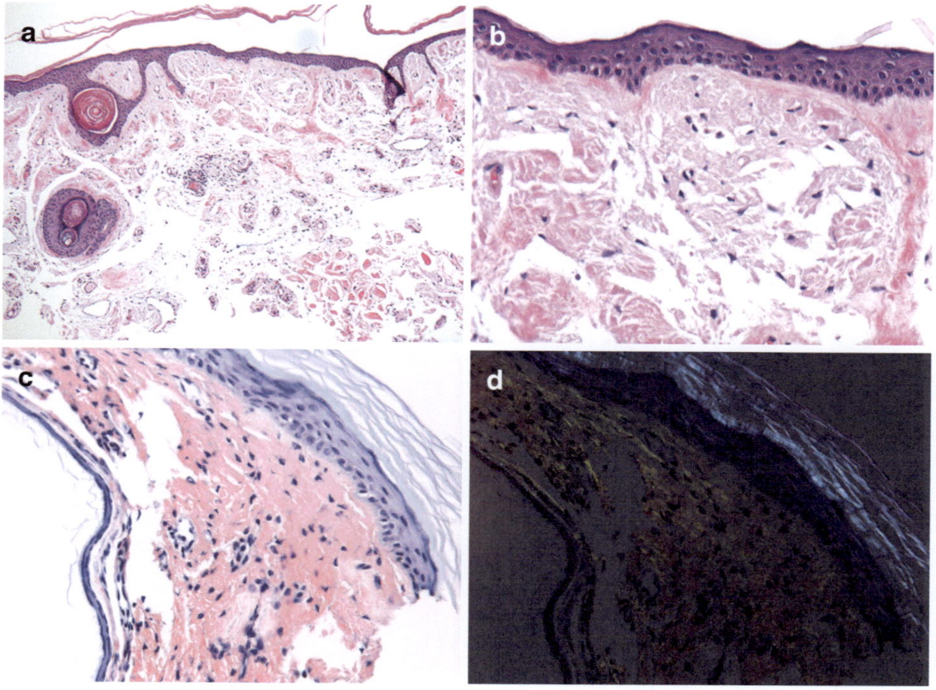

Fig. 75.2 Amyloidosis *(4x, 10x, 10x; H&E/Congo red 10x)*: (**a**) Low power evaluation of systemic amyloidosis often is subtle pink deposition within the dermis. (**b**) On higher power, deposition of pink amorphous material within the papillary dermis and surrounding blood vessels are seen. (**c**) Congo Red will highlight the deposits an orange color. (**d**) Polarization yields apple-green birefringence.

Part XI

Hospital Related Conditions

Beyond the skin diseases that lead to admission, or the secondary skin findings related to their systemic process which may evolve during hospitalization, inpatients can develop skin diseases as a result of the hospital environment. These can span the gamut from irritation due to antiseptic wipes used for surgery or line placement, to pressure ulcers due to prolonged immobility, to eruptions due to heat, friction, and sweating in the post-operative patient. This chapter discusses some of the disorders that hospitalized patients may preferentially experience and provides clinical pearls and recommended treatment for these conditions.

While these conditions may not be the primary reason for admission, they can cause significant discomfort and distress, and may sometimes lead to significant morbidity. These entities can also mimic other diseases and lead to inappropriate and sometimes unnecessary treatments if not recognized and diagnosed properly.

Decubitus ulcers can develop at any site of pressure, and it is important to recognize them rapidly—and document their presence appropriately. Better still, it is important to recognize the at-risk patient (patients in the ICU, elderly patients who are less mobile, patients with weakness, malnutrition, incontinence, or other risk factors) and to proactively recommend preventive measures such as pressure offloading, frequent turning, keeping incontinent patients dry, early use of hydrocolloid dressings to early-stage lesions, and consideration for advanced mattresses where available.

Stasis dermatitis is worth particular mention. Stasis dermatitis is due to swelling from accumulated fluid, usually in the lower legs (but it may occur in other sites, such as the pannus of the obese patient), which leads to stretch, stress, and irritation, which presents as inflammation. Red, swollen legs are unfortunately frequently diagnosed as cellulitis. Stasis dermatitis is a cause of "pseudocellulitis," and frequently is mismanaged with admission and broad spectrum IV antibiotics—and patients often improve, as, while they are admitted, they are laying flat in a hospital bed, thus offloading the lower leg oncotic pressure leading to reduced swelling, improved inflammation, and decreased redness. It is important to note that cellulitis is an acute process, almost always unilateral, and generally accompanied by fever and an elevated WBC. Bilateral cellulitis is incredibly rare, and in general indicates "pseudocellulitis," often due to stasis.

Failure to recognize (or prevent) decubitus ulcers or to diagnose stasis dermatitis can lead to hospital-related complications and re-admissions, which can be difficult for the patient, the physician, and the hospital.

Stasis Dermatitis

76

Douglas J. Pugliese

Overview

- Common chronic inflammatory skin disease of the lower extremities which develops as a consequence of increased venous pressure from chronic venous insufficiency (CVI)
- Usually the earliest cutaneous manifestation of CVI and can be a precursor to more serious complications such as lipodermatosclerosis and venous leg ulcers
- Risk factors are advanced age, pregnancy, obesity, prolonged periods of standing or sitting, history of deep venous thrombosis, knee replacement, surgery/trauma to the extremity

Clinical Presentation

- There is usually erythema from below the knee to the dorsal foot, skin hyperpigmentation from extravasated red cells' hemosiderin, and an eczematous dermatitis which may be pruritic and appear dry and scaly, or more brightly inflammatory and weepy in the acute phase (Fig. 76.1)
  - The medial ankle is most frequently involved, typically bilateral
  - Inflammation eventually encircles the ankle and extends to just below the knee
  - The skin may be warm and uncomfortable but rarely painful, symptoms improve with elevation
  - Varicose veins and edema are often present on exam but can be subtle in some early cases
  - Patients will often describe worsening edema towards the end of the day
- Cutaneous manifestations signify an underlying impediment to proper blood flow and tissue oxygenation and can result in more devastating consequences
  - Stasis can be a risk factor for the development of thromboemboli
  - Venous ulcers can develop from the fragile, edematous skin and poor circulation, which can predispose to significant wounds after minor trauma
  - Lipodermatosclerosis, or tight thickening of the skin due to chronic/persistent swelling and secondary inflammation, can lead to bound-down, 'inverted champagne bottle' legs

D. J. Pugliese, MD
Department of Dermatology, Perelman School of Medicine, Penn Presbyterian Medical Center, University of Pennsylvania, Philadelphia, PA, USA
e-mail: douglas.pugliese@uphs.upenn.edu

M. Rosenbach et al. (eds.), *Inpatient Dermatology*,
https://doi.org/10.1007/978-3-319-18449-4_76

Histopathology

- Classic histologic changes associated with venous stasis include:
  - A lobular proliferation of thick-walled blood vessels in the papillary dermis with a variable proportion of other features including extravasated red blood cells (Fig. 76.2)
  - Hemosiderin-laden macrophages
  - Dermal fibrosis (prominent dermal fibrosis and siderophages (macrophages which have consumed iron particles from local hemorrhage)
  - Epidermal acanthosis with hyperkeratosis in long-standing cases

Differential Diagnosis

- Cellulitis (should be noted that bilateral leg cellulitis is extremely rare): should come on rapidly, usually with fever and an elevated white count. Patients are frequently inappropriately admitted and treated with IV antibiotics for presumed cellulitis when they have stasis dermatitis—which also improves with hospital admission generally because patients are laying flat and offloading edema
- Deep venous thrombosis: generally unilateral and more acute, sometimes with a palpable cord
- Allergic/irritant contact dermatitis: this often compounds stasis, as patients self-medicate with topical antibiotics and develop a secondary contact reaction, which is often weepy with yellowish serous drainage and crusting
- Congestive heart failure, renal failure, liver failure: these can lead to increased edema and cause stasis dermatitis, and should be investigated as a possible culprit
- Pigmented purpuric dermatosis: usually flecks of Cayenne-pepper or reddish/orange patches scattered in vaguely annular arrays on the lower legs
- Tinea infection: should be annular with some scaling, and lack the edema of stasis
- Pretibial myxedema: often broad areas of waxy, extensive subcutaneous pitting edema and tissue hypertrophy over the anterior shins down to the foot; usually less red than stasis

Work-Up

- Biopsy is unnecessary in the majority of cases and even discouraged due to the risk of nonhealing, however may be necessary if concern for secondary malignancy
- Venous duplex ultrasound to rule out thrombosis and to evaluate for venous reflux

Treatment

- All patients should undergo leg elevation and, if tolerated, compression stockings
  - If there is concern for peripheral arterial disease or if patients develop pain with compression, vascular evaluation may be indicated
- All patients should have their total body fluid status optimized with diuresis if appropriate
- Patients should be educated about exercises, such as calf-muscle pumping, to help minimize venous pooling and maximize fluid return
- Review medication lists for potential exacerbating agents (such as calcium channel blockers)
- Mid-potency topical steroid creams or ointments can help with acute inflammation
- Topical emollient creams or ointments may help with dryness
- Referral to vascular surgery if symptomatic with obvious varicosities on exam and/or with reflux noted on venous duplex ultrasound

Suggested Readings

1. Flugman SL, et al. Stasis dermatitis. 2014. http://emedicine.medscape.com/article/1084813-overview. Accessed 1 Feb 2015.
2. Eberhardt RT, Raffetto JD. Chronic venous insufficiency. Circulation. 2014;130:333–46.

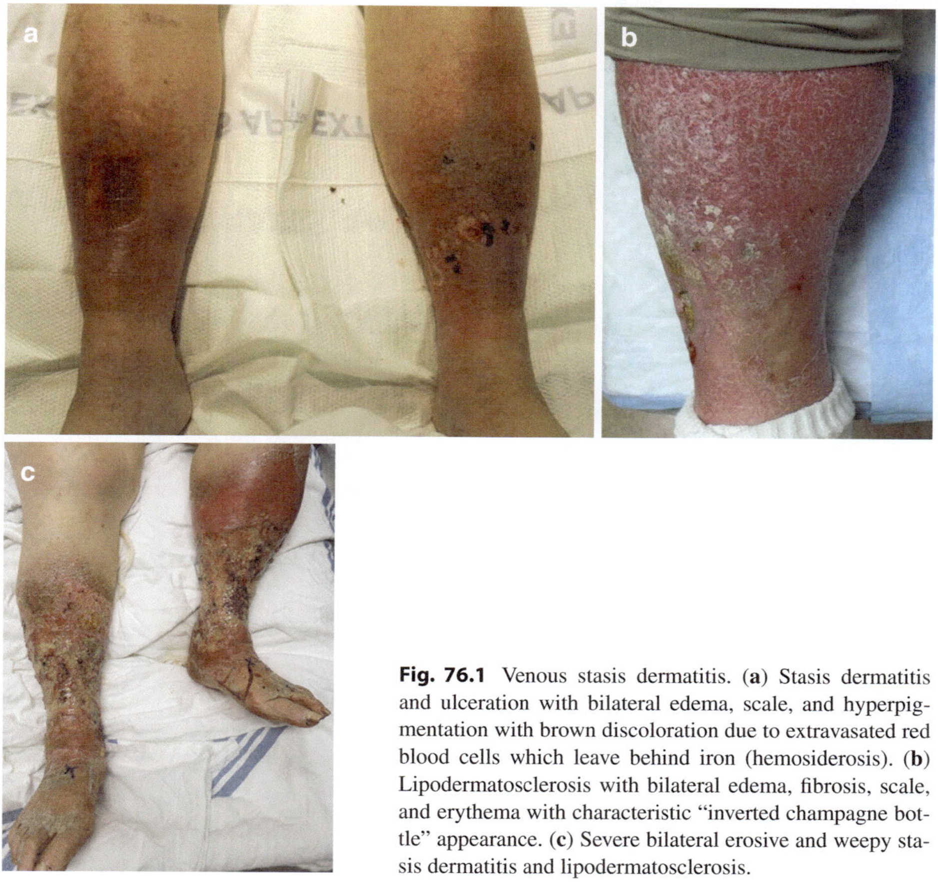

Fig. 76.1 Venous stasis dermatitis. (**a**) Stasis dermatitis and ulceration with bilateral edema, scale, and hyperpigmentation with brown discoloration due to extravasated red blood cells which leave behind iron (hemosiderosis). (**b**) Lipodermatosclerosis with bilateral edema, fibrosis, scale, and erythema with characteristic "inverted champagne bottle" appearance. (**c**) Severe bilateral erosive and weepy stasis dermatitis and lipodermatosclerosis.

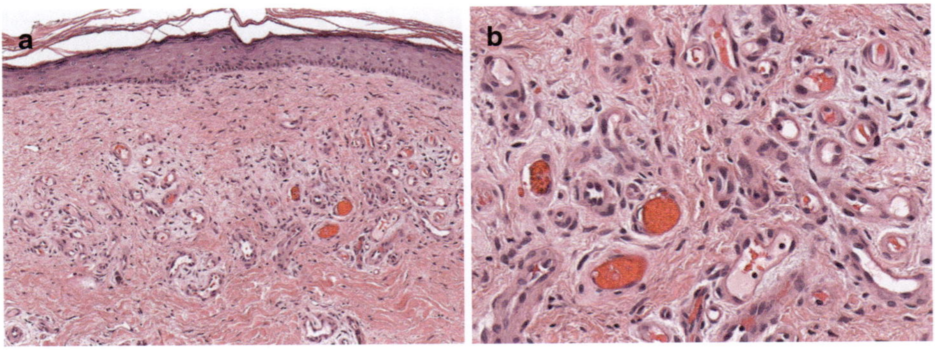

Fig. 76.2 Stasis dermatitis *(5x, 20x; H&E)*: (**a**) Ischemia secondary to poor blood circulation leads to neovascularization which can be appreciated histologically as multiple small vessels. In the superficial dermis, there are parallel oriented collagen fibers, similar to those observed in a scar, often resulting from repetitive swelling. (**b**) Vascular congestion can be observed in cases. In addition, hemosiderin deposition surrounding blood vessels is characteristic and corresponds to the brown discoloration often observed in chronic cases.

Miliaria

77

Grant Ghahramani

Overview

- Milaria, commonly known as heat rash, is a disorder of eccrine glands secondary to obstruction and retention of sweat
- There are three forms of miliaria characterized by the region of the duct or gland that is involved
  - Miliaria crystallina: superficial obstruction at the level of the stratum corneum
  - Miliaria rubra/pustulosa: mid epidermal obstruction
  - Miliaria profunda: obstruction occurs in the upper dermis
- Associated with immobility, hot/humid environments, and clothing or bedding which traps heat and perspiration preventing proper cooling
  - Commonly seen in children and neonates as sweat ducts are not fully developed
  - Also prevalent in febrile hospitalized patients who are supine for prolonged periods (e.g., post-operative patients, intubated patients) on impermeable plastic bedding
- Improves with removal of trigger and cooling, and often simply when patients move from hospital bed to sitting upright in a chair

Clinical Presentation

- Acute (days to weeks) eruption of painful and/or pruritic skin lesions not associated with hair follicles (Fig. 77.1)
- Miliaria crystallina (subtle and transient)
  - Superficial obstruction (stratum corneum) resulting in clear delicate vesicles which rupture with gentle pressure, often on the face and trunk
- Miliaria rubra/pustulosa (most common form)
  - Intermediate obstruction (mid epidermis) with pruritic erythematous papules, often excoriated, usually found on the back
- Miliaria profunda (rarely seen)
  - Deep obstruction (upper dermis) with white papules on trunk and extremities typically seen in the tropics with recurrent episodes of miliaria rubra

G. Ghahramani, MD
Cotton O'Neil Dermatology, Topeka, KS, USA

M. Rosenbach et al. (eds.), *Inpatient Dermatology*,
https://doi.org/10.1007/978-3-319-18449-4_77

Histopathology

- Obstruction of sweat ducts with inflammation at different levels may be seen with overlying keratin plug (Fig. 77.2)
  - Miliaria crystallina: intra or subcorneal vesicle associated with a sweat duct with little to no inflammation; epidermal spongiosis is often evident
  - Miliaria rubra: intrapidermal spongiosis with vesicle formation associated with a sweat duct; mild periductal and superficial perivascular dermal lymphocytic infiltrate, neutrophils may be present
  - Miliaria profunda: dermal portion of sweat duct demonstrates spongiosis with deeper lymphoplasmacytic inflammation

Differential Diagnosis

- Folliculitis: characterized by folliculocentric pustules whereas miliaria is not folliculocentric
- Corticosteroid-induced acne: monomorphic papules and pustules often also on the lateral shoulders, unlike miliaria
- Transient acantholytic dermatosis (Grover's disease): quite similar to miliaria and can be hard to distinguish, however treatment may overlap and neither represents an urgent diagnosis
- Disseminated herpes simplex or varicella zoster: often more monomorphic lesions, intact vesicles, and punched out, same-sized erosions, generally more clustered than miliaria

Work-Up

- Generally this is a clinical diagnosis and no work-up is required
- In select cases, consider biopsy to exclude alternative diagnosis if necessary
- Diagnostic testing such as polymerase chain reaction (PCR) to exclude viral etiologies if indicated

Treatment

- Self-limited disorder that will resolves in a period of days-to-weeks; if asymptomatic, does not require treatment
- Cooling patient with fans, controlling heat and humidity, treating febrile illness, remove occlusive clothing, avoidance of lying on area affected, sitting in a chair can all help
- Topical therapies include lanolin or hydrophilic ointment (they are thought to restore normal sweat function and removal of keratin plugs)
- A simple approach is to apply topical clindamycin in the morning and topical steroids in the evening, which will treat most entities on the differential and speed resolution

Suggested Readings

1. Obson RL, Lobitz WC Jr. Some histochemical observations on the human eccrine sweat glands. II. The pathogenesis of miliaria. AMA Arch Dermatol. 1957;75(5):653–66.
2. Lobitz WC Jr. Pustular miliaria; sweat retention phenomenon complicating common dermatoses. J Am Med Assoc. 1952;148(13):1097–100.

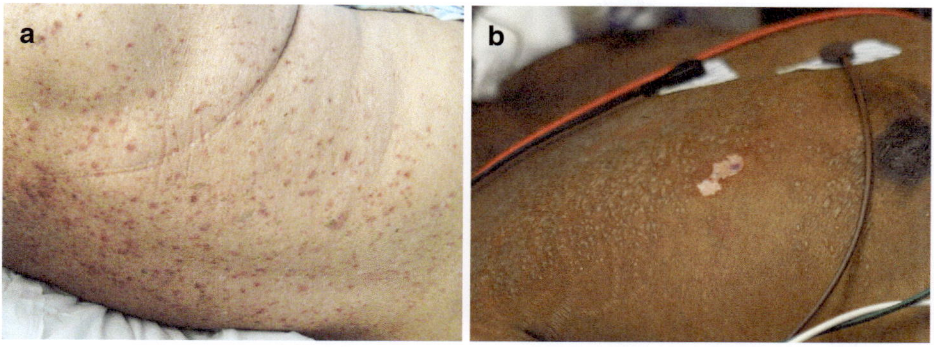

Fig. 77.1 Miliaria: (**a**) Miliaria rubra: Numerous pink, follicular papules with preference for occluded areas such as the back in a hospitalized and bed-bound patient. (**b**) Miliaria crystallina: When the obstruction is very close to the epidermis, there are superficial vesicles which are fragile and rupture with gentle pressure. This is generally seen in febrile, immobile patients in the ICU.

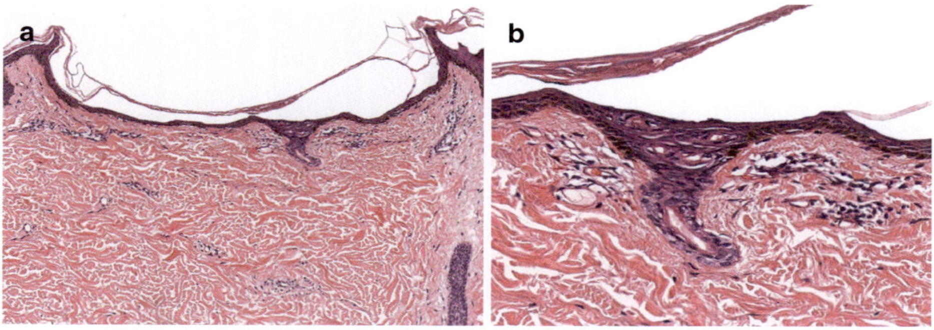

Fig. 77.2 Miliaria crystallina *(5x, 10x; H&E)*: (**a**) The subcorneal vecicle is arising in association with the underlying eccrine duct. There is a mild surrounding inflammatory infiltrate. (**b**) A superficially plugged eccrine duct results in miliara crystallina.

Decubitus Ulcers

78

Robert G. Micheletti

Overview

- Decubitus ulcers (pressure ulcers) are commonly encountered in the hospital and long-term institutional care settings and typically result from prolonged compression of soft tissue between a bony prominence and an external surface; chronic pressure leads to tissue hypoxia with skin and underlying tissue damage and necrosis
- Risk factors include severity of medical illness (such as ICU admission), immobility (e.g. hip fracture), malnutrition, reduced perfusion (e.g. hypotension, shock), sensory loss (e.g. spinal cord injury), moisture (incontinence), friction, and many others
- Decubitus ulcers account for a significant burden on the patient and the entire health care system and are considered an important patient safety issue
- Wounds may lead to a prolonged and difficult recovery period and may be life-threatening due to superinfection, resulting in cellulitis, osteomyelitis, and sepsis
- Decubitus ulcers are a frequent source of medical malpractice claims and some insurers view them as a hospital-acquired, preventable illness and will deny reimbursement for ulcer-related care for hospital-acquired ulcers

Clinical Presentation

- Decubitus ulcers most commonly occur at pressure points, most notably on the posterior lower back/sacrum, buttock, and legs, though can occur at other sites (Fig. 78.1)
- Injury severity is categorized at the time of diagnosis as:
  - Stage 1: in-tact skin with localized, non-blanchable redness
  - Stage 2: partial-thickness dermal loss; shallow ulcer with pink-red surface
  - Stage 3: full-thickness dermal loss with visible fat
  - Stage 4: exposed bone, tendon, muscle
  - Unstageable: full-thickness tissue loss; depth obscured by slough, eschar
- Wounds may also be categorized as "suspected deep tissue injury" when skin is purple and discolored, firm, boggy, and/or tender but in-tact; these may rapidly progress to Stage 3/4

R. G. Micheletti, MD
Department of Dermatology, Perelman School of Medicine, University of Pennsylvania, Philadelphia, PA, USA
e-mail: robert.micheletti@uphs.upenn.edu

M. Rosenbach et al. (eds.), *Inpatient Dermatology*,
https://doi.org/10.1007/978-3-319-18449-4_78

Histopathology

- Biopsies are not typically performed in this setting except to rule out a differential diagnosis
- Histologic findings will depend on the depth and age of the lesion; most lesions will demonstrate superficial necrosis with underlying granulation tissue consisting of highly vascularized connective tissue with an associated inflammatory infiltrate

Differential Diagnosis

- Diabetic or neuropathic ulcer: these tend to occur in sites of decreased sensation due to bone-on-skin friction that leads to an unrecognized ulcer which expands
- Ulcer due to arterial insufficiency: usually on the lateral distal lower legs not at bony prominence pressure sites
- Venous stasis ulcer: jagged, ragged ulcers on the sides of the distal lower legs with background venous stasis
- Enterocutaneous fistula: often fistulous tracks and malodorous discharge in the perianal area, not focused on a bony prominence
- Cutaneous malignancy or Marjorin ulcer: secondary malignant degeneration can occur within any chronic wound, and biopsy may be necessary to exclude malignancy

Important Work-Up

- Diagnosis of pressure ulcer is usually made clinically; when the presentation is atypical, biopsy can be considered, mainly to rule out malignancy
- Incontinence should be managed medications should be reviewed for potential triggers (e.g., laxatives avoided if possible in immobile patients if possible, and catheters may be
- Biopsy of exposed bone may be warranted to guide antibiotic therapy for osteomyelitis
- A thorough assessment of risk factors should be performed in all hospitalized patients, as prevention is key
- Regular inspection on rapid use of pressure-offloading dressings such as hydrocolloid dressings can help prevent early stage ulcers from worsening
- It is important to document the size and stage of ulcers and work with nursing staff to prevent decubiti and manage existing wounds

Treatment and Management

Prevention

- Perform risk assessment to identify patients at risk
- Correct factors which are correctable (e.g. address/treat malnutrition, incontinence, and immobility)
- Pressure redistribution using special mattresses or static overlays, cushions, wedges, and frequent turns
- Keep the skin clean and dry; use a gentle cleansing agent at regular intervals and avoid scrubbing; minimize friction and moisture

Treatment

- Reduce/eliminate contributing factors and redistribute pressure, as above
- Appropriate local wound care and debridement, as needed
  - Stage 1: cover with transparent film for protection; intensive preventive measures
  - Stage 2: semi-occlusive (transparent film) or occlusive (hydrocolloid or hydrogel) dressing; hydrocolloids may be preferable
  - Stage 3/4: debridement of necrotic tissue surgically or using collagenase; absorptive dressing (foam, alginate) for wet wounds and hydrating dressing (saline-moistened, hydrocolloid, hydrogel) for dry wounds

- Consideration for negative pressure therapy (wound vac)
- Consult with a nutritionist to optimize nutrition
- Treat clinical infection or secondary colonization with appropriate topical antimicrobials (gentle cleansing with a low concentration of acetic acid followed by application of targeted topical antimicrobials depending on the microbial flora may be helpful)
- Consideration for wound coverage (flap, graft) and diverting colostomy, if appropriate, if the patient is a good surgical candidate

Suggested Readings

1. Grey JE, Harding KG, Enoch S. Pressure ulcers. BMJ. 2006;332:472–5.
2. Reddy M, Gill SS, Kalkar SR, et al. Treatment of pressure ulcers: a systematic review. JAMA. 2008;300:2647–62.

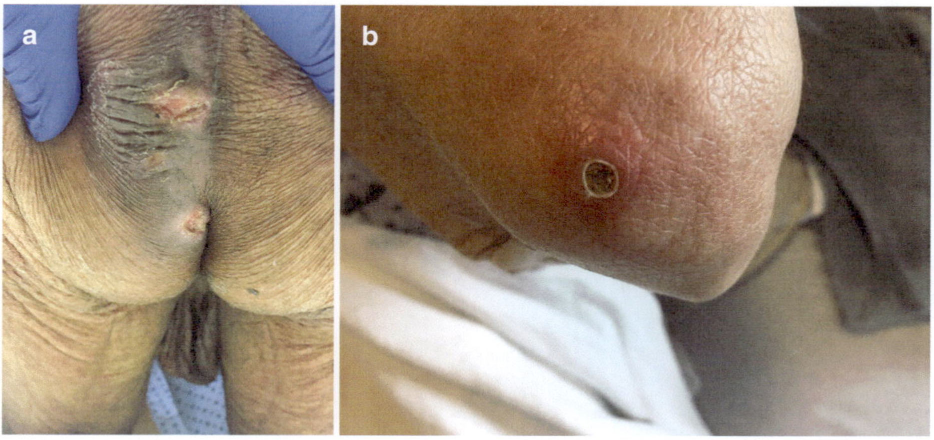

Fig. 78.1 Decubitus Ulcer: (**a**) Decubitus ulcer in patient who was partially immobilized and preferentially laying on their left side. (**b**) A pressure ulcer on the elbow in an immobile, cachectic patient.

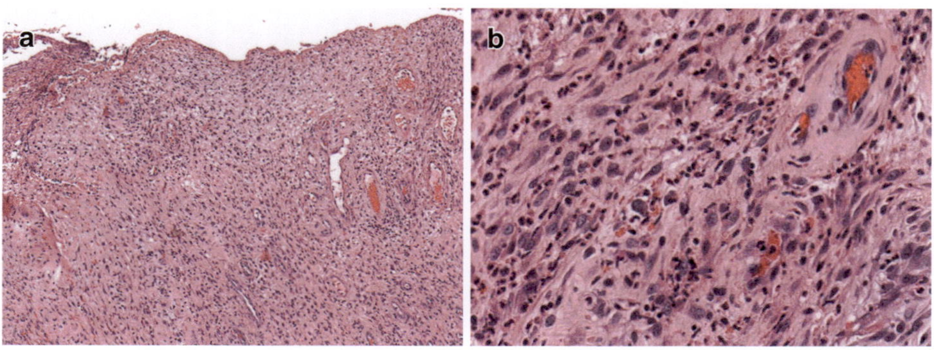

Fig. 78.2 Healing decubitus ulcer *(5x, 20x; H&E)*: (**a**) Epidermal ulceration with a dense inflammatory infiltrate and increased blood vessels are observed on low power. (**b**) Granulation tissue with an associated abundant mixed inflammatory cell infiltrate can be seen on closer inspection.

79 Intertrigo

Douglas J. Pugliese

Overview

- Superficial inflammatory dermatosis involving body folds that develops through friction of opposing skin surfaces and moisture
- The moist damaged skin is prone to secondary infections by bacteria, yeast, and/or fungi; polymicrobial skin-limited superficial infection is common
- More common in the obese, especially during hot and humid conditions
  - Elderly, bedridden, and pediatric patients are also more at risk due to reduced immunity, immobilization, and incontinence

Clinical Presentation

- Insidious onset of erythematous macerated patches of opposing skin folds; lesions may contain erosions, fissures, and exudate with involved areas often pruritic, painful, and malodorous (Fig. 79.1)
- Intertrigo primarily involves the inframammary, inguinal, abdominal, perineal, and intergluteal skin folds
  - Can also involve the retroauricular skin, folds of upper eyelids, umbilicus, creases of the neck, axillae, anticubital and popliteal areas, and the web spaces of the toes and fingers
- Acute onset or exacerbation of ongoing symptoms may be a sign of secondary infection
  - Superinfections are typically caused by *Candida*, dermatophytes, *Streptococci, Staphylococci*, *Pseudomonas*, *Corynebacteria;* combined infections are common
  - *Candida* superinfection can have satellite papules and pustules and typically involves the scrotum/groin
  - Dermatophyte superinfection may spare the scrotum/vulva and lack pustules; scale is not often seen due to the increased moisture in the body folds

D. J. Pugliese, MD
Department of Dermatology, Perelman School of Medicine, Penn Presbyterian Medical Center, University of Pennsylvania, Philadelphia, PA, USA
e-mail: douglas.pugliese@uphs.upenn.edu

M. Rosenbach et al. (eds.), *Inpatient Dermatology*,
https://doi.org/10.1007/978-3-319-18449-4_79

Histopathology

- Biopsy is rarely necessary; there are no characteristic features of intertrigo on histology, but biopsy may help eliminate entities on the differential diagnosis and may uncover occult infection

Differential Diagnosis

- Contact dermatitis: exposure history is helpful, but patients may develop allergic or irritant contact dermatitis over intertrigo due to irritating cleansers or topical antibiotics used to treat the intertrigo
- Inverse psoriasis: can be hard to distinguish clinically; signs of psoriasis elsewhere (nail pitting, scalp scaling, elbow/knee plaques) can be a helpful clue
- Erythrasma: superficial bacterial infection which affects the folds; will display fluorescence with Wood's lamp examination, and is generally more sharply demarcated than intertrigo
- Tinea/Candida: intertrigo shares common features and all three may be managed similarly in the hospital setting, making distinguishing between them often unnecessary

Work-Up

- Generally, patients are treated broadly to cover the majority of potential pathogens and improve the moist environment, and diagnostic testing is not usually required
- Tests to consider may include:
  - Potassium hydroxide preparation to evaluate for superinfection with yeast or fungi
  - Culture to evaluate for group A β-hemolytic streptococcal infection and other bacterial infections if bright red erythema and/or yellow crusting are present, or if unresponsive to treatment
  - Wood's lamp examination causes erythrasma to fluoresce a coral-pink color
  - Punch biopsy of the skin for histology and tissue culture if the rash does not respond to empiric treatment (to exclude rarer entities such as malignancies like extramammary Paget's disease or Langerhan's cell histiocytosis, genetic diseases like Hailey-Hailey, or nutritional processes such as acrodermatitis enteropathica or necrolytic migratory erythema)

Treatment

- Treatment should be directed toward eliminating friction, maceration, and any superinfection
  - Opposing skin surfaces may be separated by appropriate non-stick dressings
- Topical treatments which combine protective agents and an antimicrobial can be effective
  - A combination of low potency topical steroid and an azole antifungal, with or without a topical antibacterial agent, applied directly to the affected area followed by zinc oxide cream or ointment 1–2 times a day is a reasonable initial treatment option for rapid control; steroids should not be used for prolonged periods in skin folds
- Drying agents such as gentian violet or castellani paint can be effective in the appropriate setting
- Powder-based therapies can occasionally be useful, particularly with antifungal additives

Suggested Readings

1. Kalra MG, et al. Intertrigo and secondary skin infections. Am Fam Physician. 2014;89(7):569–73.
2. Mistiaen P, Halm-Walters MV. Prevention and treatment of intertrigo in large skin folds of adults: a systematic review. BMC Nurs. 2010;9:12.
3. James WD, et al. Andrews' diseases of the skin: clinical dermatology. 11th ed. London: Saunders/Elsevier; 2011.

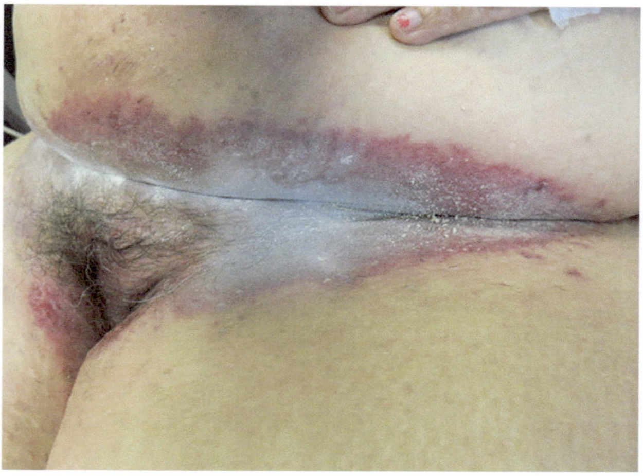

Fig. 79.1 Intertrigo: Painful, red, and eroded skin of the inguinal and abdominal folds. This can occur in any moist, occluded skin, most commonly in the skin folds, and is often a polymicrobial process.

Contact Dermatitis

80

Katherine K. Brown

Overview

- Contact dermatitis is an eczematous eruption that develops after cutaneous exposure to an irritating substance *(irritant contact dermatitis)* or allergic response to a sensitizing substance (*allergic contact dermatitis*)
- Irritant contact dermatitis (ICD) is non-immunologic and is generally cumulative after prolonged and repeated exposure, such as hand dermatitis due to over-washing, but can occur on first exposure with a caustic substance
  - Common irritants include harsh soaps and detergents; in the hospital setting, this can include skin preps used prior to line placement, intravascular procedures, dialysis, or surgeries
- Allergic contact dermatitis (ACD) is a T-cell mediated delayed-type IV hypersensitivity response to a specific allergen that will reoccur in susceptible individuals 1–2 days upon repeat exposure to the sensitizing substance, commonly caused by poison ivy and nickel
  - Some causes of ACD relevant in a hospitalized setting include topical antimicrobials, rubber accelerators, bandage adhesives, and topical antiseptics

Clinical Presentation

- Erythematous papules and plaques arranged in linear or geographic patterns, which may be intensely inflamed and develop marked edema which can lead to pseudovesicles, serous exudate, and scale crusts (Fig. 80.1)
  - Periorbital, face, neck, and hands are common sites
  - Surgical sites are commonly affect in hospitalized patients due to frequent use of topical antimicrobials perioperatively
  - Vesicles, bullae, erosions and serous crusting seen in severe cases
- Intense itching is more suggestive of ACD; symptoms of burning, stinging, irritation with mild to no itching suggest ICD
- Honey-colored crusts suggests secondary bacterial colonization or impetiginization, usually from *S. aureus*

K. K. Brown, MD
Department of Dermatology, University of Pennsylvania, Philadelphia, PA, USA
e-mail: katherine.brown@uphs.upenn.edu

M. Rosenbach et al. (eds.), *Inpatient Dermatology*,
https://doi.org/10.1007/978-3-319-18449-4_80

Histopathology

- Acute: variable degrees of spongiosis with intraepidermal vesicle formation which may contain clusters of Langerhans cells; lymphistiocytic infiltrate in the dermis with variable eosinophils both within the spongiotic epidermis and dermis (Fig. 80.2)
- Chronic: prominent acanthosis, hyperkeratosis, mild spongiosis, sparse inflammatory infiltrate

Differential Diagnosis

- Atopic dermatitis: history of atopy, symmetrical involvement of flexural creases, lack of geometric plaques and no clear exposure history
- Dyshidrotic eczema: pinpoint deep-seated vesicles on the hands and lateral fingers without a history of exposure
- Dermatophytosis: more annular with rounded edges and prominent scale in most cases
- Drug eruption: usually more diffuse, with deeper erythema and less epidermal involvement

Work-Up

- Generally, a clinical diagnosis based on history and physical exam
- Can be confirmed with skin patch-testing as an outpatient
- Most important is a careful thorough history of all patient's cutaneous exposures, including personal care products and over the counter topical medicaments; for hospitalized patients special thought should be given to recent procedures, line placement, or ancillary tests which involve topical agents.
- Hospitalized patients with contact dermatitis frequently have a history of topical antimicrobial agent use, which may not appear on standard medication lists; careful history-taking is essential
- Biopsy rarely required; may be considered in a new onset dermatitis that is difficult to control, particularly in an adult without prior history of atopic disease

Treatment

- Diligent avoidance is the mainstay of treatment of ACD
  - Patient education and counseling on how to avoid potential allergens is imperative
  - It may take up to 12 weeks to fully clear after removal of offending agent
- For active dermatitis, topical therapy includes various strengths of topical steroids
- Frequent use of thick cream or ointment based emollients to repair skin barrier
- Consider oral prednisone for severe flares; often 3 weeks of a tapering dose is necessary to avoid rebound of dermatitis
- Oral antibiotics may be required for impetiginized cases

Suggested Readings

1. Rietschel RL, Fowler JF, editors. Fisher's contact dermatitis. Philadelphia: Lippincott Williams & Wilkins; 2008. p. 6e.
2. Cashman MW, Reutemann PA, Ehrlich A. Contact dermatitis in the United States: epidemiology, economic impact, and workplace prevention. Dermatol Clin. 2012;30(1):87–98.
3. Renner R, Simon JC, Treudler R. Contact sensitization to modern wound dressings in 70 patients with chronic leg ulcers. Dermatitis. 2013;24(2):60–3.

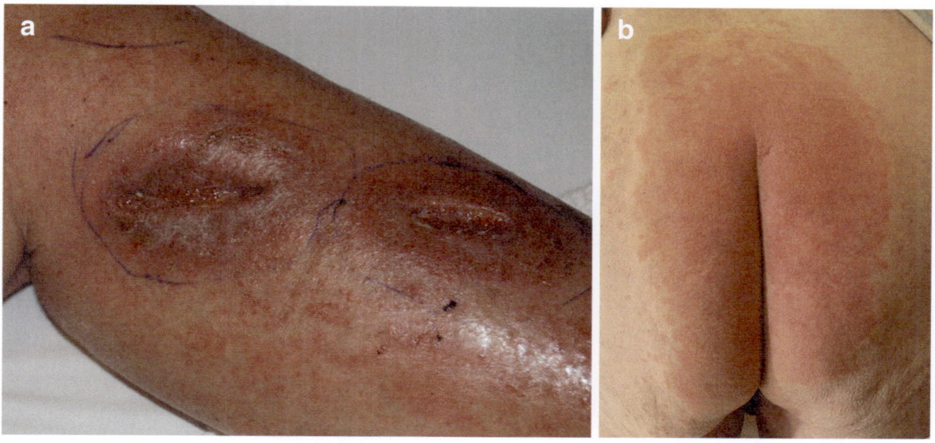

Fig. 80.1 Contact dermatitis: (**a**) Allergic contact dermatitis to neosporin: Erythematous and eczematous contact dermatitis localized to sites of neosporin application following vein harvest. (**b**) Allergic contact dermatitis to propylene glycol: Geometric erythema localized around the intergluteal cleft due to propylene glycol in wet wipes. The patient received intravenous antibiotics and was hospitalized for an inappropriate diagnosis of cellulitis.

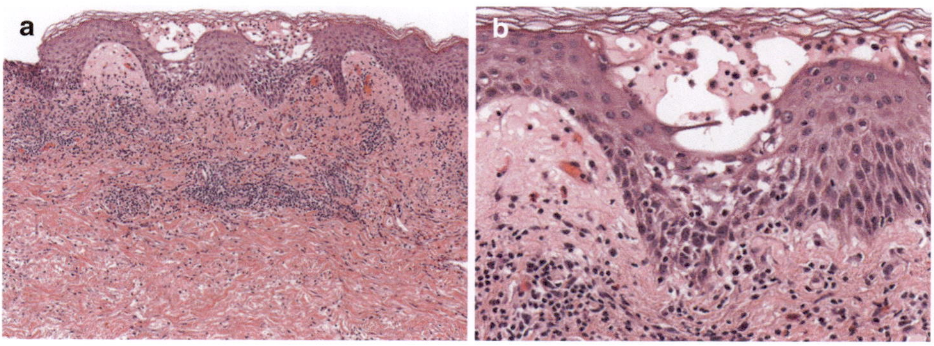

Fig. 80.2 Contact dermatitis (*5×, 20×; H&E*): (**a**) There is prominent spongiosis within the epidermis with resultant vesicle formation and a dense superficial inflamamtory infiltrate. (**b**) Within the spongiotic epidermis, there is associated serum and lymphocyte exocytosis. The superficial dermis contains a lymphohistocytic and eosinophilic infiltrate.

Edema Blisters

81

Nkanyezi N. Ferguson

Overview

- Tense cutaneous bullae occurring after an acute exacerbation of swelling/edema, often in a patient with baseline edema or anasarca
- Most commonly effects the elderly and immobile patient, or acutely ill patients (such as those with sepsis after early goal directed therapy and large volume IVF resuscitation); potential underlying etiologies include decompensated hepatic, cardiac, or renal disease, or acute venous outflow obstruction
- Often involves the lower extremities with tendency towards involvement of the dorsal foot and ankle; can also frequently affect the underside of the upper extremities in the setting of anasarca
- Management and control of edema results in resolution of symptoms

Clinical Presentation

- The hallmark is large bullae without any surrounding erythema (Fig. 81.1)
- The tense, fluid-filled bullae (which can vary in size from pinpoint to extensive) typically develop on an edematous, often anasarcic site with gradual enlargement over a period of days; often non-inflammatory but can be on background of acute stasis dermatitis
- Associated surrounding edema, often pitting and weeping with evidence of acute or chronic stasis dermatitis

Histopathology

- Epidermal spongiosis often prominent; subepidermal bullae may be evident (Fig. 81.2)
- Marked edema present in the dermis causing generous spacing between collagen bundles
- Evidence of stasis changes characterized by dilated vessels with surrounding fibrosis
- Chronic lymphocytic and histiocytic inflammatory infiltrate
- If DIF is performed it will be negative

N. N. Ferguson, MD
University of Iowa Hospital and Clinics, Iowa City, IA, USA
e-mail: nkanyezi-ferguson@uiowa.edu

M. Rosenbach et al. (eds.), *Inpatient Dermatology*,
https://doi.org/10.1007/978-3-319-18449-4_81

Differential Diagnosis

- Allergic contact dermatitis: smaller, more numerous bullae, with more pruritus, erythema, and serous drainage and crust
- Diabetic bullae: can look quite similar, though usually on the lower legs of patients with poorly controlled diabetes
- Pseudoporphyria: similar appearing bland bullae, often seen in patients with ESRD or after use of certain medications (e.g. NSAID)
- Bullous pemphigoid: usually will demonstrate some urticarial inflammation around the bullae, and more numerous bullae, not associated with edema
- Bullous cellulitis: unilateral, acute, with bright inflammation and signs of infection; can be hemorrhagic

Work-Up

- A thorough history and physical examination is warranted
- Evaluation for underlying etiology of acute edema
- Histological and immunofluorescence studies are generally not required unless diagnosis is in question

Treatment

- Control of underlying edema (varies depending on etiology) and optimization of total body fluid and nutritional status is essential
- Compression garments (e.g. compression hosiery or bandaging, sequential compression devices, lymphatic massage with physical therapy, etc.)
- Extremity elevation
- If tender, the bullae can be drained by creating a small window with a sterile needle or #11 blade with overlying blister top left in place to act as a biologic dressing
- Fluid re-accumulation can be prevented by compression dressings

Suggested Readings

1. Bhushan M, Chalmers RJ, Cox NH. Acute oedema blisters: a report of 13 cases. Br J Dermatol. 2001;144(3):580–2.

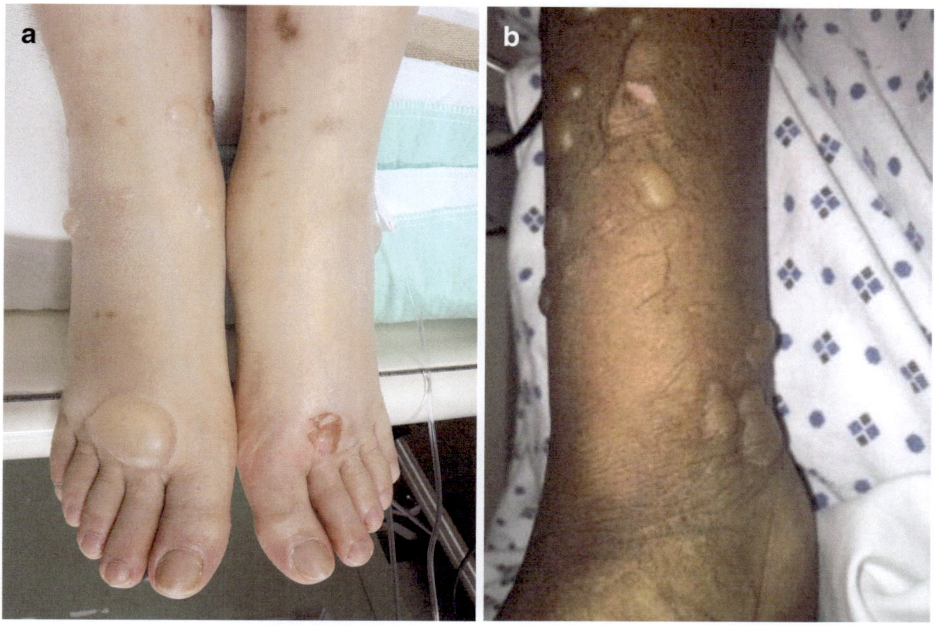

Fig. 81.1 Edema bullae: (**a**, **b**) non-inflammatory tense bullae in areas of dependent edema. The lack of erythema is important in making this diagnosis.

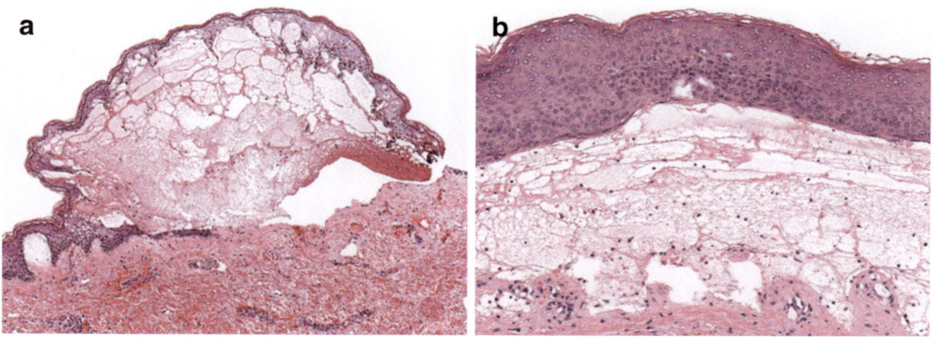

Fig. 81.2 Edema bullae (*5×, 10×; H&E*): (**a**, **b**) Two different examples of edema bullae: There is prominent dermal papillary edema with associated blister formation. Associated prominent epidermal spongiosis also can be observed in some cases.

Steroid Acne

82

Juliana K. Choi

Overview

- Patients develop a monomorphic eruption of inflammatory follicular papules and small pustules commonly on the chest, back, and shoulders after several weeks of corticosteroid therapy
  - Characteristically appears after systemic corticosteroid administration, but can occur on skin after chronic topical or inhaled corticosteroid use
- All age groups can be affected but most commonly seen in early adulthood, with an increased susceptibility in patients with current or previous acne
- Incidence increasing as systemic steroids are used in autoimmune disease, allograft transplant rejection, oncologic treatments, and intra- and post-operative neurosurgical patients
- While most cases of drug induced acne are related to systemic steroid use, less common causes include isoniazid, lithium, phenytoin and other agents

Clinical Presentation

- Abrupt onset of monomorphic 1–3 mm flesh-colored to pink-to-red, dome-shaped follicular papules and papulo-pustules which typically develop after 1–4 weeks of steroid use (Fig. 82.1)
  - More specific timeline depends on dose and route of corticosteroid administration
- Inflammatory papules may later be replaced by comedones, but comedones are often absent during the initial eruption
- Most commonly affected areas are the chest and upper back, shoulders, lateral upper arms, with less common involvement of the face

Histopathology

- Early lesions demonstrate focal necrosis of a segment of the follicle with neutrophils and lymphocytes forming a perifollicular abscess (Fig. 82.2)

J. K. Choi, MD
Department of Dermatology, University of Pennsylvania, Philadelphia, PA, USA

Department of Dermatology, Veteran Affairs Medical Center, Philadelphia, PA, USA
e-mail: juliana.choi@uphs.upenn.edu

M. Rosenbach et al. (eds.), *Inpatient Dermatology*,
https://doi.org/10.1007/978-3-319-18449-4_82

- The abscess is encapsulated and a comedo is formed
- This is the opposite of acne vulgaris in which the formation of a comedo is followed by an inflammatory lesion

Differential Diagnosis

- Acne vulgaris (heterogeneous): almost always on the face, with comedones, and without a history of steroid use
- Drug eruption: more erythematous macules, more diffuse, may be accentuated under elastic bands or sites of pressure and dependent areas
- Folliculitis: often larger pustules with more liquid than the firmer small papules and pustules of steroid acne, and more diffuse versus the localization to chest/back/shoulders
- Pityrosporum folliculitis: clinically identical to steroid acne, and may require biopsy to distinguish
- Other drug-induced acneiform eruptions: (Epidermal growth factor receptor (EGFR) inhibitors; halogenated compounds (iodides, radiopaque contrast, bromides); antiepileptic drugs; lithium; isoniazid; hormonal agents (growth hormone, contraceptive drugs, anabolic steroids); cyclosporine: exposure history is essential in distinguishing these entities

Work-Up

- Biopsy is typically not indicated in this setting; biopsy and culture (± sensitivity profile) of a pustule can be performed if atypical or infectious causes of folliculitis are being considered as well as in the setting of resistance to therapy
- Diagnosis based on monomorphic nature of lesions and history of corticosteroid use

Treatment

- Discontinuation of corticosteroids if possible
- Resolution occurs 2–6 weeks after onset if corticosteroids have been discontinued
- If due to systemic corticosteroids which can't be discontinued:
  - Oral antibiotics may be utilized, but the eruption often persists as long as steroids are being used
  - Low-dose isotretinoin can also be used in select cases but is rarely indicated
- If due to topical corticosteroids:
  - Low-strength topical retinoid
  - Topical antibiotics are not helpful

Suggested Readings

1. Plewig G, Kligman AM. Acne and rosacea. Berlin: Springer; 2000.
2. Hurwitz RM. Steroid acne. J Am Acad Dermatol. 1989;21(6):1179–81.
3. Dessinioti C, Antoniou C, Katsambas A. Acneiform eruptions. Clin Dermatol. 2014;32(1):24–34.

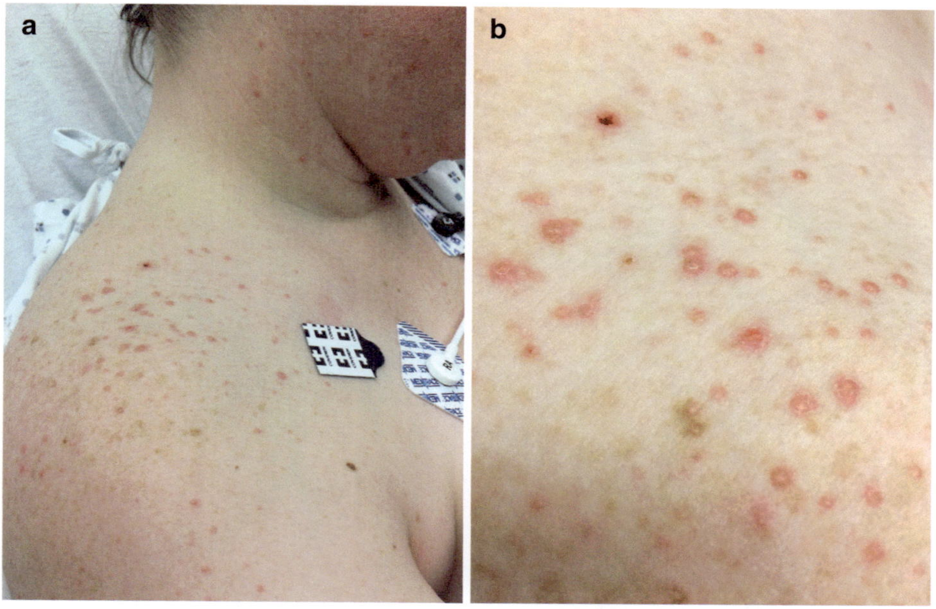

Fig. 82.1 Steroid acne (**a**, **b**): Monomorphic acneiform papules involving the upper trunk, shoulders, and face.

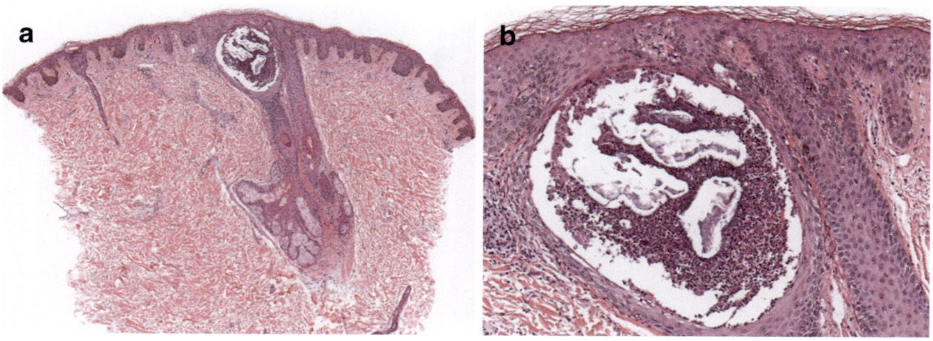

Fig. 82.2 Steroid folliculitis *(2.5X, 10X; H&E)*: Biopsy often is not necessary but can help exclude other entities. (**a**) A superficial intrafollicular pustule with mild surrounding inflammation is observed. (**b**) The intrafollicular pustules demonstrates abundant neutrophils without any organisms. Although the etiology of the acute folliculitis cannot be determined by H&E alone, clinical correlation with recent high-dose steroids can help make the diagnosis of steroid folliculitis.

Index

M. Rosenbach et al. (eds.), *Inpatient Dermatology*,
https://doi.org/10.1007/978-3-319-18449-4

MIX
Papier aus verantwortungsvollen Quellen
Paper from responsible sources
FSC® C105338

If you have any concerns about our products,
you can contact us on
ProductSafety@springernature.com

In case Publisher is established outside the EU,
the EU authorized representative is:
Springer Nature Customer Service Center GmbH
Europaplatz 3, 69115 Heidelberg, Germany

Printed by Libri Plureos GmbH
in Hamburg, Germany